CRITICAL CARE NURSING IN A FLASH

Wolters Kluwer Health | Lippincott Williams & Wilkins
Philadelphia • Baltimore • New York • London
Buenos Aires • Hong Kong • Sydney • Tokyo

STAFF

Executive Publisher
Judith A. Schilling McCann, RN, MSN

Editorial Director
H. Nancy Holmes

Clinical Director
Joan M. Robinson, RN, MSN

Art Director
Elaine Kasmer

Editorial Project Managers
Sean Webb, Deborah Grandinetti

Clinical Project Manager
Kate Stout, RN, MSN, CCRN

Copy Editors
Kimberly Bilotta (supervisor), Jeannine Fielding, Amy Furman, Linda Hager, Dona Perkins, Dorothy P. Terry

Designers
Matie Anne Patterson, BJ Crim, Lynn Foulk

Digital Composition Services
Diane Paluba (manager), Joyce Rossi Biletz, Donna S. Morris

Associate Manufacturing Manager
Beth J. Welsh

Editorial Assistants
Karen J. Kirk, Jeri O'Shea, Linda K. Ruhf

Indexer
Pat Perrier, BSN

The clinical procedures described and recommended in this publication are based on research and consultation with nursing, medical, pharmaceutical, and legal authorities. To the best of our knowledge, these procedures reflect currently accepted practice; nevertheless, they can't be considered absolute and universal recommendations. For individual application, all recommendations must be considered in light of the patient's clinical condition and, before the administration of new or infrequently used drugs, in light of the latest package-insert information. The authors and publisher disclaim responsibility for adverse effects resulting directly or indirectly from the suggested procedures, from undetected errors, or from the reader's misunderstanding of the text.

CCNIAF010608—030311

Library of Congress Cataloging-in-Publication Data

Critical care nursing in a flash.
p. ; cm.
Includes bibliographical references and index.
1. Intensive care nursing—Handbooks, manuals, etc.
[DNLM: 1. Critical Care—methods—Handbooks. 2. Critical Illness—nursing—Handbooks. WY 49 C9337 2009]
RT120.I5C762 2009
616.02'8—dc22
ISBN-13: 978-0-7817-9284-4 (alk. paper)
ISBN-10: 0-7817-9284-3 (alk. paper)
2008006859

Contents

Contributors and consultants

Susan W. Bowers, RN-BC, MSN
Education Coordinator–Coordinator of Progressive Care School
Cape Fear Valley Health System
Fayetteville, N.C.

Cheryl L. Brady, RN, MSN
Assistant Professor
Kent State University
Salem, Ohio

Maurice H. Espinoza, RN, MSN
Critical Care Clinical Nurse Specialist
University of California Irvine Medical Center
Orange

Evan Klein, RN, BSN, CCRN
Staff Nurse, Intensive Care Unit
Atlanta (Ga.) Medical Center

Virginia La Fleur, RN, MSN
Clinical Instructor–Adjunct
Rio Hondo College
Whittier, Calif.
Mount San Antonio College
Walnut, Calif.

Marcella A. Mikalaitis, RN, MSN, CCRN
Staff Nurse, Cardiovascular Intensive Care Unit
Doylestown (Pa.) Hospital

Beth Spence, RN, CEN, CFRN, EMT-PT
Critical Care Ground Transport Nurse
Sunstar Paramedics
Largo, Fla.

Belinda L. Spencer, RN, MSN, ACNP-BC, CCRN
Chief Inspections
Army Medical Command
Fort Sam Houston, Tex.

Tamara Zupanc, RN, BSN, CCRN
Critical Care Nurse Educator
Saint Joseph's Hospital
Marshfield, Wis.

Assessment

Evaluating a symptom

Ask the patient about what symptom is bothering him.

Form a first impression. Does the patient's condition alert you to an emergency?

Yes

Take a brief history to gather more clues.

Perform a focused physical examination to quickly determine the severity of the patient's condition.

No

Take a thorough history to get an overview of the patient's condition. Ask him about other signs or symptoms.

Thoroughly examine the patient to evaluate the chief sign or symptom and to detect additional signs and symptoms.

Evaluate your findings. Are emergency signs or symptoms present?

Yes

Based on your findings, intervene appropriately to stabilize the patient. Notify the doctor immediately of the assessment findings and carry out the doctor's orders.

After the patient's condition is stabilized, review your findings to consider possible causes.

No

Evaluate your findings to consider possible causes.

Develop an appropriate care plan.

Height and weight conversions

Height conversion

To convert a patient's height from inches to centimeters, multiply the number of inches by 2.54. To convert a patient's height from centimeters to inches, multiply the number of centimeters by 0.394.

Imperial	Inches	Metric (cm)
4′ 8″	56	142.2
4′ 9″	57	144.8
4′ 10″	58	147.3
4′ 11″	59	149.9
5′	60	152.4
5′ 1″	61	154.9
5′ 2″	62	157.5
5′ 3″	63	160
5′ 4″	64	162.6
5′ 5″	65	165.1
5′ 6″	66	167.6
5′ 7″	67	170.2
5′ 8″	68	172.7
5′ 9″	69	175.3
5′ 10″	70	177.8
5′ 11″	71	180.3
6′	72	182.9
6′ 1″	73	185.4
6′ 2″	74	188
6′ 3″	75	190.5

Weight conversion

To convert a patient's weight from pounds to kilograms, divide the number of pounds by 2.2 kg; to convert a patient's weight from kilograms to pounds, multiply the number of kilograms by 2.2 lb.

Pounds	Kilograms
10	4.5
20	9.1
30	13.6
40	18.2
50	22.7
60	27.3
70	31.8
80	36.4
90	40.9
100	45.5
110	50
120	54.5
130	59.1
140	63.6
150	68.2
160	72.7
170	77.3
180	81.8
190	86.4
200	90.9
210	95.5
220	100
230	104.5
240	109.1
250	113.6
260	118.2

Temperature conversion

To convert Fahrenheit to Celsius, subtract 32 from the temperature in Fahrenheit and then divide by 1.8; to convert Celsius to Fahrenheit, multiply the temperature in Celsius by 1.8 and then add 32.

$$(F - 32) \div 1.8 = \text{degrees Celsius}$$
$$(C \times 1.8) + 32 = \text{degrees Fahrenheit}$$

Degrees Fahrenheit (°F)	Degrees Celsius (°C)	Degrees Fahrenheit (°F)	Degrees Celsius (°C)
89.6	32	100.8	38.2
91.4	33	101	38.3
93.2	34	101.2	38.4
94.3	34.6	101.4	38.6
95.0	35	101.8	38.8
95.4	35.2	102	38.9
96.2	35.7	102.2	39
96.8	36	102.6	39.2
97.2	36.2	102.8	39.3
97.6	36.4	103	39.4
98	36.7	103.2	39.6
98.6	37	103.4	39.7
99	37.2	103.6	39.8
99.3	37.4	104	40
99.7	37.6	104.4	40.2
100	37.8	104.6	40.3
100.4	38	104.8	40.4
		105	40.6

Performing auscultation

Auscultation of body sounds—particularly those produced by the heart, lungs, blood vessels, stomach, and intestines—detects both high-pitched and low-pitched sounds. You can perform auscultation directly over a body area using only your ears, but you'll typically perform it indirectly, using a stethoscope.

Assessing high-pitched sounds

To properly assess high-pitched sounds, such as breath sounds and first and second heart sounds, use the diaphragm of the stethoscope. Make sure you place the entire surface of the diaphragm firmly on the patient's skin. If the area is excessively hairy, you can improve diaphragm contact and reduce background noise by applying water or water-soluble jelly to the skin before auscultating.

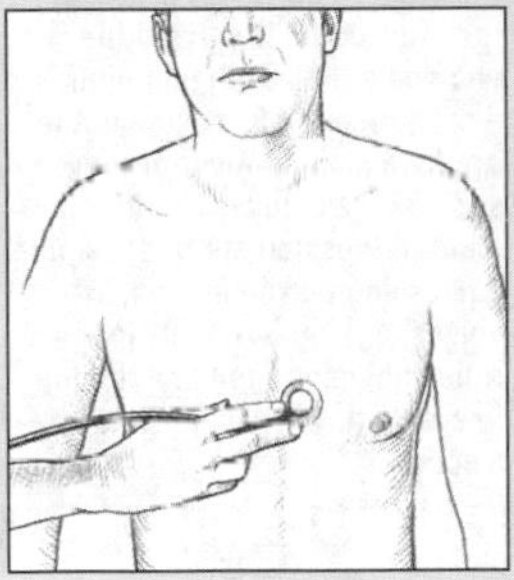

Assessing low-pitched sounds

To assess low-pitched sounds, such as heart murmurs and third and fourth heart sounds, lightly place the bell of the stethoscope on the appropriate area. Don't exert pressure. If you do, the patient's chest will act as a diaphragm and you will miss low-pitched sounds. If the patient is extremely thin or emaciated, use a stethoscope with a pediatric chest piece.

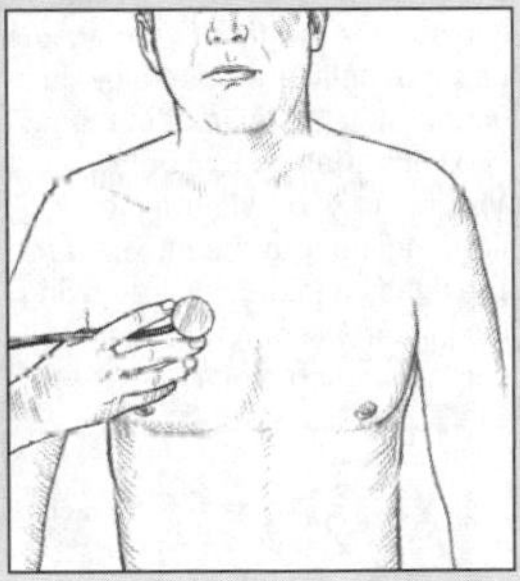

Performing percussion

Percussion has two basic purposes: to produce percussion sounds and to elicit tenderness. It involves three types: indirect, direct, and blunt.

Indirect percussion

The most common method, indirect percussion, produces clear, crisp sounds when performed correctly. To perform indirect percussion, use the second finger of your nondominant hand as the pleximeter (the mediating device used to receive the taps) and the middle finger of your dominant hand as the plexor (the device used to tap the pleximeter). Place the pleximeter finger firmly against a body surface, such as the upper back or abdomen. With your wrist flexed loosely, use the tip of your plexor finger to deliver a crisp blow just beneath the distal joint of the pleximeter (as shown below). Make sure you hold the plexor perpendicular to the pleximeter. Tap lightly and quickly, removing the plexor as soon as you have delivered each blow.

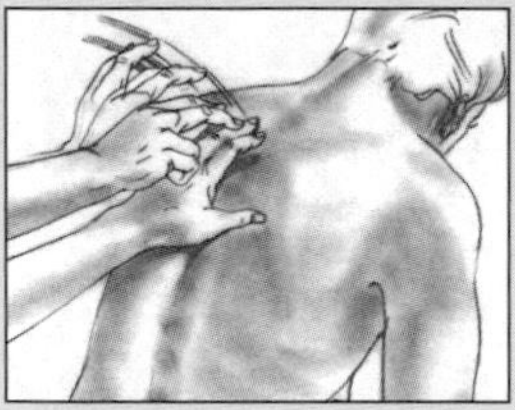

Direct percussion

To perform direct percussion, tap your hand or fingertip directly against the body surface (as shown below). This method helps assess an adult's sinuses for tenderness.

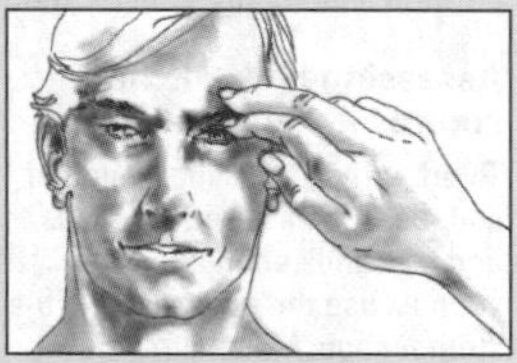

Blunt percussion

To perform blunt percussion, strike the ulnar surface of your fist against the body surface. Alternatively, use both hands. Place one palm over the area to be percussed. Make a fist with the other hand; use it to strike the back of the first hand (as shown below). Both techniques aim to elicit tenderness—not to create a sound—over organs such as the kidneys. Another blunt percussion method, used in a neurologic examination, involves tapping a rubber-tipped reflex hammer against a tendon to create a reflexive muscle contraction.

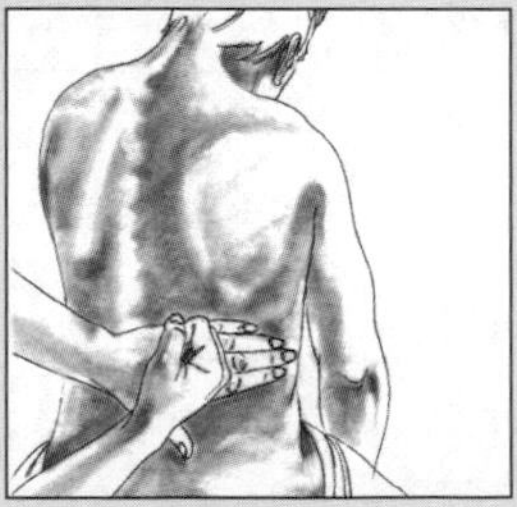

Performing palpation

Palpation uses pressure to assess structure size, placement, pulsation, and tenderness. Ballottement, a variation, involves bouncing tissues against the hand to assess rebound of floating structures. Ballottement can be used to assess a mass in a patient with ascites.

Light palpation

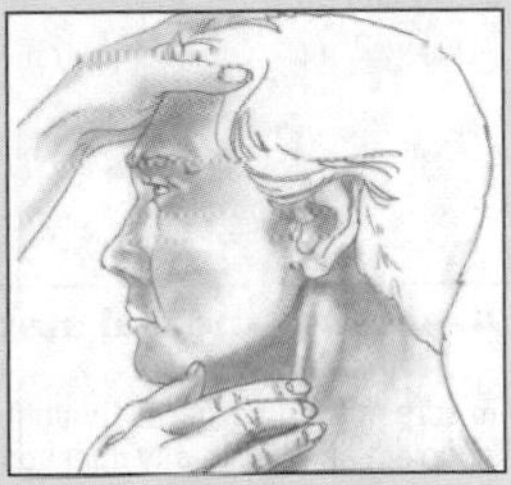

To perform light palpation, press gently on the skin, indenting it 1½" to 3½" (4 to 9 cm) (as shown at right). Use the lightest touch possible; too much pressure blunts your sensitivity. Close your eyes to concentrate on feeling.

Deep palpation

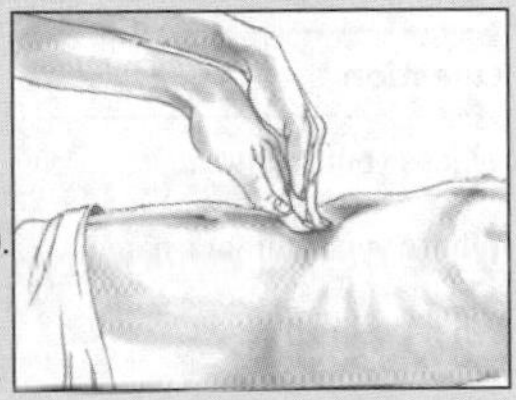

To perform deep palpation, indent the skin about 1½" (4 cm). Place your other hand on top of the palpating hand to control and guide your movements (as shown at right). To perform deep palpation that allows you to pinpoint an inflamed area, push down slowly and deeply, then lift your hand away quickly. If the patient complains of increased pain as you release the pressure, you have identified rebound tenderness.

Use both hands (bimanual palpation) to trap a deep, hard-to-palpate organ (such as the kidney or spleen) or to fix or stabilize an organ (such as the uterus) while palpating with the other hand.

ALERT Don't perform deep palpation if the patient complains of acute abdominal pain.

Light ballottement

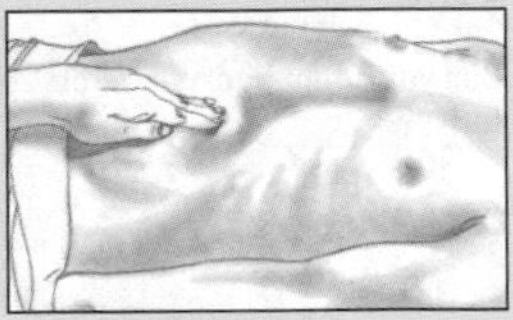

To perform light ballottement, apply light, rapid pressure from quadrant to quadrant of the patient's abdomen. Keep your hand on the surface of the skin to detect tissue rebound (as shown at right).

(continued)

Performing palpation *(continued)*

Deep ballottement

To perform deep ballottement, apply abrupt, deep pressure; then release, but maintain contact (as shown at right).

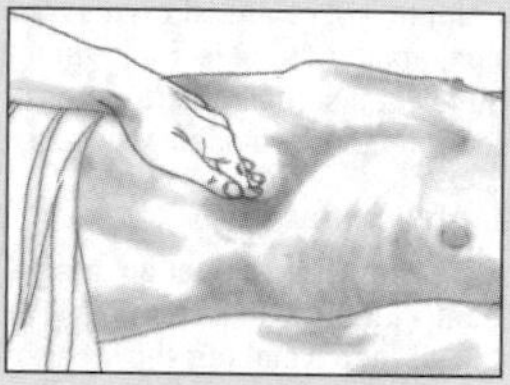

Assessing mental status

To screen for disordered thought processes, ask these questions. An incorrect answer to any question may indicate the need for a complete mental status examination.

Question	Function screened
What's your name?	Orientation to person
What's your mother's name?	Orientation to other people
What year is it?	Orientation to time
Where are you now?	Orientation to place
How old are you?	Memory
When were you born?	Remote memory
What did you have for breakfast?	Recent memory
Who's the President of the United States?	General knowledge
Can you count backward from 20 to 1?	Attention span and calculation skills

Comparing delirium and dementia

This chart highlights distinguishing characteristics of delirium and dementia.

Clinical feature	Delirium	Dementia
Onset	Acute, sudden	Gradual
Course	Short, diurnal fluctuations in symptoms; worse at night, in darkness, and on awakening	Lifelong; symptoms progressive and irreversible
Progression	Abrupt	Slow but uneven
Duration	Hours, to less than 1 month; seldom longer	Months to years
Awareness	Reduced	Clear
Alertness	Fluctuates from lethargic to hypervigilant	Generally normal
Attention	Decreased	Generally normal
Orientation	Generally impaired, but reversible	May be impaired as disease progresses
Memory	Recent and immediate, impaired	Recent and remote impaired
Thinking	Disorganized, distorted, fragmented; incoherent speech, either slow or accelerated	Difficulty with abstraction; thoughts impoverished; judgment impaired; words difficult to find
Perception	Distorted: illusions, delusions, and hallucinations; difficulty distinguishing between reality and misperceptions	Misperceptions usually absent

(continued)

Comparing delirium and dementia *(continued)*

Clinical feature	Delirium	Dementia
Speech	Incoherent	Dysphasia as disease progresses; aphasia
Psychomotor behavior	Variable: hypokinetic, hyperkinetic, and mixed	Normal; may have apraxia
Sleep and wake cycle	Altered	Fragmented
Affect	Variable affective anxiety, restlessness, irritability; reversible	Typically superficial, inappropriate, and labile; attempts to conceal deficits in intellect; possible personality changes, aphasia, agnosia; lack of insight
Mental status testing	Distracted from task; numerous errors	Failings highlighted by family; frequent "near miss" answers, struggles with test, great effort to find an appropriate reply; frequent requests for feedback on performance

Neurologic stages of altered arousal

This table highlights the six stages of altered arousal. An alert patient responds to voice and has purposeful movement and appropriate spontaneous activity.

Stage	Manifestations
Confusion	• Loss of ability to think rapidly and clearly • Impaired judgment and decision making
Disorientation	• Beginning loss of consciousness • Disorientation to time progressing to disorientation to place • Impaired memory • Lack of recognition of self (last symptom)
Lethargy	• Limited spontaneous movement or speech • Easily aroused by normal speech or touch • Possible disorientation to time, place, or person
Obtundation	• Mild to moderate reduction in arousal • Limited responsiveness to environment • Ability to fall asleep easily without verbal or tactile stimulation • Minimum response to questions
Stupor	• State of deep sleep or unresponsiveness • Arousable with difficulty (motor or verbal response only to vigorous and repeated stimulation) • Withdrawal or grabbing response to stimulation
Coma	• Lack of motor or verbal response to external environment or stimuli • No response to noxious stimuli such as deep pain • Can't be aroused by any stimulus

Glasgow Coma Scale

A decreased score in one or more categories may signal an impending neurologic crisis. The best response is scored.

Test	Score	Patient's response
Eye opening		
Spontaneously	4	Opens eyes spontaneously
To speech	3	Opens eyes to verbal command
To pain	2	Opens eyes to painful stimulus
None	1	Doesn't open eyes in response to stimulus
Motor response		
Obeys	6	Reacts to verbal command
Localizes	5	Identifies localized pain
Withdraws	4	Flexes and withdraws from painful stimulus
Abnormal flexion	3	Assumes a decorticate position
Abnormal extension	2	Assumes a decerebrate position
None	1	Doesn't respond; just lies flaccid
Verbal response		
Oriented	5	Is oriented and converses
Confused	4	Is disoriented and confused
Inappropriate words	3	Replies randomly with incorrect words
Incomprehensible	2	Moans or screams
None	1	Doesn't respond
Total score		

Grading pupil size

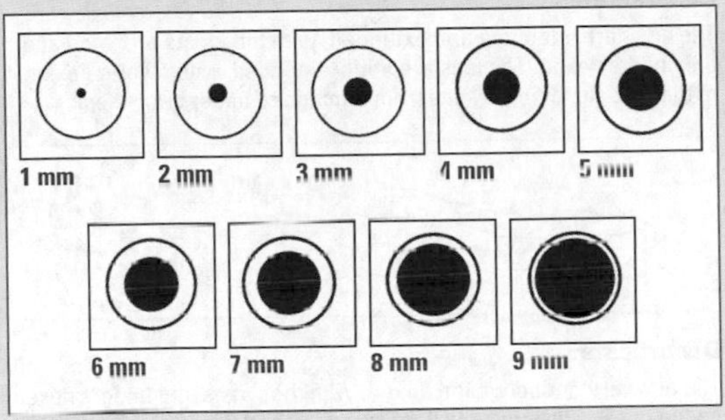

Babinski's reflex

Stroking the lateral aspect of the sole of the foot with a thumbnail or another moderately sharp object normally elicits flexion of all toes (a negative Babinski's reflex), as shown below left. In a positive Babinski's reflex, the great toe dorsiflexes and the other toes fan out, as shown below right.

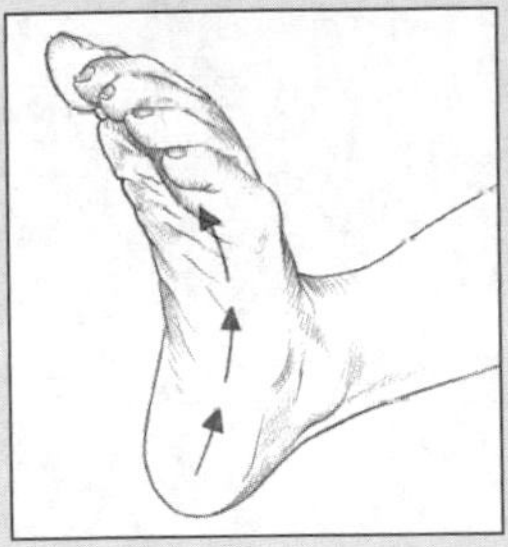

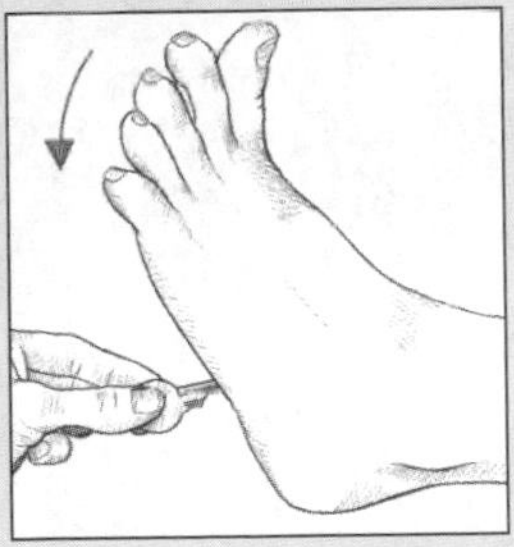

Decerebrate and decorticate postures

Decerebrate

The arms are adducted and extended, with the wrists pronated and the fingers flexed. The legs are stiffly extended, with plantar flexion of the feet. Condition results from damage to upper brain stem.

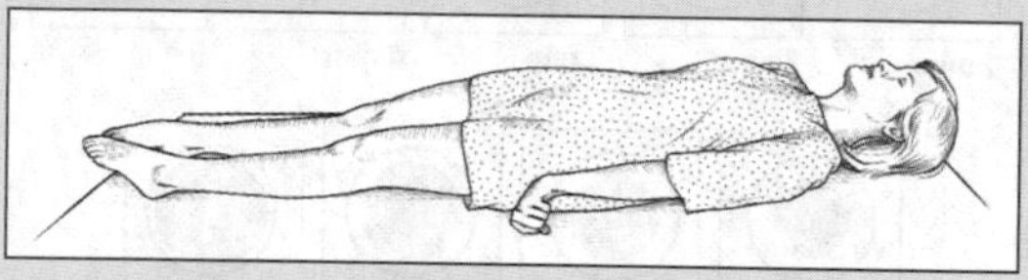

Decorticate

The arms are adducted and flexed, with the wrists and fingers flexed on the chest. The legs are stiffly extended and internally rotated, with plantar flexion of the feet. Condition results from damage to one or both corticospinal tracts.

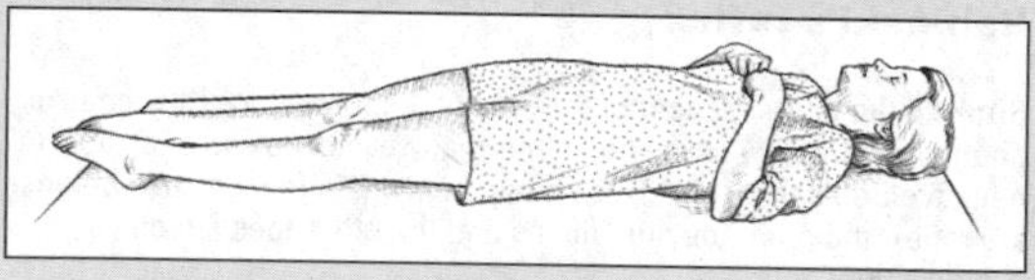

Detecting increased ICP

The earlier you can recognize the signs of increased intracranial pressure (ICP), the more quickly you can intervene and better the patient's chance of recovery. By the time late signs appear, interventions may be useless.

	Early signs	Late signs
Level of consciousness	• Requires increased stimulation • Subtle orientation loss • Restlessness and anxiety • Sudden quietness	Unarousable
Pupils	• Pupil changes on side of lesion • One pupil constricts but then dilates (unilateral hippus) • Sluggish reaction of both pupils • Unequal pupils	Pupils fixed and dilated
Motor response	• Sudden weakness • Motor changes on side opposite the lesion • Positive pronator drift; with palms up, one hand pronates	Profound weakness
Vital signs	• Intermittent increases in blood pressure	Increased systolic pressure, profound bradycardia, abnormal respirations (Cushing's syndrome)

ICP waveforms

Three waveforms—A, B, and C—are used to monitor ICP.

Normal waveform

A normal ICP waveform (below) typically shows a steep upward systolic slope followed by a downward diastolic slope with a dicrotic notch. In most cases, this waveform occurs continuously and indicates an ICP between 0 and 15 mm Hg—normal pressure.

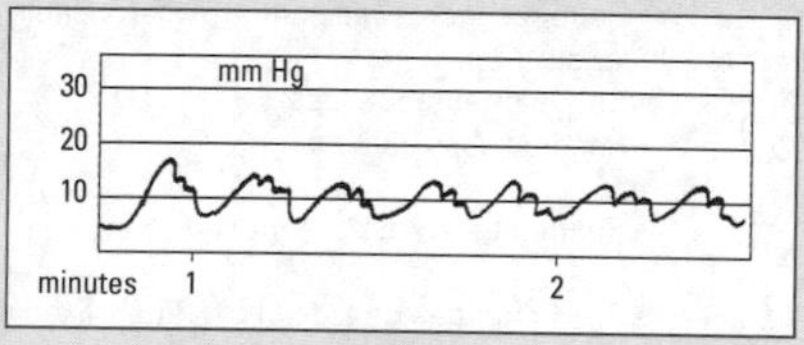

A waves

The most clinically significant ICP waveforms are A waves (shown below), which may reach elevations of 50 to 100 mm Hg, persist for 5 to 20 minutes, then drop sharply—signaling exhaustion of the brain's compliance mechanisms. Certain activities, such as sustained coughing or straining during defecation, can cause temporary elevations in thoracic pressure.

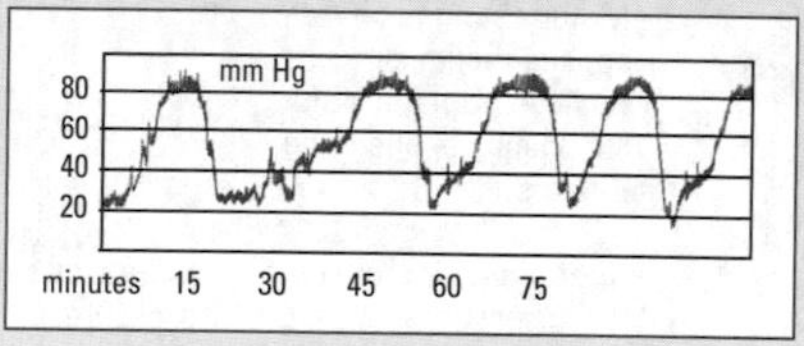

B waves

B waves, which appear sharp and rhythmic with a sawtooth pattern (shown below), occur every 1½ to 2 minutes and may reach elevations of 50 mm Hg. The clinical significance of B waves isn't clear, but the waves correlate with respiratory changes and may occur more often with decreasing compensation.

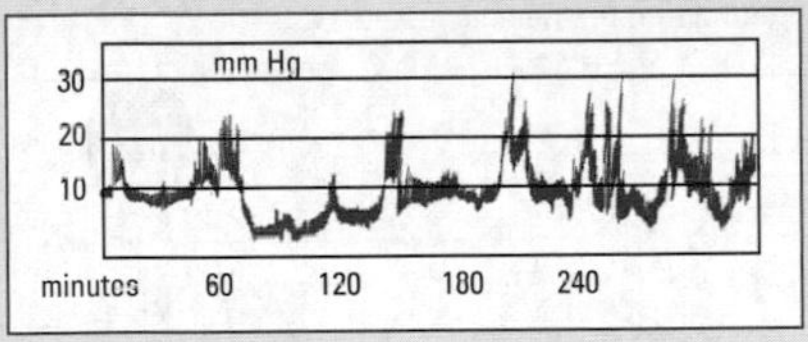

C waves

Like B waves, C waves (shown below) are rapid and rhythmic, but they aren't as sharp. They're clinically insignificant and may fluctuate with respirations or systemic blood pressure changes.

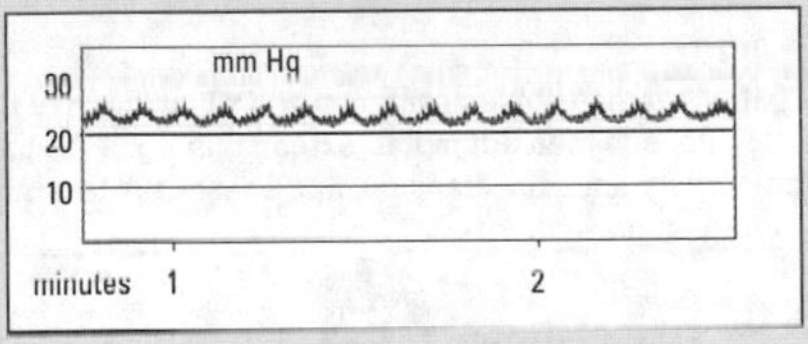

Brudzinski's and Kernig's signs

Positive Brudzinski's and Kernig's signs indicate meningeal irritation. Follow these guidelines to test for these two signs.

Brudzinski's sign

With the patient in the supine position, place your hand under his neck and flex it forward, chin to chest. The test is positive if he flexes his ankles, knees, and hips bilaterally. The patient typically complains of pain when the neck is flexed.

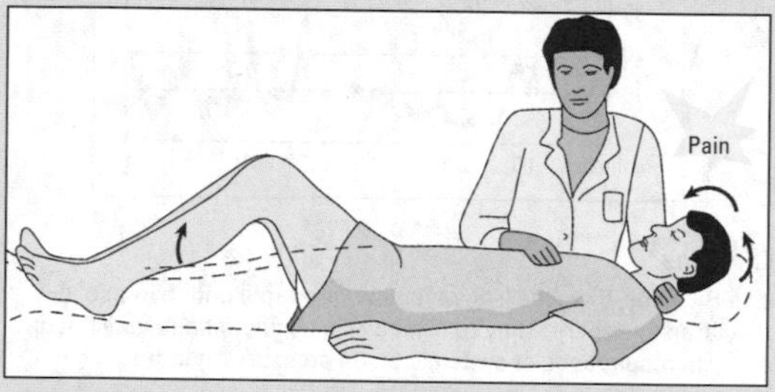

Kernig's sign

With the patient in the supine position, flex his hip and knee to form a 90-degree angle, and then attempt to extend this leg. If the patient exhibits pain, resistance to extension, and spasm, the test is positive.

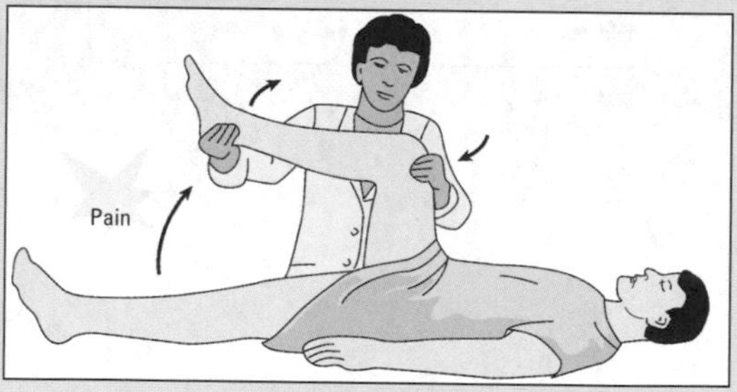

Cranial nerves

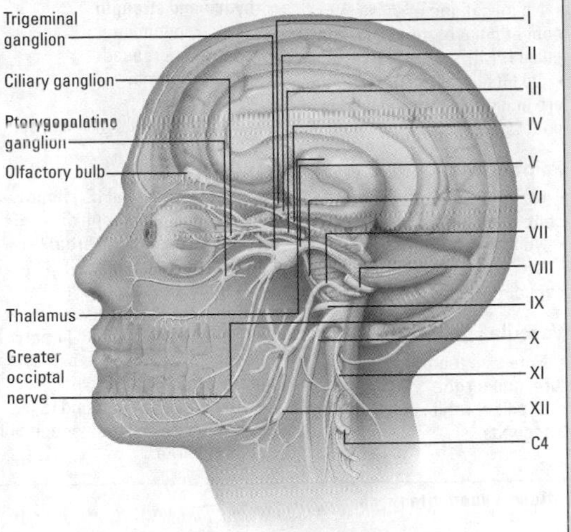

Cranial nerve function

CN I: Olfactory—Smell
CN II: Optic—Vision
CN III: Oculomotor—Extraocular movement, pupillary constriction, upper eyelid elevation, lens shape change
CN IV: Trochlear—Downward and inward eye movement
CN V: Trigeminal—Chewing, corneal reflex, face and scalp sensations
CN VI: Abducens—Lateral eye movement
CN VII: Facial—Expressions in forehead, eye, and mouth; taste
CN VIII: Acoustic—Hearing and balance
CN IX: Glossopharyngeal—Swallowing, salivating, taste
CN X: Vagus—Swallowing, gag reflex, talking; sensations of throat, larynx, and abdominal viscera
CN XI: Spinal accessory—Shoulder movement, head rotation
CN XII: Hypoglossal—Tongue movement

Cardiovascular assessment

Inspection

- No pulsations are visible except at point of maximum impulse (PMI).
- No lifts (heaves) or retractions are evident in four valve areas of chest wall.

Palpation

- No vibrations or thrills are evident.
- No lifts or heaves are evident.
- No pulsations are visible except at PMI and epigastric area.

Vascular palpation

- Note skin temperature, texture, and turgor.
- Capillary refill is no more than 3 seconds.
- Pulses should be regular in rhythm and strength.

  4+ = bounding
  3+ = increased
  2+ = normal
  1+ = weak
  0 = absent

Auscultation

- First heart sound (S_1) heard best with stethoscope diaphragm over mitral area.
- Second heart sound (S_2) heard best with stethoscope diaphragm over aortic area.
- Third heart sound (S_3) heard best with stethoscope bell over mitral area.
- Additional heart sound (S_4) heard best with stethoscope bell at mitral area.

Heart sound sites

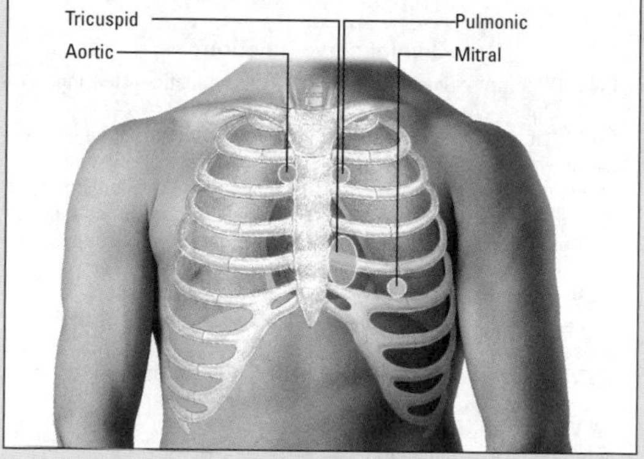

Edema scale

0	None observed
+1	Minimal (< 2 mm)
+2	Depression 2 to 4 mm
+3	Depression 5 to 8 mm
+4	Depression > 8 mm

Classifying blood pressure readings

These categories are based on the average of two or more readings taken on separate visits after an initial screening. They apply to adults age 18 and older.

Category	Systolic		Diastolic
Normal	< 120 mm Hg	and	< 80 mm Hg
Prehypertension	120 to 139 mm Hg	or	80 to 89 mm Hg
Hypertension			
Stage 1	140 to 159 mm Hg	or	90 to 99 mm Hg
Stage 2	≥ 160 mm Hg	or	≥ 100 mm Hg

Arterial pressure monitoring

Normal arterial blood pressure produces a characteristic waveform representing ventricular systole and diastole. The waveform has five distinct components: the anacrotic limb, systolic peak, dicrotic limb, dicrotic notch, and end diastole.

The *anacrotic limb* marks the waveform's initial upstroke, which results as blood is rapidly ejected from the ventricle through the open aortic valve into the aorta. The rapid ejection causes a sharp rise in arterial pressure, which appears as the waveform's highest point. This is called the *systolic peak.*

As blood continues into the peripheral vessels, arterial pressure falls and the waveform begins a downward trend. This part is called the *dicrotic limb.* Arterial pressure usually continues to fall until pressure in the ventricle is less than pressure in the aortic root. When this occurs, the aortic valve closes. This event appears as a small notch on the waveform's downside, known as the *dicrotic notch.*

When the aortic valve closes, diastole begins, progressing until the aortic root pressure gradually descends to its lowest point. On the waveform, this is known as *end diastole.*

Normal arterial waveform

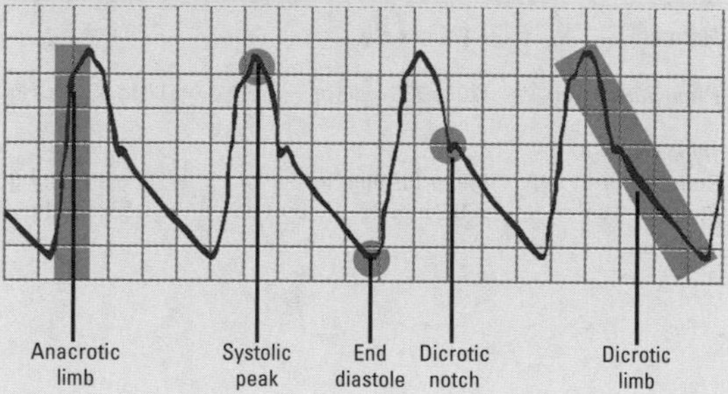

Implications of abnormal heart sounds

Upon detecting an abnormal heart sound, you must accurately identify the sound as well as its location and timing in the cardiac cycle. This information will help you identify the possible cause of the sound. This chart lists abnormal heart sounds with their possible causes.

Abnormal heart sound	Timing	Possible causes
Accentuated S_1	Beginning of systole	Mitral stenosis; fever
Diminished S_1	Beginning of systole	Mitral insufficiency; severe mitral regurgitation with calcified immobile valve; heart block
Accentuated S_2	End of systole	Pulmonary or systemic hypertension
Diminished or inaudible S_2	End of systole	Aortic or pulmonic stenosis
Persistent S_2 split	End of systole	Delayed closure of the pulmonic valve, usually from overfilling of the right ventricle, causing prolonged systolic ejection time
Reversed or paradoxical S_2 split that appears on expiration and disappears on inspiration	End of systole	Delayed ventricular stimulation; left bundle-branch block or prolonged left ventricular ejection time
S_3 (ventricular gallop)	Early diastole	Normal in children and young adults; overdistention of ventricles in rapid-filling segment of diastole; mitral insufficiency or ventricular failure

(continued)

Implications of abnormal heart sounds *(continued)*

Abnormal heart sound	Timing	Possible causes
S_4 (atrial gallop or presystolic extra sound)	Late diastole	Forceful atrial contraction from resistance to ventricular filling late in diastole; left ventricular hypertrophy; pulmonic stenosis; hypertension; coronary artery disease; and aortic stenosis
Pericardial friction rub (grating or leathery sound at left of sternal border; usually muffled, high-pitched, and transient)	Throughout systole and diastole	Pericardial inflammation
Click	Early systole or midsystole	Aortic stenosis; aortic dilation; hypertension; chordae tendineae damage of the mitral valve
Opening snap	Early diastole	Mitral or tricuspid valve abnormalities
Summation gallop	Diastole	Tachycardia

Identifying heart murmurs

Timing	Quality and pitch	Location	Possible causes
Midsystolic (systolic ejection)	Harsh, rough with medium to high pitch	Pulmonic	Pulmonic stenosis
	Harsh, rough with medium to high pitch	Aortic and suprasternal notch	Aortic stenosis
Holosystolic (pansystolic)	Harsh with high pitch	Tricuspid	Ventricular septal defect
	Blowing with high pitch	Mitral, lower left sternal border	Mitral insufficiency
	Blowing with high pitch	Tricuspid	Tricuspid insufficiency
Early diastolic	Blowing with high pitch	Midleft sternal edge (not aortic area)	Aortic insufficiency
	Blowing with high pitch	Pulmonic	Pulmonic insufficiency
Middiastolic to late diastolic	Rumbling with low pitch	Apex	Mitral stenosis
	Rumbling with low pitch	Tricuspid, lower right sternal border	Tricuspid stenosis

Grading murmurs

Murmurs are graded on a scale of 1 to 6. Use the system outlined below to describe the intensity of a murmur:

- Grade I is a barely audible murmur.
- Grade II is audible but quiet and soft.
- Grade III is moderately loud, without a thrust or thrill.
- Grade IV is loud, with a thrill.
- Grade V is very loud, with a palpable thrill.
- Grade VI is loud enough to be heard before the stethoscope comes into contact with the chest.

When recording your findings, use Roman numerals as part of a fraction, always with VI as the denominator. For instance, a grade III murmur would be recorded as "grade III/VI."

Interpreting rhythm strips

Interpreting a rhythm strip is a skill developed through practice. You can use one of several methods, as long as you're consistent. Rhythm strip analysis requires a sequential and systematic approach. The eight-step method outlined below provides just that.

Eight-step method

1. Determine the rhythm.
2. Determine the rate.
3. Evaluate the P wave.
4. Measure the PR interval.
5. Determine the QRS duration.
6. Examine the T waves.
7. Measure the QT interval.
8. Check for ectopic beats and other abnormalities.

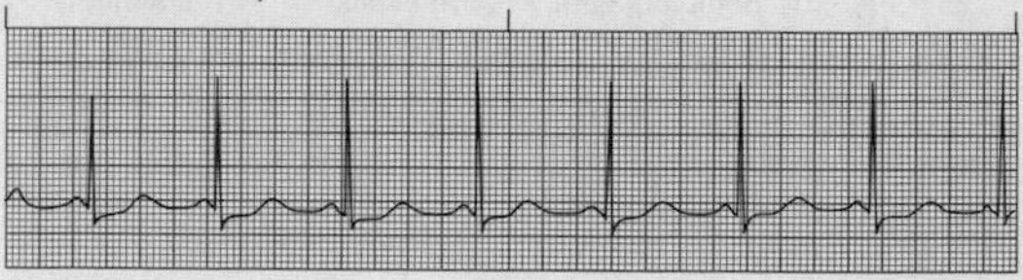

Normal sinus rhythm

Rhythm	Regular
Rate	60 to 100 beats/minute
P wave	Normal, upright
PR interval	0.12 to 0.20 second
QRS complex	0.06 to 0.10 second

Types of cardiac arrhythmias

This chart reviews many common cardiac arrhythmias and outlines their features.

Sinus tachycardia

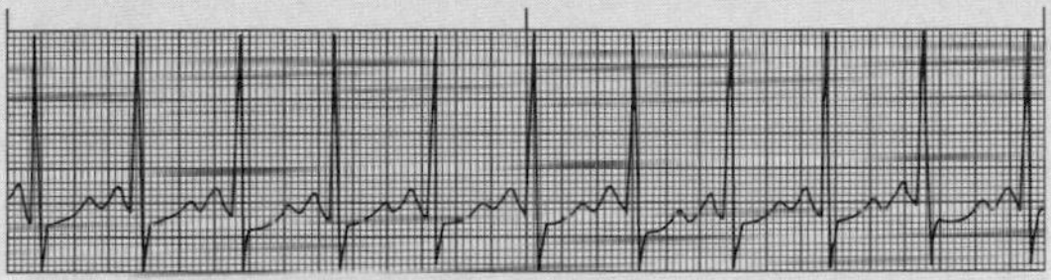

- Atrial and ventricular rhythms regular
- Rate > 100 beats/minute; rarely, > 160 beats/minute
- Normal P wave preceding each QRS complex

Sinus bradycardia

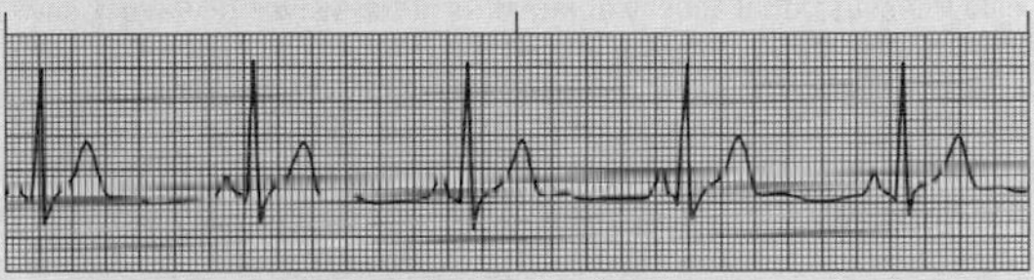

- Atrial and ventricular rhythms regular
- Rate < 60 beats/minute
- Normal P waves preceding each QRS complex

Paroxysmal supraventricular tachycardia

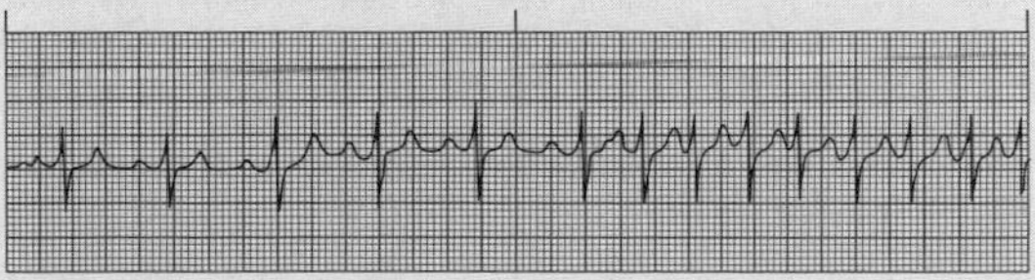

- Atrial and ventricular rhythms regular
- Heart rate > 160 beats/minute; rarely exceeds 250 beats/minute
- P waves regular but aberrant; difficult to differentiate from preceding T wave

(continued)

Types of cardiac arrhythmias *(continued)*

Paroxysmal supraventricular tachycardia (continued)

- P wave preceding each QRS complex
- Sudden onset and termination of arrhythmia

Atrial flutter

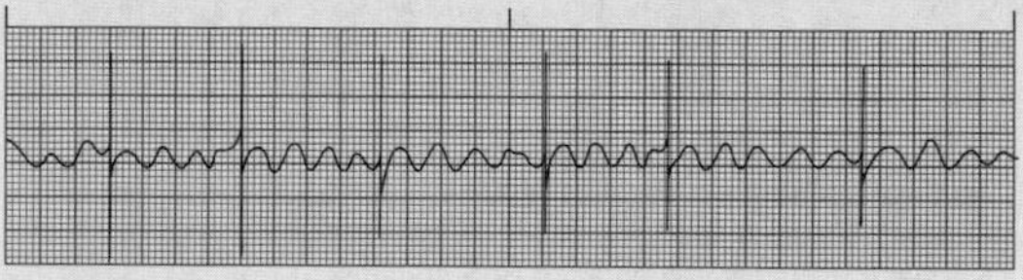

- Atrial rhythm regular; rate 250 to 400 beats/minute
- Ventricular rate variable, depending on degree of AV block (usually 60 to 100 beats/minute)
- No P waves; atrial activity appears as flutter waves (F waves); saw-tooth configuration common in lead II
- QRS complexes uniform in shape, but usually irregular in rate

Atrial fibrillation

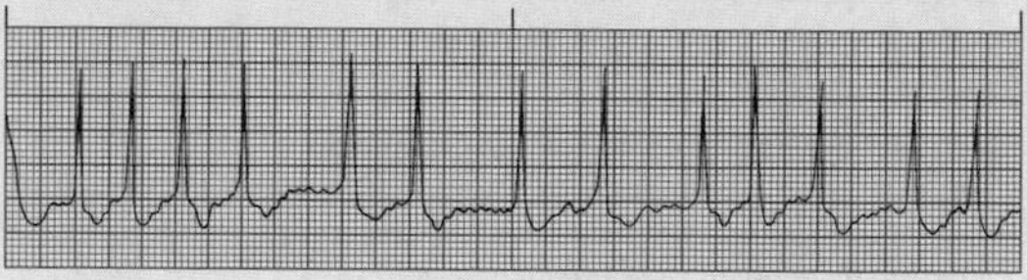

- Atrial rhythm grossly irregular; rate > 400 beats/minute
- Ventricular rhythm grossly irregular
- QRS complexes of uniform configuration and duration
- PR interval indiscernible
- No P waves; atrial activity appears as erratic; irregular, baseline fibrillatory waves (f waves)

Types of cardiac arrhythmias *(continued)*

Junctional rhythm

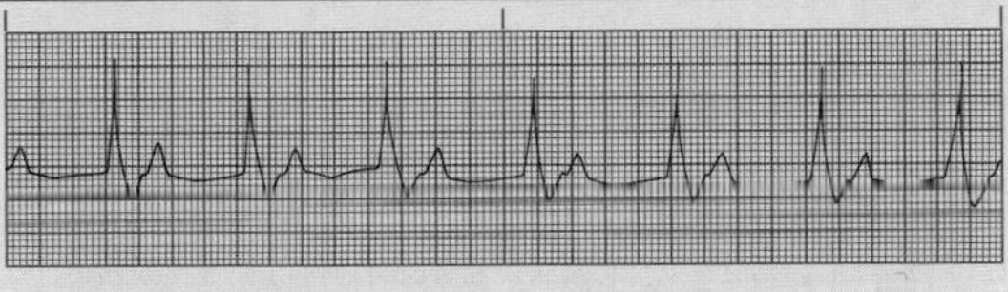

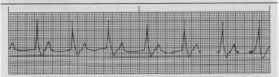

- Atrial and ventricular rhythms regular; atrial rate 40 to 60 beats/minute; ventricular rate usually 40 to 60 beats/minute (60 to 100 beats/minute is accelerated junctional rhythm)
- P waves preceding, hidden within (absent), or after QRS complex; usually inverted if visible
- PR interval (when present) < 0.12 second
- QRS complex configuration and duration normal, except in aberrant conduction

First-degree AV block

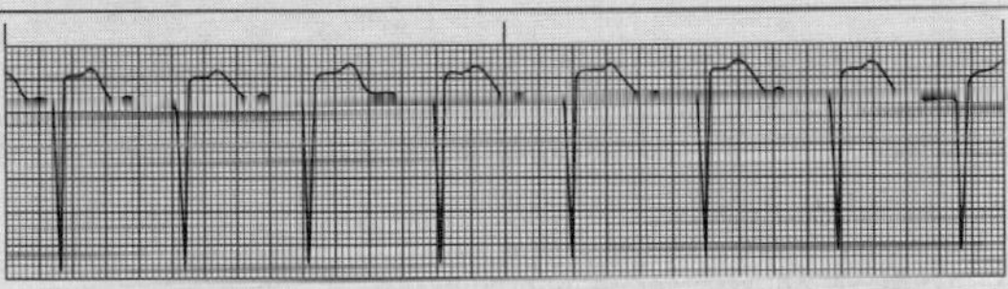

- Atrial and ventricular rhythms regular
- PR interval > 0.20 second
- P wave precedes QRS complex
- QRS complex normal

(continued)

Types of cardiac arrhythmias *(continued)*

Second-degree AV block Mobitz I (Wenckebach)

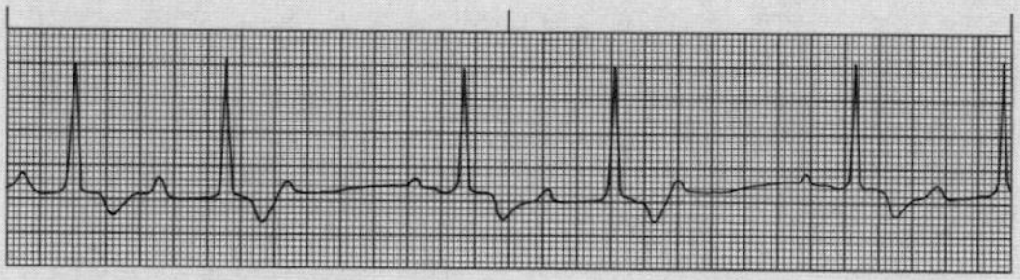

- Atrial rhythm regular
- Ventricular rhythm irregular
- Atrial rate exceeds ventricular rate
- PR interval progressively longer with each cycle until QRS complex disappears (dropped beat); PR interval shorter after dropped beat

Second-degree AV block Mobitz II

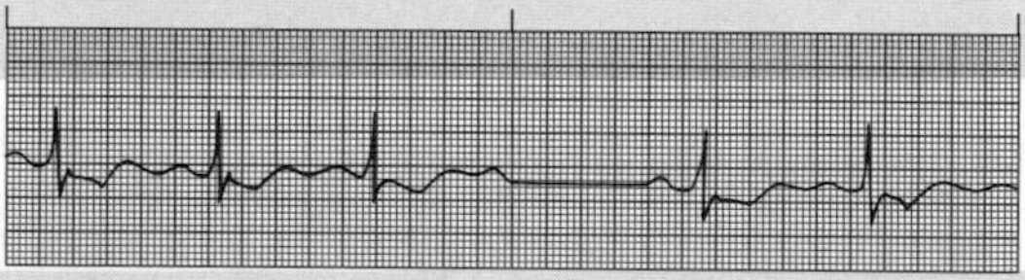

- Atrial rhythm regular
- Ventricular rhythm regular or irregular, with varying degree of block
- P-R interval constant for conducted beats
- P waves normal size and configuration, but some P waves not followed by a QRS complex

Third-degree AV block (complete heart block)

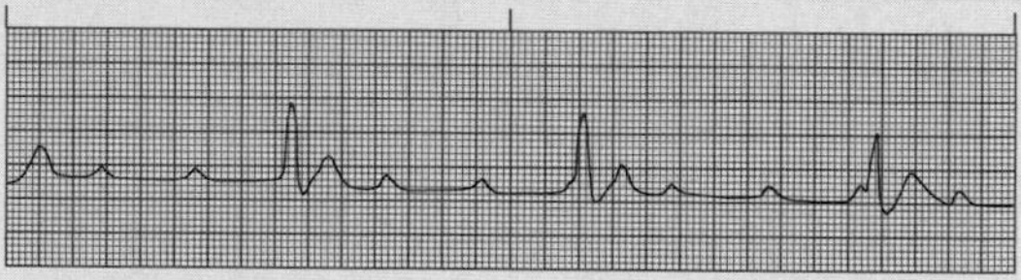

- Atrial rhythm regular
- Ventricular rhythm regular and rate slower than atrial rate
- No relation between P waves and QRS complexes

Types of cardiac arrhythmias *(continued)*

Third-degree AV block (complete heart block) (continued)

- No constant PR interval
- QRS duration normal (junctional pacemaker) or wide and bizarre (ventricular pacemaker)

Premature ventricular contraction (PVC)

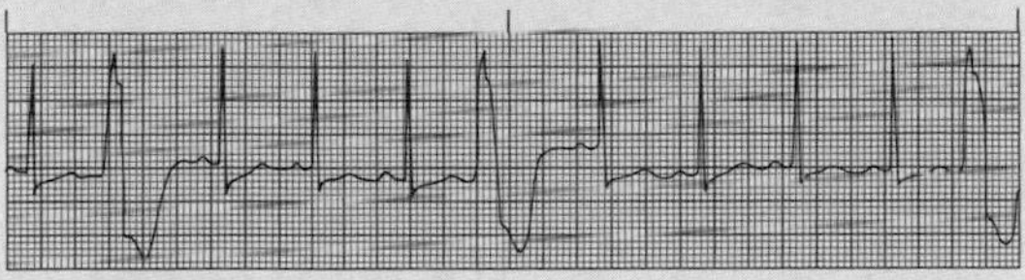

- Atrial rhythm regular
- Ventricular rhythm irregular
- QRS complex premature, usually followed by a complete compensatory pause
- QRS complex wide and distorted, usually > 0.12 second
- Premature QRS complexes occurring alone, in pairs, or in threes, alternating with normal beats; focus from one or more sites
- Ominous when clustered, multifocal, or with R wave on T pattern

Ventricular tachycardia

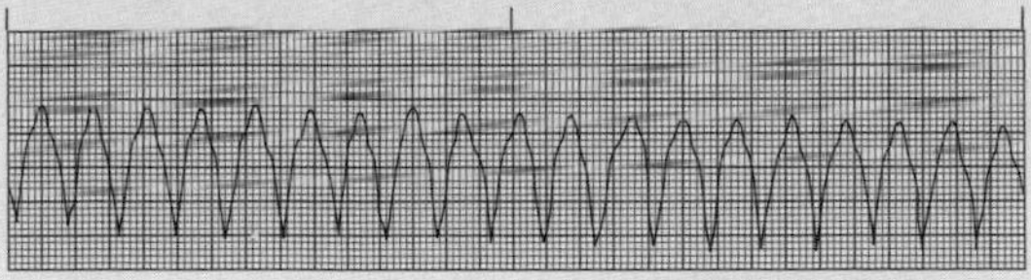

- Ventricular rate 100 to 220 beats/minute, rhythm usually regular
- QRS complexes wide, bizarre, and independent of P waves
- P waves not discernible
- May start and stop suddenly

(continued)

Types of cardiac arrhythmias *(continued)*

Ventricular fibrillation

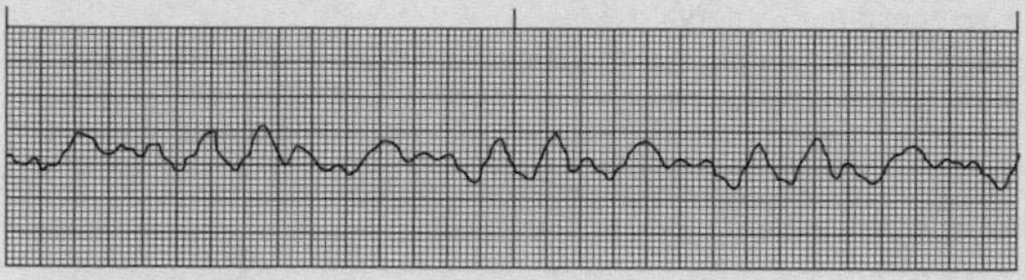

- Ventricular rhythm and rate chaotic and rapid
- QRS complexes wide and irregular; no visible P waves

Asystole

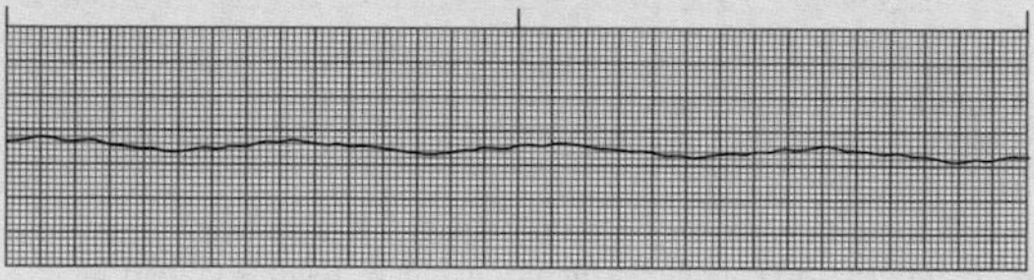

- No atrial or ventricular rate or rhythm
- No discernible P waves, QRS complexes, or T waves

Normal pulmonary artery waveforms

Right atrium

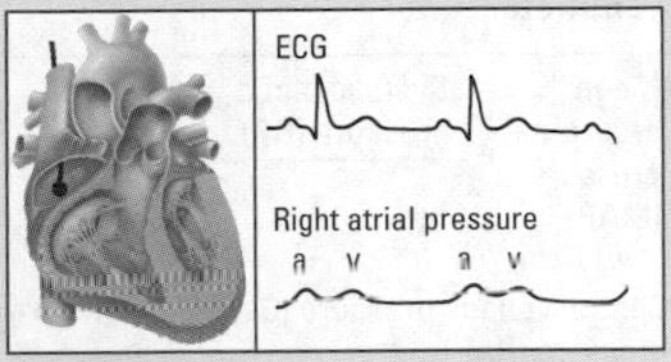

When the catheter tip enters the right atrium, a waveform like the one shown at right appears on the monitor. The *a* waves represent right ventricular end-diastolic pressure; the *v* waves, right atrial filling.

Right ventricle

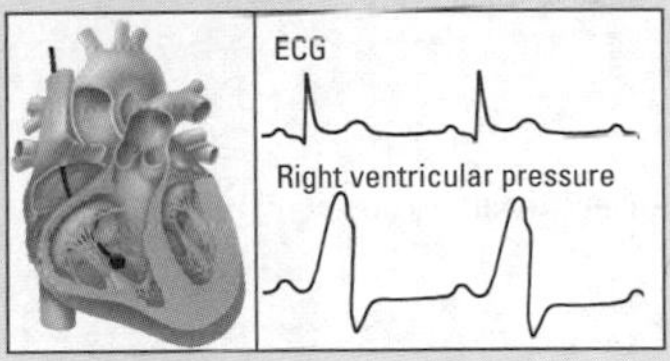

As the catheter tip reaches the right ventricle, you'll see a waveform with sharp systolic upstrokes and lower diastolic dips.

Pulmonary artery

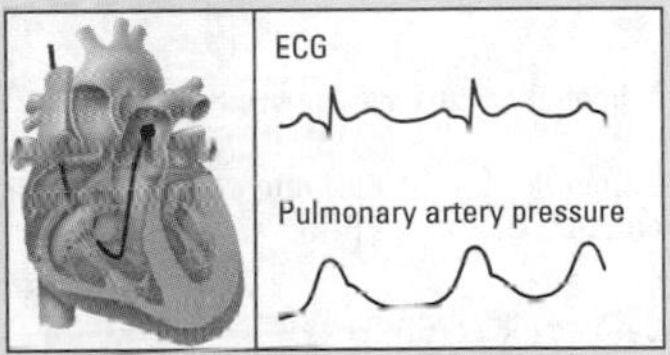

The catheter then floats into the pulmonary artery, causing a waveform like the one shown at right. Note that the upstroke here is smoother than the one on the right ventricular waveform. The dicrotic notch indicates pulmonic valve closure.

PAWP

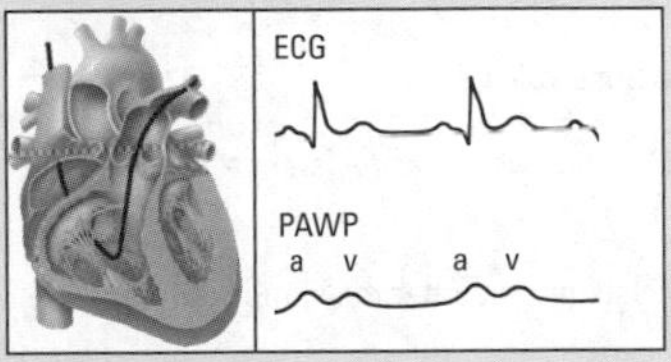

Floating into a distal branch of the pulmonary artery, the balloon wedges where the vessel becomes too narrow for it to pass. The monitor now shows a pulmonary artery wedge pressure (PAWP) waveform. The *a* waves represent left ventricular end-diastolic pressure; the *v* waves represent left atrial filling.

Hemodynamic variables

Parameter	Normal value
Mean arterial pressure (MAP) $= \dfrac{\text{Systolic blood pressure (BP)} + 2\,(\text{diastolic BP})}{3}$	70 to 105 mm Hg
Central venous pressure (CVP); right atrial pressure (RAP)	2 to 6 cm H_2O; 2 to 8 mm Hg
Right ventricular pressure	20 to 30 mm Hg (systolic) 0 to 8 mm Hg (diastolic)
Pulmonary artery pressure (PAP)	20 to 30 mm Hg (systolic; PAS) 8 to 15 mm Hg (diastolic; PAD) 10 to 20 mm Hg (mean; PAM)
Pulmonary artery wedge pressure (PAWP)	4 to 12 mm Hg
Cardiac output (CO) $=$ Heart rate (HR) $\times$ stroke volume (SV)	4 to 8 L/min
Cardiac index (CI) $= \dfrac{\text{CO}}{\text{Body surface area}}$	2.5 to 4 L/min/m^2
Stroke volume (SV) $= \dfrac{\text{CO}}{\text{HR}}$	60 to 100 ml/beat
Stroke volume index	30 to 60 ml/beat/m^2
Systemic vascular resistance	900 to 1,200 dynes/sec/cm^{-5}
Systemic vascular resistance index	1,360 to 2,200 dynes/sec/cm^{-5}/m^2

$S\bar{v}o_2$ monitoring

The mixed venous oxygen saturation ($S\bar{v}o_2$) monitoring system consists of a flow-directed pulmonary artery catheter with fiber-optic filaments, an optical module, and a co-oximeter. The co-oximeter displays a continuous digital $S\bar{v}o_2$ value; the strip recorder prints a permanent record.

Normal $S\bar{v}o_2$ waveform

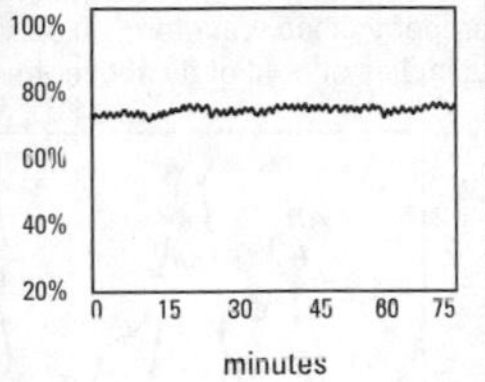

$S\bar{v}o_2$ with patient activities

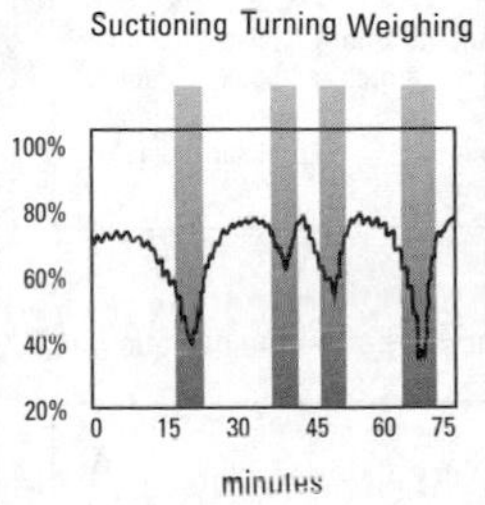

$S\bar{v}o_2$ with PEEP and Fio_2 changes

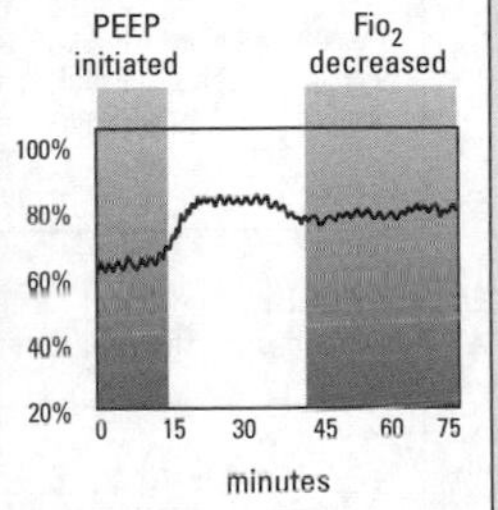

Intra-aortic balloon waveforms

Normal inflation-deflation timing

Balloon inflation occurs after aortic valve closure; deflation, during isovolumetric contraction, just before the aortic valve opens. In a properly timed waveform, like the one shown below, the inflation point lies at or slightly above the dicrotic notch.

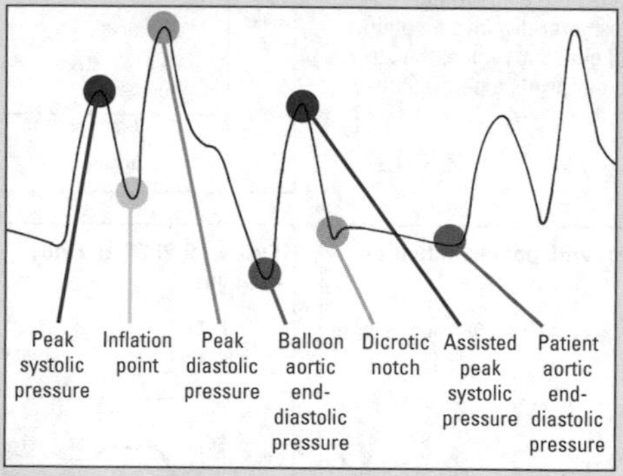

Early inflation

With *early inflation,* the inflation point lies before the dicrotic notch.

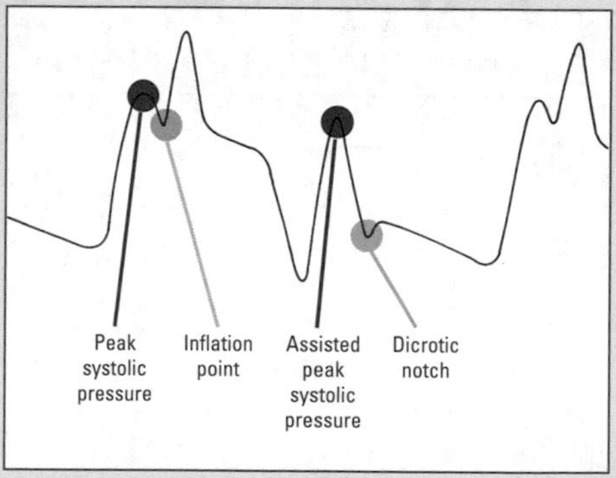

Intra-aortic balloon waveforms *(continued)*

Early deflation

With *early deflation,* a U shape appears and peak systolic pressure is less than or equal to assisted peak systolic pressure.

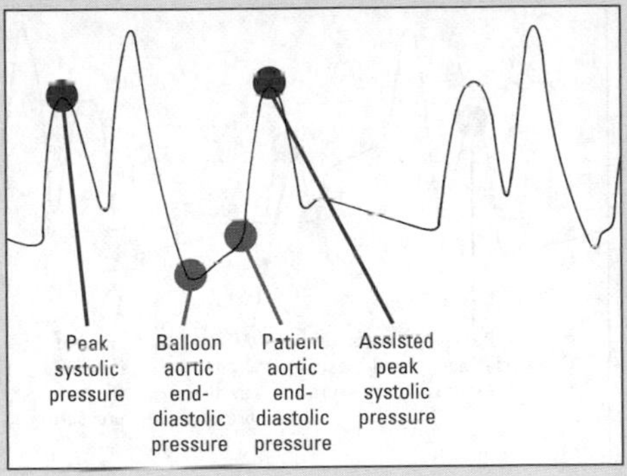

Late inflation

With *late inflation,* the dicrotic notch precedes the inflation point, and the notch and the inflation point create a W shape.

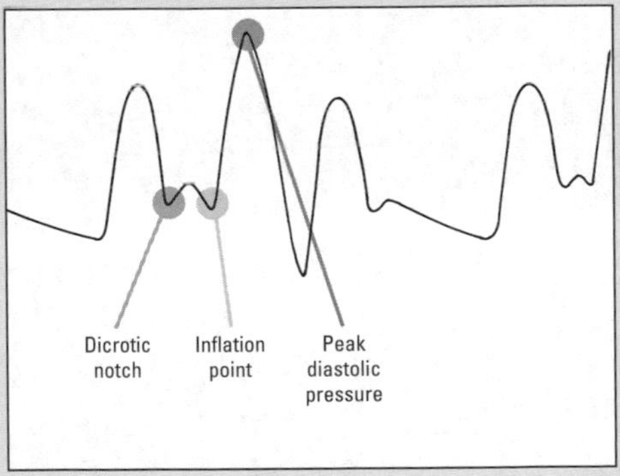

(continued)

Intra-aortic balloon waveforms *(continued)*

Late deflation

With *late deflation,* peak systolic pressure exceeds assisted peak systolic pressure.

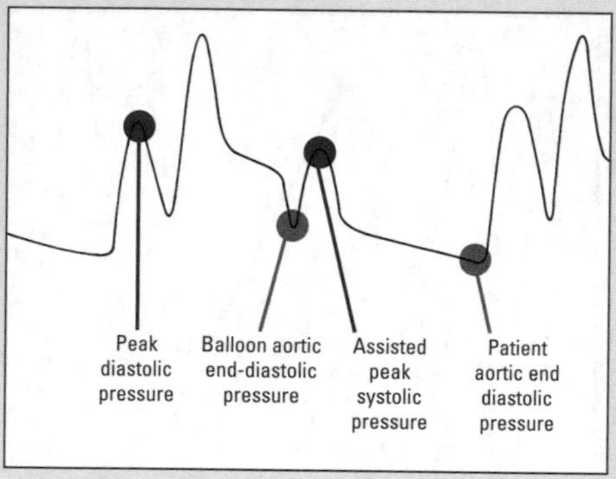

Respiratory assessment

Inspection	Chest configuration, tracheal position, chest symmetry, skin condition, nostril flaring, accessory muscle use, respiratory rate and pattern, cyanosis, clubbing of fingers
Palpation	Crepitus, pain, tactile fremitus, scars, lumps, lesions, ulcerations, chest wall symmetry and expansion
Percussion	Resonance (normal), hyperresonance, dullness, tympany
Auscultation	Four types of breath sounds over normal lungs: Tracheal, bronchial, bronchovesicular, and vesicular

Abnormal breath sounds

Sound	Description
Crackles	Light cracking, popping, intermittent, nonmusical sounds; like hairs rubbed together; heard on inspiration or expiration
Pleural friction rub	Low-pitched, continual, superficial, squeaking or grating sound; like pieces of sandpaper being rubbed together; heard on inspiration and expiration
Rhonchi	Low-pitched, snoring, monophonic sounds heard primarily on expiration; may be heard throughout the respiratory cycle
Stridor	High-pitched, monophonic crowing sound heard on inspiration; louder in the neck than chest wall
Wheezes	High-pitched, continual, musical or whistling sound heard on expiration; may be heard on inspiration and expiration

Auscultation sequence

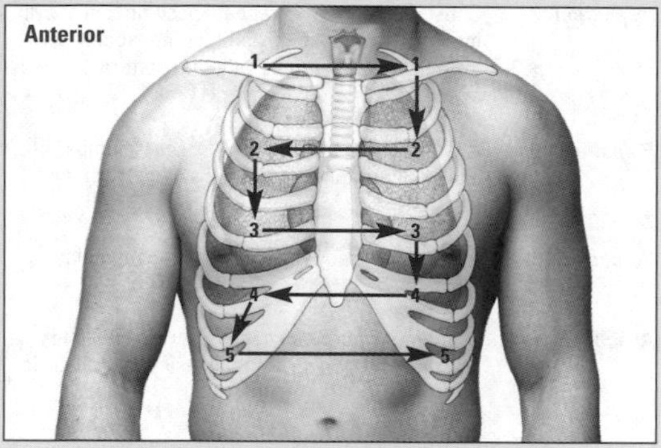

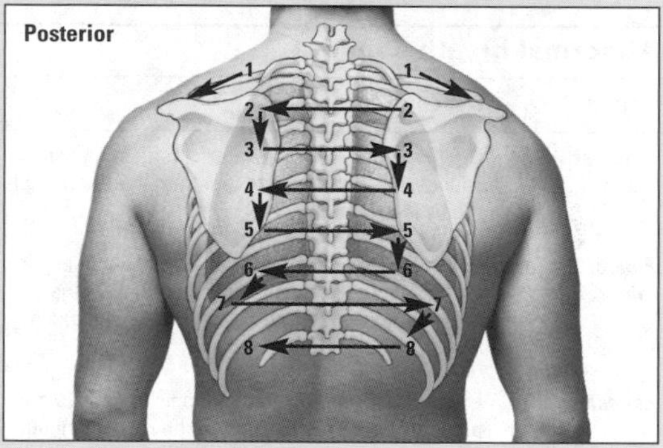

GI and GU assessment

Inspection

- *GI:* Abdominal symmetry, shape, contour, bumps, bulges, bruises, masses, striae, dilated veins, scars, movement and pulsations, distention, skin tightness, and glistening
- *GU:* Inflammation or discharge from urethral meatus

Auscultation

- *GI:* Bowel motility, underlying vessels and organs, bowel sounds (normal, hypoactive, or hyperactive), bruits, venous hum, or friction rub
- *GU:* Renal arteries (with bell in left and right upper abdominal quadrants)

Percussion

- *GI:* Tympany, dullness, size and location of abdominal organs, excessive accumulation of fluid and air (Don't percuss if abdominal aortic aneurysm or transplanted abdominal organ is present.)
- *GU:* Kidneys for tenderness; bladder for position and contents

Palpation

- *GI:* Abdominal size, shape, position; tenderness of major organs; masses and fluid accumulation
- *GU:* Kidneys and bladder

Abdominal quadrants

Right upper quadrant

- Right lobe of liver
- Gallbladder
- Pylorus
- Duodenum
- Head of the pancreas
- Hepatic flexure of the colon
- Portions of the ascending and transverse colon

Left upper quadrant

- Left lobe of the liver
- Stomach
- Body of the pancreas
- Splenic flexure of the colon
- Portions of the transverse and descending colon

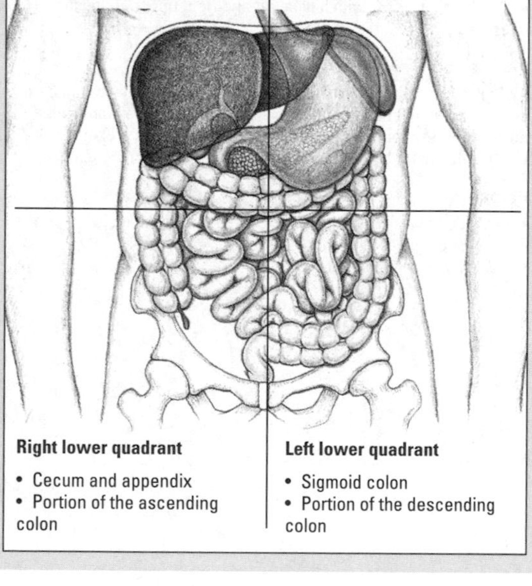

Right lower quadrant

- Cecum and appendix
- Portion of the ascending colon

Left lower quadrant

- Sigmoid colon
- Portion of the descending colon

Interpreting abnormal abdominal sounds

Sound and description	Location	Possible causes
Abnormal bowel sounds		
Hyperactive sounds (unrelated to hunger)	Any quadrant	Diarrhea, laxative use, or early intestinal obstruction
Hypoactive, then absent, sounds	Any quadrant	Paralytic ileus or peritonitis
High-pitched tinkling sounds	Any quadrant	Intestinal fluid and air under tension in a dilated bowel
High-pitched rushing sounds accompanied by abdominal cramps	Any quadrant	Intestinal obstruction
Systolic bruits		
Vascular blowing sounds	Over abdominal aorta	Aneurysm, partial arterial obstruction or turbulent blood flow
	Over renal artery	Renal artery stenosis
	Over iliac artery	Iliac artery occlusion
Venous hum		
Continuous, medium-pitched tone created by blood flow in a large, engorged vascular organ	Epigastric and umbilical regions	Increased collateral circulation between portal and systemic venous systems, as in cirrhosis
Friction rub		
Harsh, grating sound	Over liver and spleen	Inflammation of the peritoneal surface of liver

Musculoskeletal assessment

Inspection
- No gross deformities
- Symmetrical body parts
- Good body alignment
- No involuntary movements
- Smooth gait
- Active range of motion (ROM) with no pain in all muscles and joints
- No swelling or inflammation in joints or muscles
- Equal bilateral limb length and symmetrical muscle mass

Palpation
- Normal muscle mass shape, with no swelling or tenderness
- Equal bilateral muscle tone, texture, and strength
- No involuntary contractions or twitching
- Equally strong bilateral pulses

Grading muscle strength

Grade muscle strength on a scale of 0 to 5, as follows.

5/5	Normal	Patient moves joint through full ROM and against gravity with full resistance.
4/5	Good	Patient completes ROM against gravity with moderate resistance.
3/5	Fair	Patient completes ROM against gravity only.
2/5	Poor	Patient completes ROM with gravity eliminated (passive motion).
1/5	Trace	Patient's attempt at muscle contraction is palpable but without joint movement.
0/5	None	No evidence of muscle contraction is present.

Testing muscle strength

Biceps strength

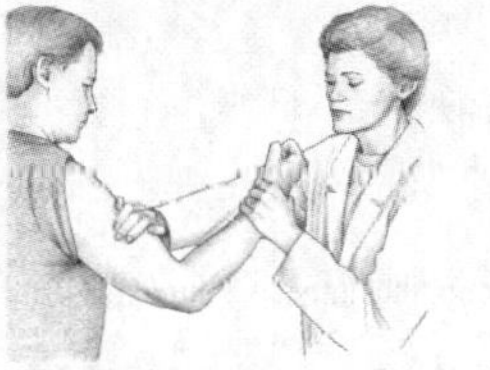

Ankle strength: Plantar flexion

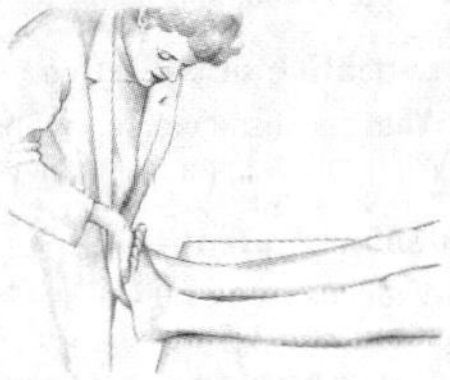

Triceps strength

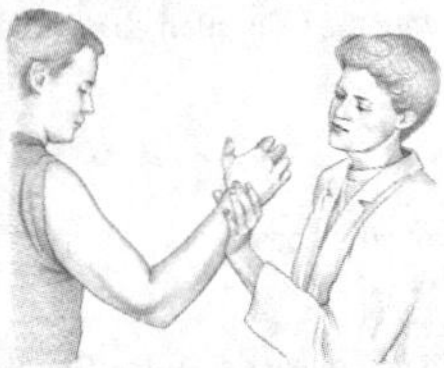

Ankle strength: Dorsiflexion

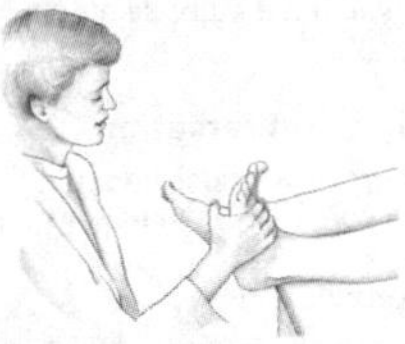

The 5 P's of musculoskeletal injury

Pain

Ask the patient whether he feels pain. If he does, assess its location, severity, and quality.

Paresthesia

Assess the patient for loss of sensation by touching the injured area with the tip of an open safety pin. Abnormal sensation or loss of sensation indicates neurovascular involvement.

Paralysis

Assess whether the patient can move the affected area. If he can't, he might have nerve or tendon damage.

Pallor

Paleness, discoloration, and coolness on the injured side may indicate neurovascular compromise.

Pulse

Check all pulses distal to the injury site. If a pulse is decreased or absent, blood supply to the area is reduced.

PQRST: The alphabet of pain assessment

Use the PQRST mnemonic device to obtain more information about the patient's pain. Asking the questions below helps identify important details about his pain.

Provocative or palliative

- What causes or worsens your pain?
- What relieves the pain or makes it subside?

Quality or quantity

- What does the pain feel like? Is it aching, intense, knifelike, burning, or cramping?
- Are you having pain right now? If so, is it more or less severe than usual?
- To what degree does the pain affect your normal activities?
- Do you have other symptoms along with the pain, such as nausea or vomiting?

Region and radiation

- Where is your pain located?
- Does the pain radiate to other parts of your body?

Severity

- How severe is your pain? How would you rate it on a 0-to-10 scale, with 0 being no pain and 10 being the worst pain imaginable?
- How would you describe the intensity of your pain when it's least severe? When it's most severe? Right now?

Timing

- When did your pain begin?
- At what time of day is your pain least severe? At what time is it most severe?
- Is the onset sudden or gradual?
- Is the pain constant or intermittent?

Numerical rating scale

A numerical rating scale can help the patient quantify his pain. Have him choose a number from 0 (indicating no pain) to 10 (indicating the worst pain imaginable) to reflect his current pain level. He can either circle the number on the scale itself or verbally state the number that best describes his pain (as shown below).

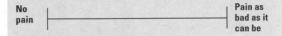

No pain	**0**	**1**	**2**	**3**	**4**	**5**	**6**	**7**	**8**	**9**	**10**	**Pain as bad as it can be**

Visual analog scale

To use the visual analog scale, ask the patient to place a mark on the scale to indicate his current level of pain as shown below.

No pain |————————————————| **Pain as bad as it can be**

Wong-Baker FACES pain rating scale

A pediatric patient or an adult patient with language difficulties may not be able to express the pain he's feeling. In such cases, use the pain intensity scale below. Ask the patient to choose the face that best represents the severity of his pain on a scale from 0 to 10.

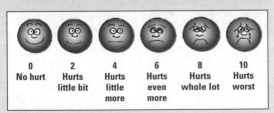

0	**2**	**4**	**6**	**8**	**10**
No hurt	**Hurts little bit**	**Hurts little more**	**Hurts even more**	**Hurts whole lot**	**Hurts worst**

From Wong, D.L., et al. *Wong's Essentials of Pediatric Nursing*, 6th ed. St. Louis: Mosby, 2001. Reprinted with permission.

Comparing types of chest pain

What the pain feels like	Where the pain is located
Aching, squeezing, burning pain as well as pressure and heaviness; usually subsides within 10 minutes	Substernal; may radiate to jaw, neck, arms, or back
Tightness or pressure; burning, aching pain, possibly accompanied by shortness of breath, diaphoresis, weakness, anxiety, or nausea; sudden onset; lasts 30 minutes to 2 hours	Typically across chest but may radiate to jaw, neck, arms, or back
Sharp and continuous; may be accompanied by friction rub; sudden onset	Substernal; may radiate to neck or left arm
Excruciating, tearing pain; may be accompanied by blood pressure difference between right and left arm; sudden onset	Retrosternal, upper abdominal, or epigastric; may radiate to back, neck, or shoulders
Sudden, stabbing pain; possibly cyanosis, dyspnea, or cough with hemoptysis	Over lung area
Sudden, severe pain; may experience dyspnea, increased pulse rate, decreased breath sounds, or deviated trachea	Lateral thorax

What makes it less painful?	What makes it more painful?	What causes the pain?
Rest, nitroglycerin (Note: Unstable angina appears even at rest.)	Eating, physical effort, smoking, cold weather, stress, anger, hunger, lying down	Angina pectoris
Opioid analgesics, such as morphine and nitroglycerin	Exertion, anxiety	Acute MI
Sitting up, leaning forward, anti-inflammatory drugs	Deep breathing, supine position	Pericarditis
Analgesics, surgery	Not applicable	Dissecting aortic aneurysm
Analgesics	Inspiration	Pulmonary embolus
Analgesics, chest tube insertion	Normal respiration	Pneumothorax

Comparing types of abdominal pain

Description	Location	Possible causes
Visceral: Originates in an abdominal organ; caused by stretching of nerve fibers around the organ; may be cramping, gassy, colicky, intermittent; may vary in intensity	Periumbilical	Appendicitis, cholecystitis, gastroenteritis, bowel obstruction, renal colic
Parietal or somatic: Caused by chemical or bacterial irritation; often rapid onset; sharp, steady, and severe in intensity	Localized	Viral or bacterial peritonitis, late appendicitis, gastroenteritis
Referred: Caused by irritation of shared dermatomes of affected organ	Distant from site of pathology	MI, angina, pancreatitis, renal colic, abdominal aortic aneurysm

Skin assessment

Color
- Bruising
- Discoloration
- Erythema
- Pallor
- Duskiness
- Jaundice
- Cyanosis

Texture
- Thickness
- Mobility
- Roughness
- Smoothness
- Fragility
- Thinness

Turgor
- Returns to regular shape after the skin on the forearm is squeezed: normal; doesn't return to regular shape, returns slowly, or leaves a tented shape: abnormal

Moisture
- Excessive dryness
- Excessive moisture
- Diaphoresis

Temperature
- Generalized or localized coolness or warmth

Lesions
- Vascular changes
- Hemangiomas
- Telangiectases
- Petechiae
- Purpura
- Ecchymosis
- Other lesions

Wound age

When determining wound age, you need to first determine if the wound is acute or chronic. Be careful—you can't base your determination solely on time because there isn't a set time frame before an acute wound becomes a chronic wound.

Wound type	Characteristics
Acute	• A new or relatively new wound • Occurs suddenly • Healing progresses in a timely, predictable manner • Typically heals by primary intention • Examples: surgical and traumatic wounds
Chronic	• May develop over time • Healing has slowed or stopped • Typically heals by secondary intention • Examples: pressure, vascular and diabetic ulcers • More susceptible to infection

Measuring wound depth

To measure the depth of a wound, you'll need gloves, a cotton-tipped swab, and a disposable measuring device. You can also use this method to measure wound tunneling or undermining.

Put on gloves, and then gently insert the swab into the deepest portion of the wound.

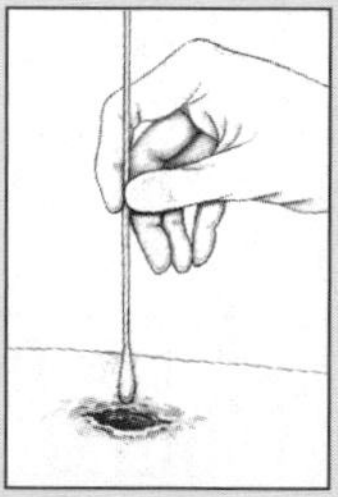

Grasp the swab with your fingers at the point that corresponds to the wound's margin. You can carefully mark the swab where it meets the edge of the skin.

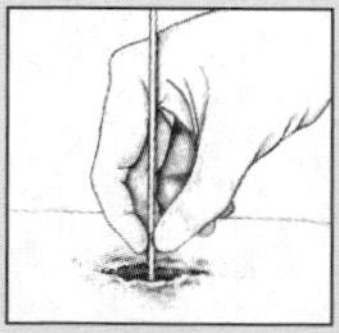

Remove the swab and measure the distance from your fingers or from the mark on the swab to the end of the swab to determine the depth.

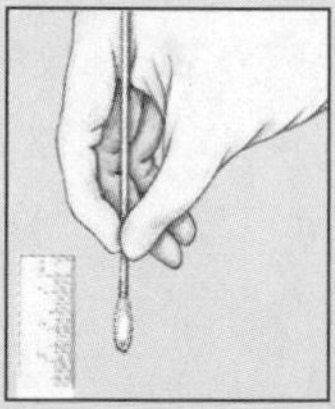

Disorders

Acute respiratory distress syndrome

Disorders

Description

- Severe form of alveolar or acute lung injury resulting in damage to alveolar capillary membrane.
- Pulmonary edema in the absence of cardiac failure.
- Hallmark sign: hypoxemia despite increased supplemental oxygen
- Also called *adult respiratory distress syndrome; ARDS;* and *shock, stiff, wet,* or *Da Nang lung* (see *Understanding ARDS*)

Causes

- Acute miliary tuberculosis
- Anaphylaxis
- Aspiration of gastric contents
- Coronary artery bypass grafting
- Disseminated intravascular coagulation
- Drug overdose
- Idiosyncratic drug reaction
- Indirect or direct lung trauma (most common)
- Massive blood transfusions
- Near drowning
- Oxygen toxicity
- Pancreatitis
- Pulmonary infection
- Sepsis
- Thoracic trauma
- Toxic inhalation of noxious gases and vapors
- Venous air embolism, fat embolism

Signs and symptoms

Stage I

- Shortness of breath, especially on exertion
- Normal to increased respiratory and pulse rates
- Anxiety, restlessness

Stage II

- Respiratory distress
- Thick, frothy sputum; bloody, sticky secretions
- Bibasilar crackles
- Cool, clammy skin; tachycardia; elevated blood pressure

Stage III

- Respiratory rate more than 30 breaths/minute, productive cough, crackles, and rhonchi
- Tachycardia with arrhythmias, labile blood pressure, pale, cyanotic skin

SNAPSHOT
Understanding ARDS

Phase 1. Injury reduces normal blood flow to the lungs. Platelets aggregate and release neutrophils (N), histamine (H), serotonin (S), and bradykinin (B).

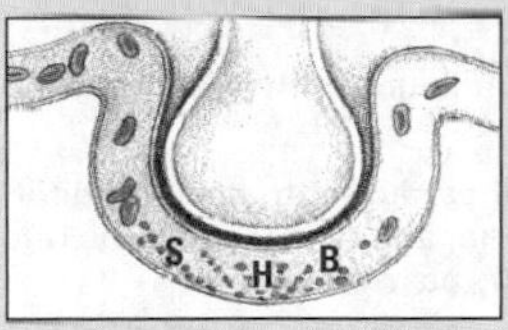

Phase 2. The released substances inflame and damage the alveolar capillary membrane, increasing capillary permeability. Fluids then shift into the interstitial space.

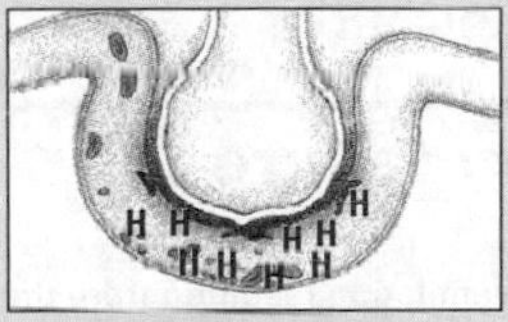

Phase 3. Capillary permeability increases and proteins and fluids leak out, increasing interstitial osmotic pressure and causing pulmonary edema.

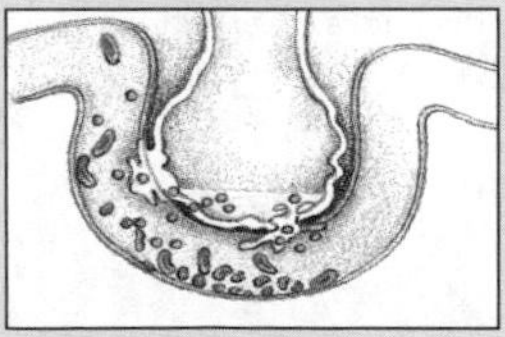

Phase 4. Decreased blood flow and fluids in the alveoli damage surfactant and impair the cell's ability to produce more. The alveoli then collapse, impairing gas exchange, casing pulmonary edema and decreased lung compliance.

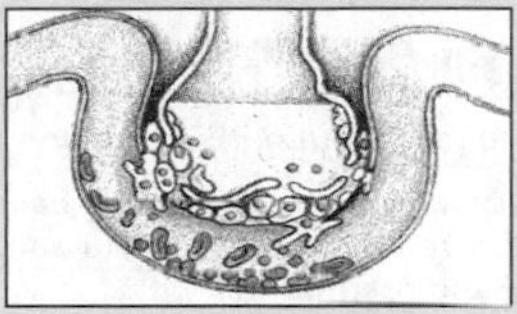

Phase 5. Oxygenation is impaired, but carbon dioxide (CO_2) easily crosses the alveolar capillary membrane and is expired. Blood oxygen (O_2) and CO_2 levels are low.

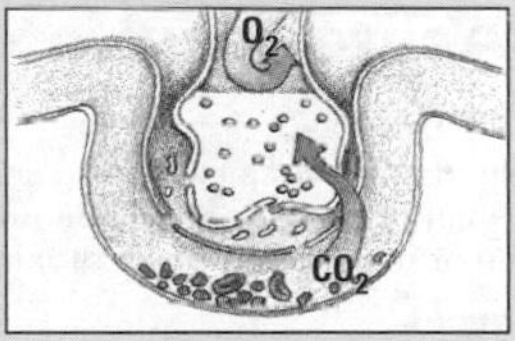

Phase 6. Pulmonary edema worsens and inflammation leads to fibrosis. Gas exchange is further impeded.

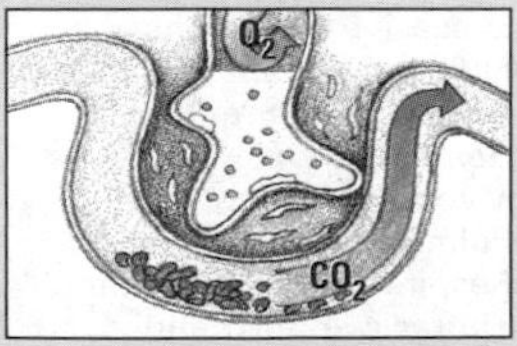

Disorders

- Mental status changes

Stage IV

- Acute respiratory failure with severe hypoxia
- Metabolic and respiratory acidosis
- Deteriorating mental status
- Pale, cyanotic skin
- Cardiac arrhythmias; hypotension
- Potential multi-organ failure

Management

- Oxygen therapy, mechanical ventilation with positive end-expiratory pressure (PEEP)

ALERT PEEP may lower cardiac output, so monitor for hypotension, tachycardia, and decreased urine output. To maintain PEEP, suction only as needed.

- Treatment of underlying cause
- Correction of electrolyte and acid-base imbalances
- Fluid restriction
- Tube feedings or parenteral nutrition
- Medications: antimicrobials, bronchodilators, mucolytics, corticosteroids, diuretics, fluids, neuromuscular blockers, opioids, sedatives, and vasopressors
- Frequent repositioning
- Frequent mouth care

Acute respiratory failure

Description

- Inadequate gas exchange and ventilation resulting from the inability of the lungs to adequately maintain arterial oxygenation or eliminate carbon dioxide

Causes

- Airway irritants
- Bronchospasm
- Central nervous system depression
- Chronic obstructive pulmonary disease exacerbation
- Endocrine or metabolic disorders
- Excessive secretions
- Fluid overload
- Gas exchange failure
- Heart failure
- Myocardial infarction
- Pulmonary emboli
- Respiratory tract infection
- Thoracic abnormalities
- Ventilatory failure

Signs and symptoms

- Cyanosis of the oral mucosa, lips, and nail beds
- Ashen skin; cold, clammy skin
- Use of accessory muscles; pursed-lip breathing
- Nasal flaring; rapid breathing
- Asymmetrical chest movement
- Anxiety, restlessness
- Hyperresonance
- Diminished or absent breath sounds
- Wheezes (with asthma)
- Rhonchi (with bronchitis)
- Crackles (with pulmonary edema)

Management

- Oxygen therapy with mechanical ventilation
- Fluid restriction (with heart failure)
- Medications: antacids, antibiotics, bronchodilators, corticosteroids, diuretics, histamine-receptor antagonists, positive inotropic drugs, vasopressors
- Frequent repositioning
- Frequent mouth care

Disorders

Anaphylaxis

Description

- Dramatic, acute atopic reaction to an allergen marked by sudden onset of rapidly progressive urticaria and respiratory distress
- Earlier signs and symptoms more severe after exposure to the antigen
- Severe reactions possibly initiating vascular collapse, leading to systemic shock and, possibly, death (see *Understanding anaphylaxis,* pages 58 and 59)

Causes

- Systemic exposure to:
  - blood transfusions
  - contrast media
  - foods (especially shellfish)
  - insect venom
  - latex
  - other specific antigens
  - sensitizing drugs

Signs and symptoms

- Anxiety
- Hives
- Angioedema

(Text continues on page 60.)

SNAPSHOT

Understanding anaphylaxis

1. Response to antigen

Imunoglobulins (Ig) M and G recognize and bind to antigen.

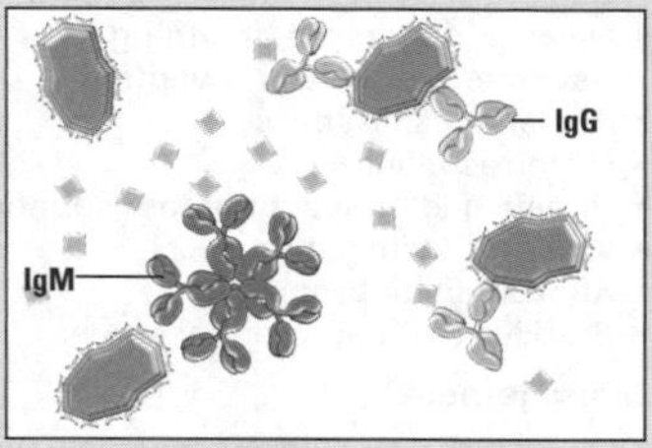

Complement cascade

2. Release of chemical mediators

Activated IgE on basophils promotes release of mediators: histamine, serotonin, and leukotrienes.

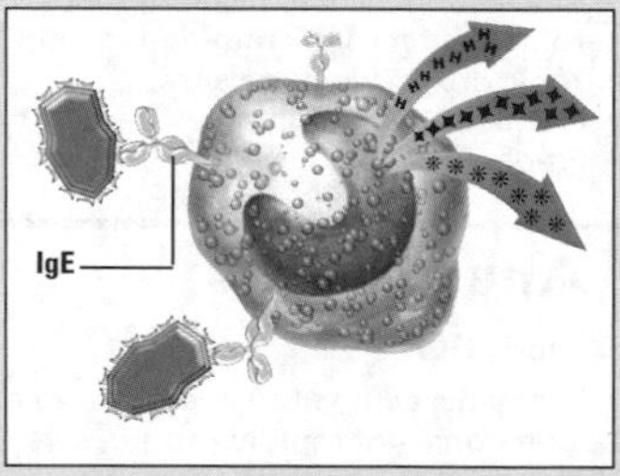

Histamine H Serotonin ◆ Leukotrienes ✳

3. Intensified response

Mast cells release more histamine and eosinophil chemotactic factor of anaphylaxis (ECF-A), which create venule-weakening lesions.

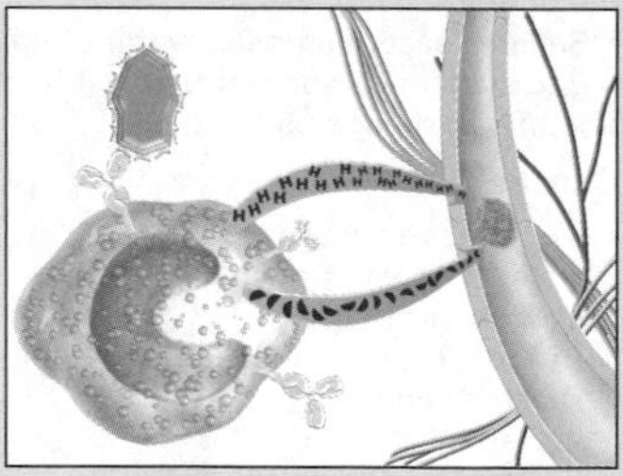

ECF-A ◖ Histamine H

Disorders

4. Respiratory distress

In the lungs, histamine causes endothelial cell destruction and fluid leakage into alveoli.

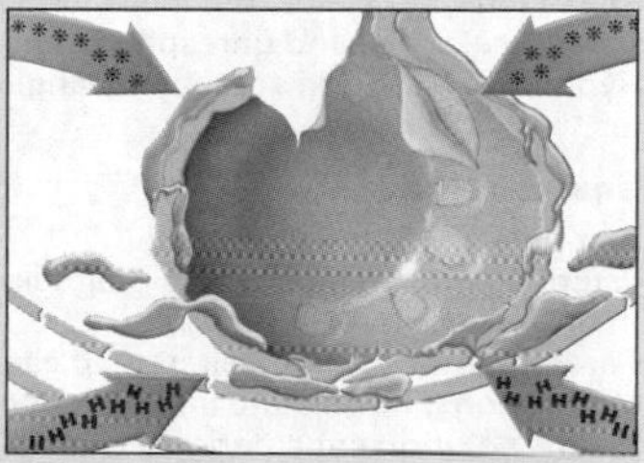

Leukotrienes ✲ Histamine H

5. Deterioration

Meanwhile, mediators increase vascular permeability, causing fluid to leak from the vessels.

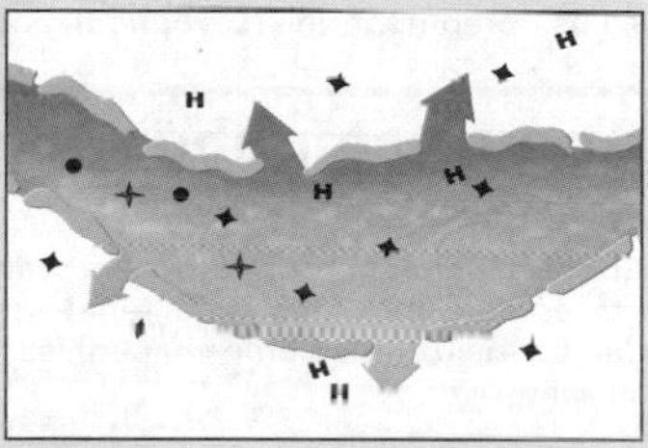

Bradykinin ● Prostaglandins ✦
Histamine H Serotonin ◆

6. Failure of compensatory mechanisms

Endothelial cell damage causes basophils and mast cells to release heparin and mediator-neutralizing substances. However, anaphylaxis is now irreversible.

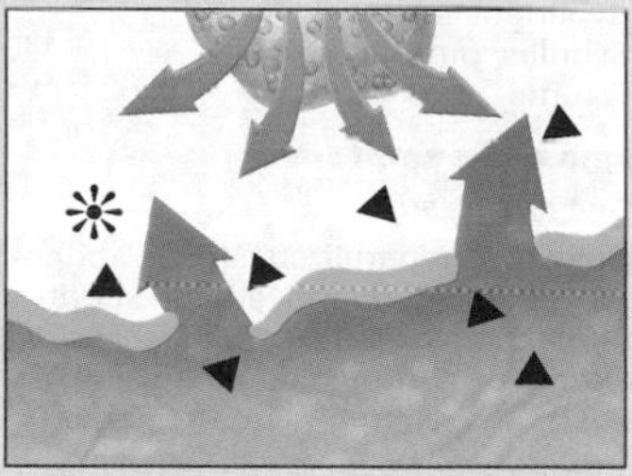

Leukotrienes ✲ Heparin ▲

• Hoarseness or stridor; wheezing
• Severe abdominal cramps, nausea, diarrhea
• Urinary urgency and incontinence
• Altered mental status, dizziness, drowsiness, headache, restlessness, seizures, and unresponsiveness
• Hypotension, shock; sometimes angina and cardiac arrhythmias

Management

• Removal of offending antigen
• Patent airway (establish and maintain); endotracheal intubation or tracheostomy, if indicated
• Cardiopulmonary resuscitation, if cardiac arrest occurs
• Medications: immediate injection of epinephrine 1:1,000 aqueous solution subcutaneously or I.V; corticosteroids; antihistamines, such as diphenhydramine (Benadryl); bronchodilators; volume expander infusions as needed; vasopressors, such as norepinephrine (Levophed), and dopamine (Intropin).

Aneurysm, abdominal aortic

Description

• Abnormal dilation from a weakness in the arterial wall of the aorta, commonly between the renal arteries and iliac branches
• Can be fusiform (spindle-shaped), saccular (pouch like), or dissecting

Causes

• Arteriosclerosis or atherosclerosis (95%)
• Connective tissue disorders
• Hypertension
• Syphilis; other infections
• Trauma

Signs and symptoms

Intact aneurysm

• Gnawing, generalized, steady abdominal pain; lower back pain unaffected by movement; sudden onset of severe abdominal pain or lumbar pain with radiation to flank and groin
• Gastric or abdominal fullness
• Possible pulsating mass in the periumbilical area

Ruptured aneurysm

• Into the peritoneal cavity: severe, persistent abdominal and back pain; into the duodenum: GI bleeding with massive hematemesis and melena
• Mottled to cyanotic skin, poor distal perfusion, absent peripheral distal pulses

- Decreased level of consciousness, syncope, diaphoresis, hypotension, tachycardia, oliguria
- Distended abdomen, ecchymosis or hematoma in the abdominal, flank, or groin area
- Systolic bruit over the aorta

Management

- Control of hypertension; fluid and blood replacement with rupture
- Medications: analgesics, antibiotics, antihypertensives, beta-adrenergic blockers
- Endovascular grafting or surgical resection for those that produce symptoms; bypass procedures for poor perfusion distal to aneurysm; graft replacement for repair of ruptured aneurysm

ALERT If rupture does occur, surgery must be done immediately. A pneumatic antishock garment may be used while transporting the patient to surgery.

After surgery

- Pulse assessment
- Blood pressure maintenance

Aneurysm, cerebral

Description

- Weakness in the wall of a cerebral artery causing localized dilation
- Berry aneurysm (most common form); saclike outpouching in a cerebral artery
- Usually occurs at an arterial junction in the Circle of Willis, the circular anastomosis forming the major cerebral arteries at the base of the brain
- Commonly ruptures, causing subarachnoid hemorrhage

Causes

- Congenital defect, degenerative process, or combination (see *How a cerebral aneurysm develops,* page 62)
- Trauma

Signs and symptoms

- Based on the site and amount of bleeding
- Vision defects
- Grade I (minimal bleeding): no neurologic deficit; possibly having slight headache and nuchal rigidity

SNAPSHOT

How a cerebral aneurysm develops

In an intracranial (cerebral) aneurysm, weakness in the wall of a cerebral artery causes localized dilation. Blood flow exerts pressure against the wall, stretching it like a balloon and making it likely to rupture. Cerebral aneurysms usually arise at the arterial bifurcation in the Circle of Willis and its branches. This illustration shows the most common sites around this circle.

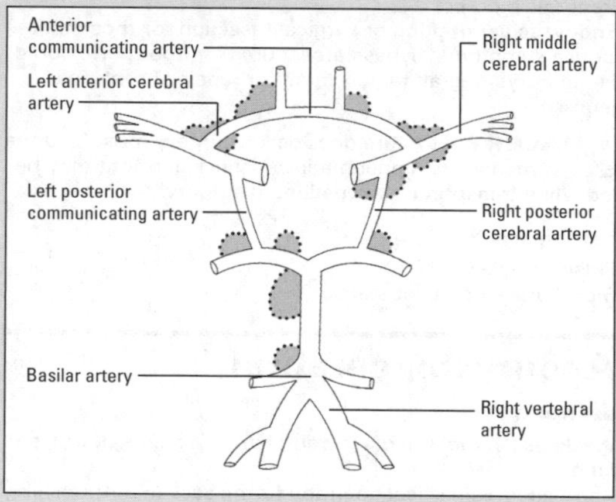

- Grade II (mild bleeding): alert with a mild to severe headache and nuchal rigidity; possibly having third-nerve palsy
- Grade III (moderate bleeding): altered mental status, with nuchal rigidity and, possibly, a mild focal deficit
- Grade IV (severe bleeding): stuporous with nuchal rigidity and possibly mild to severe hemiparesis
- Grade V (moribund; commonly fatal): deep coma or decerebrate

Management

- Aneurysm precautions (bed rest in a quiet, darkened room, keeping the head of the bed flat or less than 30 degrees, as ordered; limited visitation; avoidance of strenuous physical activity and straining with bowel movements; and restricted fluid intake)

- Avoidance of coffee, other stimulants, and aspirin
- Medications: aminocaproic acid, analgesics, anticonvulsants, antihypertensives, calcium channel blockers, corticosteroids, sedatives
- Surgical repair by clipping, ligation, or wrapping (before or after rupture)

Arterial occlusive disease

Description

- An obstruction or narrowing of the lumen of the aorta and its major branches; may affect the carotid, vertebral, innominate, subclavian, femoral, iliac, renal, mesenteric, and celiac arteries
- Prognosis dependent on location of the occlusion and development of collateral circulation that counteracts reduced blood flow

Causes

- Atheromatous debris (plaques)
- Atherosclerosis
- Direct blunt or penetrating trauma
- Embolism
- Fibromuscular disease
- Immune arteritis
- Indwelling arterial catheter
- Raynaud's disease
- Thromboangiitis obliterans
- Thrombosis

Signs and symptoms

- Narrowing of lumen may be present; may not cause symptoms
- Trophic changes and diminished or absent pulses of involved arm or leg, pallor with elevation of arm or leg, dependent rubor, ischemic ulcers
- Arterial bruit, hypertension
- Pain, pallor, pulselessness distal to the occlusion, paralysis and paresthesia occurring in the affected arm or leg, poikilothermy
- Sensory or motor deficits, expressive or receptive aphasia, vision disturbances

Management

- General: smoking cessation; hypertension, diabetes, and dyslipidemia control; foot and leg care; weight control; low-fat, low-cholesterol, high-fiber diet; regular walking program

• Medications: anticoagulants, antihypertensives, antiplatelets, hypoglycemics, lipid-lowering drugs, niacin or vitamin B complex, thrombolytics
• Surgery: embolectomy, endarterectomy, atherectomy, laser surgery or angioplasty, endovascular stent placement, percutaneous transluminal angioplasty, patch or bypass grafting, lumbar sympathectomy, amputation, bowel resection
• For chronic arterial occlusive disease use preventive measures, such as minimal pressure mattresses, heel protectors, a foot cradle, or a footboard.
• Preoperative care during an acute episode: circulatory status and pulse monitoring
• Frequent repositioning
• Avoid elevating or applying heat to the affected leg.

Disorders

After surgery

• Pulse and circulation assessment
• With mesenteric artery occlusion: nasogastric decompression
• Maintaining fluid and electrolyte balance

Cardiac arrhythmias

Description

• Variations in the normal pattern of electrical conduction of the heart
• Vary in severity, from mild, producing no symptoms and requiring no treatment to catastrophic, requiring immediate resuscitation (see *Comparing normal and abnormal conduction,* pages 66 and 67)
• Classified according to their origin (atrial, junctional, ventricular or supraventricular); clinical significance determined by effect on cardiac output and blood pressure, partially affected by site of origin

Causes

• Acid-base imbalances
• Cellular hypoxia
• Congenital defects
• Connective tissue disorders
• Degeneration of the conductive tissue
• Drug toxicity
• Electrolyte imbalances
• Emotional stress
• Hyperthyroidism
• Hypertrophy of the heart muscle
• Idiopathic or a combination of causes
• Myocardial infarction or ischemia

- Organic heart disease
- Valvular heart disease

Signs and symptoms

- Circulatory failure along with an absence of pulse and respirations with asystole, ventricular fibrillation and, occasionally, with ventricular tachycardia; reduced urine output
- Pallor, cold and clammy extremities, hypotension
- Dyspnea
- Weakness, chest pain, dizziness, syncope (with severely impaired cerebral circulation)
- Palpitations

Management

- Supportive measures: cardiopulmonary resuscitation, defibrillation, adherence to ACLS protocols
- Medications: antiarrhythmics, electrolyte replacements
- Cardioversion
- Temporary or permanent placement of a pacemaker
- Implantable cardioverter-defibrillator (if indicated)
- Ablation therapy for atrial arrhythmias
- Surgical removal or cryotherapy of an irritable ectopic focus to prevent recurring arrhythmias
- Treatment of the underlying disorder
- ECG monitoring

Cardiac tamponade

Description

- Rapid increase in intrapericardial pressure caused by fluid accumulation in the pericardial sac
- Impaired diastolic filling of the heart (see *Understanding cardiac tamponade,* page 68)

Causes

- Acute myocardial infarction
- Acute pericarditis
- Acute rheumatic fever (rare)
- Bacterial infections
- Cardiac catheterization
- Cardiac surgery
- Chronic renal failure (rare)
- Connective tissue disorders (rare)
- Drug reaction
- Effusion in cancer
- Hemorrhage (nontraumatic cause)
- Idiopathic
- Radiation therapy

Disorders

SNAPSHOT

Comparing normal and abnormal conduction

Normal cardiac conduction

The conduction system of the heart, shown below, begins at the heart's pacemaker, the sinoatrial (SA) node. When an impulse leaves the SA node, it travels through the atria along Bachmann's bundle and the internodal pathways to the atrioventricular (AV) node and then down the bundle of His, along the bundle branches and, finally, down the Purkinje fibers to the ventricles.

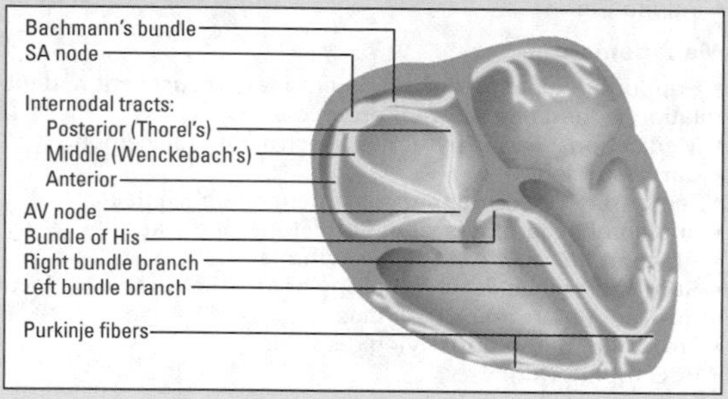

Abnormal cardiac conduction

Altered automaticity, irritability, reentry, or conduction disturbances may cause cardiac arrhythmias.

Altered automaticity

Altered automaticity is the result of partial depolarization, which may increase the intrinsic rate of the SA node or latent pacemakers, or may induce ectopic pacemakers to reach threshold and depolarize.

- Trauma
- Thrombolytic therapy
- Tuberculosis
- Viral pericarditis

Signs and symptoms

- Anxiety and restlessness, diaphoresis, pallor, or cyanosis
- Beck's triad (jugular vein distention, hypotension, muffled heart sounds); edema; rapid, weak pulses; increased central venous pressure; pulsus paradoxus; narrow pulse pressure

Automaticity may be altered by such drugs as epinephrine, atropine, and digoxin (Lanoxin), and by such conditions as acidosis, alkalosis, hypoxia, myocardial infarction (MI), hypokalemia, hypermagnesemia, and hypocalcemia. Examples of arrhythmias caused by altered automaticity include atrial fibrillation and flutter, supraventricular tachycardia, ventricular tachycardia and fibrillation, accelerated idioventricular and junctional rhythms, and premature atrial, junctional, and ventricular complexes.

Reentry

Reentry occurs when ischemia or deformation causes an abnormal circuit to develop within conductive fibers. Although current flow is blocked in one direction within the circuit, the descending impulse can travel in the other direction. By the time the impulse completes the circuit, the previously depolarized tissue within the circuit is no longer refractory to stimulation.

Conditions that increase the likelihood of reentry include hyperkalemia, myocardial ischemia, and the use of certain antiarrhythmic drugs. Reentry may be responsible for such arrhythmias as paroxysmal supraventricular tachycardia, ventricular tachycardia, and premature atrial, junctional, and ventricular complexes.

An alternative reentry mechanism depends on the presence of a congenital accessory pathway linking the atria and the ventricles outside the AV junction; for example, Wolff-Parkinson-White syndrome.

Conduction disturbances

Conduction disturbances occur when impulses are conducted too quickly or too slowly. Possible causes include trauma, drug toxicity, myocardial ischemia, MI, and electrolyte abnormalities. The AV blocks occur as a result of conduction disturbances.

- Chest pain
- Hepatomegaly

Management

- Pericardiocentesis, if necessary
- Medications: inotropic drugs, intravascular volume expansion, oxygen
- Surgery: pericardiocentesis, pericardial window, subxiphoid pericardiotomy, complete pericardectomy, thoracotomy

SNAPSHOT

Understanding cardiac tamponade

The pericardial sac, which surrounds and protects the heart, is composed of several layers. The fibrous pericardium is the tough outermost membrane; the inner membrane, called the serous membrane, consists of the visceral and parietal layers. The visceral layer clings to the heart and is also known as the epicardial layer of the heart. The parietal layer lies between the visceral layer and the fibrous pericardium. The pericardial space—between the visceral and parietal layers—contains 10 to 30 ml of pericardial fluid. This fluid lubricates the layers and minimizes friction when the heart contracts.

Normal heart and pericardium

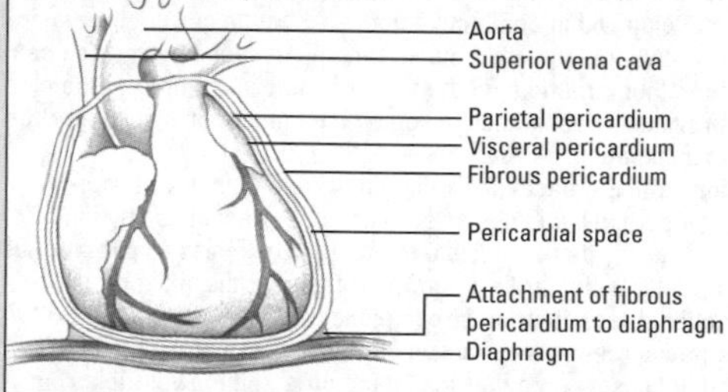

In cardiac tamponade, blood or fluid fills the pericardial space, compressing the heart chambers, increasing intracardiac pressure, and obstructing venous return. As blood flow into the ventricles falls, so does cardiac output. Without prompt treatment, low cardiac output can be fatal.

Cardiac tamponade

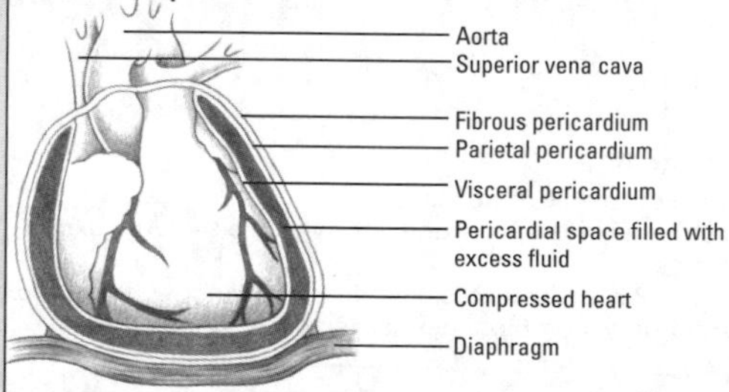

Disorders

Cerebral contusion

Description
- Ecchymosis of brain tissue resulting from injury to the head

Causes
- Acceleration-deceleration or coup-contrecoup injuries
- Head trauma

ALERT Complications may include intracranial hemorrhage, hematoma, tentorial herniation, and increased intracranial pressure (ICP).

Signs and symptoms
- Unconscious patient: pale and motionless; altered vital signs
- Conscious patient: drowsy or easily disturbed
- Scalp wound
- Possible involuntary evacuation of bowel and bladder; hemiparesis

Management
- Establishment of a patent airway and adequate oxygenation and circulation
- Administration of I.V. fluids

ALERT Dextrose 5% in water should be avoided because it may increase cerebral edema.

- Minimization of environmental stimuli
- Nothing by mouth until fully conscious
- Medications: nonopioid analgesics
- Surgery: craniotomy, depending on severity or location
- Neurologic status monitoring
- Seizure precautions, if indicated

Diabetic ketoacidosis

Description
- Acute complication of hyperglycemic crisis possibly occurring in the patient with diabetes
- If not treated properly, may result in coma or death (see *What happens in diabetic ketoacidosis,* pages 70 and 71)
- Also called *DKA*

Causes
- Autoimmune dysfunction
- Failure to take insulin or pump failure for those with insulin pumps

(Text continues on page 72.)

SNAPSHOT

What happens in diabetic ketoacidosis

This flowchart highlights the pathophysiologic events that occur in diabetic ketoacidosis.

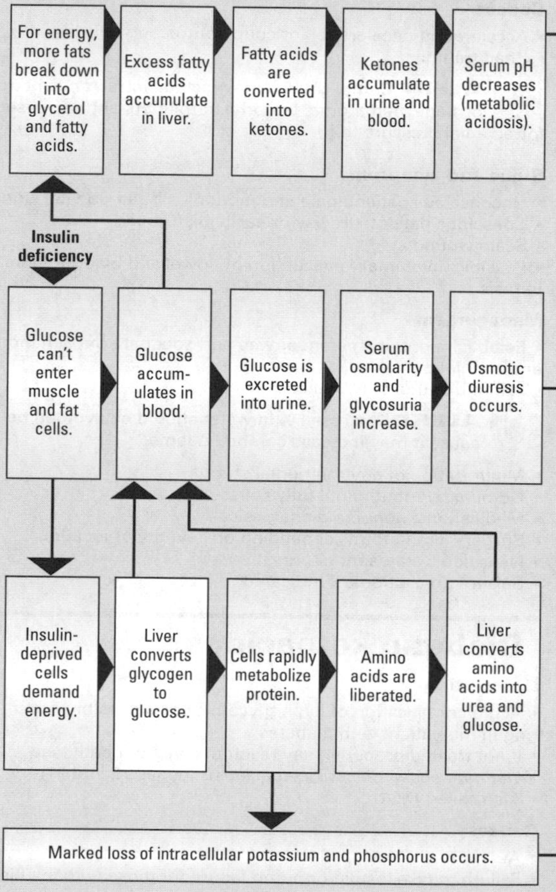
For energy, more fats break down into glycerol and fatty acids.
Excess fatty acids accumulate in liver.
Fatty acids are converted into ketones.
Ketones accumulate in urine and blood.
Serum pH decreases (metabolic acidosis).
Insulin deficiency
Glucose can't enter muscle and fat cells.
Glucose accumulates in blood.
Glucose is excreted into urine.
Serum osmolarity and glycosuria increase.
Osmotic diuresis occurs.
Insulin-deprived cells demand energy.
Liver converts glycogen to glucose.
Cells rapidly metabolize protein.
Amino acids are liberated.
Liver converts amino acids into urea and glucose.
Marked loss of intracellular potassium and phosphorus occurs.

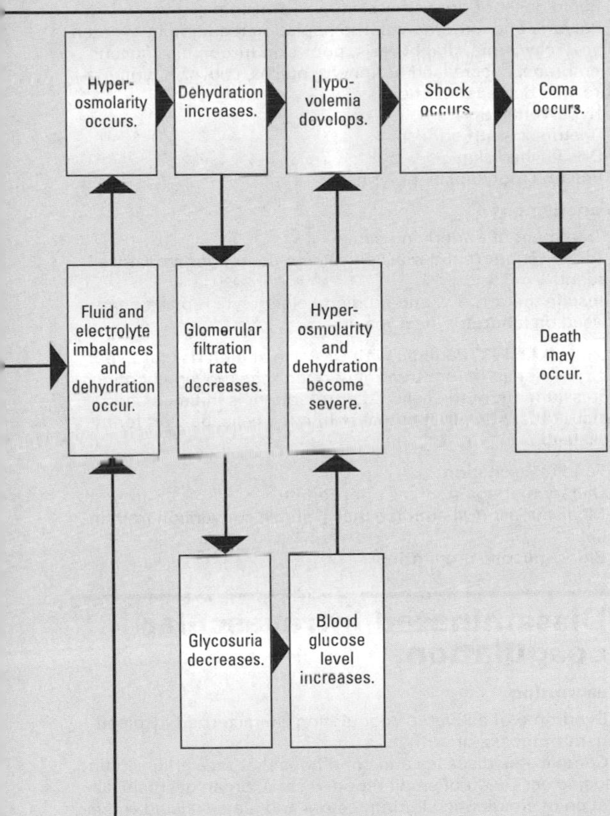
Hyper-osmolarity occurs.
Dehydration increases.
Hypo-volemia develops.
Shock occurs.
Coma occurs.
Fluid and electrolyte imbalances and dehydration occur.
Glomerular filtration rate decreases.
Hyper-osmolarity and dehydration become severe.
Death may occur.
Glycosuria decreases.
Blood glucose level increases.

Disorders

• Illness
• Other endocrine disease
• Recent stress or trauma
• Severe viral infection
• Use of drugs that increase blood glucose levels

Signs and symptoms

• Rapid onset of drowsiness, stupor, and coma
• Polyuria and extreme volume depletion resulting in hypotension, tachycardia, diaphoresis, poor skin turgor, dry mucous membranes, decreased peripheral pulses, cool skin temperature, and decreased reflexes
• Hyperventilation
• Acetone breath odor
• Dry, flushed skin
• Polyuria, polydipsia, polyphagia

Management

• Treatment of underlying cause
• Airway support and mechanical ventilation (for comatose patient)
• Insulin therapy, I.V. and fluid and electrolyte replacements (based on laboratory test results)

ALERT Patients with DKA are at high risk for hyperkalemia before treatment due to the movement of potassium out of the cells. After treatment is initiated and potassium begins to move back into the cells, be alert for hypokalemia.

• Fluid resuscitation
• Dietary management, as appropriate
• Medications: oral antidiabetics if stable conversion from insulin
• Blood glucose monitoring

Disseminated intravascular coagulation

Description

• Syndrome of activated coagulation characterized by bleeding, thrombosis, or both
• Complicates diseases and conditions that accelerate clotting, causing occlusion of small blood vessels, organ necrosis, depletion of circulating clotting factors and platelets, and activation of the fibrinolytic system (see *How disseminated intravascular coagulation happens*)

SNAPSHOT

How disseminated intravascular coagulation happens

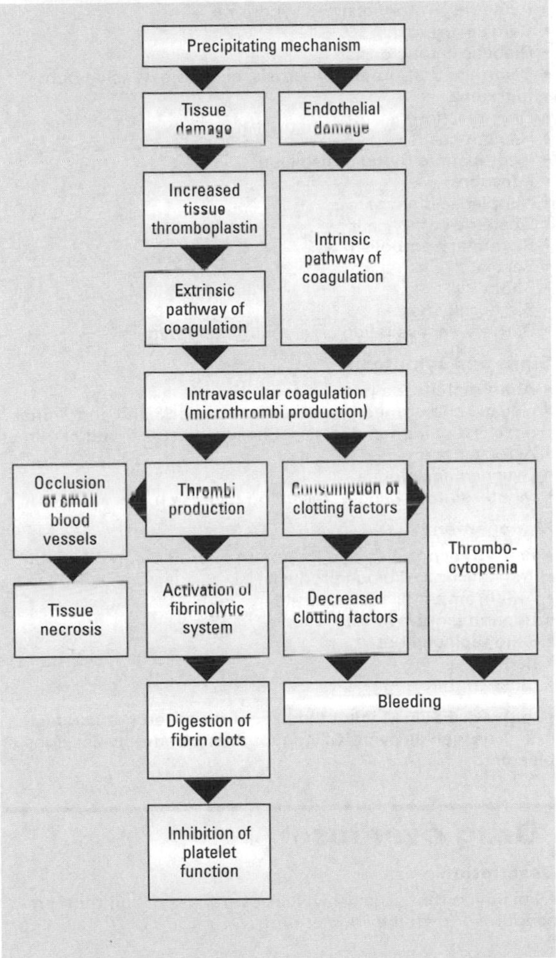

• Also called *DIC, consumption coagulopathy,* and *defibrination syndrome*

Causes

• Acute respiratory distress syndrome
• Cardiac arrest
• Diabetic ketoacidosis
• Disorders that produce necrosis, such as extensive burns and trauma
• Drug reactions
• Heatstroke
• Incompatible blood transfusion
• Infection
• Neoplastic disease
• Obstetric complications
• Pulmonary embolism
• Sepsis
• Shock
• Sickle cell anemia
• Surgery necessitating cardiopulmonary bypass

Signs and symptoms

• Abnormal bleeding
• Nausea and vomiting; severe muscle, back, and abdominal pain; chest pain; hemoptysis; epistaxis; seizures; and oliguria
• Acrocyanosis
• Dyspnea, tachypnea
• Mental status changes, including confusion

Management

• Prompt recognition and treatment of underlying condition
• Transfusions of blood products
• Antithrombin III and gabexate
• Heparin (controversial)
• Fluid replacement
• Bed rest
• Close monitoring

ALERT Monitor the patient for covert (intracranial) as well as overt (GI, genitourinary, hemoptysis) signs of bleeding.

Drug overdose

Description

• Poisoning that usually involves overdoses of common prescription or over-the-counter drugs

• Commonly ingested substances: illegal drugs, chemicals in the home or workplace, plants, and food
• Other sources of exposure: inhalation, injection, and direct absorption (skin and mucous membranes)
• Factors influencing signs and symptoms: type and amount of substance ingested, patient's tolerance to the toxin, number of toxins ingested, and time between ingestion and treatment
• Synergistic effects when drug combinations produce an effect that's greater than the sum of the effect of the two drugs
• Antagonistic effects when a drug combination produces an effect that's less than the sum of the drugs acting alone

Causes
• Accidental or intentional drug or chemical ingestion
• Ammonia, carbon dioxide, chlorine, hydrogen sulfide, and nitrogen dioxide
• Ingestion of salicylates (aspirin), cleaning agents, cosmetics, insecticides, paints, and plants (accidental in children)
• Ingestion of, or skin contamination from plants (such as azalea, dieffenbachia, mistletoe, philodendron)

Signs and symptoms
• Vary depending on what substance was taken, when it was taken, how much was taken, the time since it was taken, and the route (ingested, injected, inhaled)
• Altered mental status
• Seizures
• Constricted or dilated pupils
• Tachypnea, bradypnea, Kussmaul's respirations, or apnea
• Cardiac arrhythmia or arrest
• Dry mouth, diarrhea, nausea, vomiting, or hematemesis

Management
• Supportive measures: cardiopulmonary resuscitation, defibrillation, adherence to ACLS protocols
• Antidote administration; activated charcoal, gastric lavage, inducement of vomiting

ALERT Inducing vomiting is contraindicated when corrosive acid poisoning is suspected or if the patient has an altered level of consciousness or an impaired gag reflex. Gastric lavage is recommended for patients with ingestion of a potentially lethal amount of drug or toxin who present within 1 hour of ingestion.

• Close monitoring of neurologic, cardiac, and respiratory status
• I.V. fluid therapy
• Aspiration precautions

ALERT To prevent aspiration in the unconscious patient, an ET tube should be in place before performing lavage.

- Dialysis

Gastrointestinal bleeding

Description

- May occur anywhere in the GI tract
- Upper GI bleeding that occurs above the ligament of Treitz (where the duodenum meets the jejunum) includes bleeding in the esophagus, stomach, and duodenum
- Bleeding below Treitz ligament considered lower GI bleeding, with the most common site being the colon
- Also called *GI bleeding*

Causes

Lower GI bleeding

- Arteriovenous malformation (AVM)
- Diverticulitis or inflammatory bowel disease
- Polyps or neoplasms

Upper GI bleeding

- Angiodysplasias
- AVM
- Erosive gastritis
- Esophagitis and esophageal ulcers
- Mallory-Weiss syndrome
- Peptic ulcer disease (common)
- Rupture of esophageal varices

Signs and symptoms

- Bright red blood or coffee ground nasogastric tube drainage or vomitus, melena (upper GI bleed)
- Bright red blood from the rectum (lower GI bleed)
- Signs and symptoms of hypovolemic shock (cool, clammy skin; pallor; restlessness, apprehension; tachycardia; diaphoresis; hypotension; and syncope)

Management

- Fluid volume replacement with crystalloid solutions initially, followed by colloids and blood component therapy

ALERT When massive bleeding occurs, lactated Ringer's solution is preferred for fluid volume replacement because its use minimizes the risk of electrolyte imbalances.

- Respiratory support as indicated
- Gastric intubation with gastric lavage
- Medications: antacids, histamine-2 receptor antagonists, sucralfate (Carafate), misoprostol (Cytotec), and omeprazole (Prilosec)
- Endoscopic or surgical repair of bleeding sites
- Monitoring of hematologic lab tests
- Parenteral nutrition possible

Guillain-Barré syndrome

Description

- Form of polyneuritis that manifests as acute, rapidly progressive, and potentially fatal
- Occurs in three phases: acute beginning from first symptom, ending in 1 to 3 weeks; plateau lasting several days to 2 weeks; and recovery, which coincides with remyelination and axonal process regrowth; extending over 4 to 6 months and possibly taking up to 2 to 3 years; recovery possibly not complete

Causes

- Risk factors: Hodgkin's disease or another malignant disease, lupus erythematosus, rabies or swine influenza vaccination, surgery, or viral illness
- Unknown

ALERT Complications include thrombophlebitis, pressure ulcers, contractures, muscle wasting, aspiration, respiratory tract infections, and life-threatening respiratory and cardiac compromise.

Signs and symptoms

- History of minor febrile illness 1 to 4 weeks before current symptoms
- Tingling and numbness (paresthesia) in the legs with progression of symptoms to arms, trunk and, finally, the face
- Stiffness and pain in the calves
- Muscle weakness (the major neurologic sign)
- Sensory loss, usually in the legs (spreading to arms)
- Difficulty talking, chewing, and swallowing; paralysis of the ocular, facial, and oropharyngeal muscles
- Loss of position sense
- Diminished or absent deep tendon reflexes

Management

- Symptomatic and supportive care
- Possible endotracheal (ET) intubation or tracheotomy

- Fluid volume replacement
- Plasmapheresis
- Possible tube feedings with ET intubation
- Exercise program
- Maintenance of skin integrity
- Medications: I.V. beta-adrenergic blockers, parasympatholytics, I.V. immune globulin
- Surgery: possible tracheostomy, gastrostomy, or jejunostomy feeding tube insertion
- Frequent repositioning
- Frequent mouth care

Heart failure

Description

- Fluid buildup in the ventricles of the heart due to a weak myocardium that can't provide sufficient cardiac output
- Usually occurs in a damaged left ventricle, but may happen in the right ventricle primarily, or secondary to left-sided heart failure; failure of one ventricle eventually leading to failure of the other ventricle (see *What happens in left- and right-sided heart failure*)
- Also called *cardiac insufficiency* or *ventricular failure*

Causes

- Anemia
- Arrhythmias
- Atherosclerosis with myocardial infarction
- Constrictive pericarditis
- Emotional stress
- Hypertension
- Increased salt or water intake
- Infections
- Mitral or aortic insufficiency
- Mitral stenosis secondary to rheumatic heart disease, constrictive pericarditis, or atrial fibrillation
- Myocarditis
- Pregnancy
- Pulmonary embolism
- Thyrotoxicosis
- Ventricular and atrial septal defects

Signs and symptoms

- Dyspnea or paroxysmal nocturnal dyspnea
- Pink, frothy sputum
- Bibasilar crackles, rhonchi, and expiratory wheezing
- Peripheral edema, ascites
- Severe fatigue, weakness, insomnia

SNAPSHOT

What happens in left- and right-sided heart failure

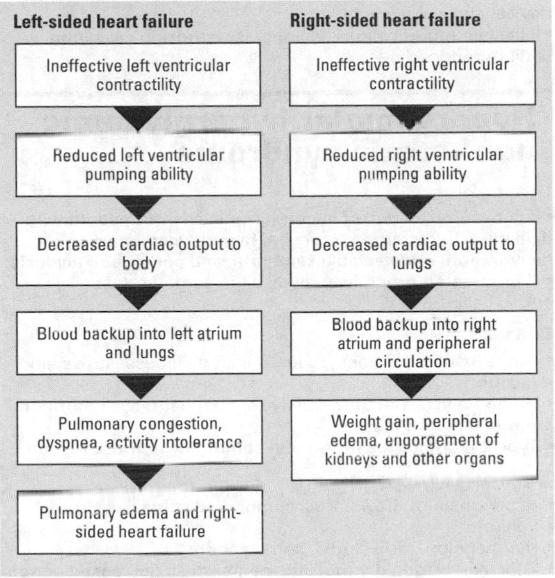

- Anorexia, nausea, sense of abdominal fullness (particularly in right-sided heart failure)
- Cyanosis of the lips and nail beds; pale, cool, clammy skin; diaphoresis
- Jugular vein distention, hepatomegaly and, possibly, splenomegaly (particularly in right-sided failure)
- Tachycardia, pulsus alternans, decreased pulse pressure, third and fourth heart sounds; decreased urinary output

Management

- Oxygen therapy with mechanical ventilation, if indicated
- Medications: diuretics, human B-type natriuretic peptide, inotropic drugs, vasodilators, angiotensin converting enzyme inhibitors, angiotensin receptor blockers, cardiac glycosides, potassium supplements, beta-adrenergic blockers, anticoagulants

- Fluid restriction (200 ml)
- Antiembolism stockings and elevation of lower extremities
- Sodium-restricted diet; calorie and fat restriction if indicated
- Valve replacement, heart transplantation, ventricular assist device, stent placement
- Lifestyle modifications: weight loss, smoking cessation, sodium reduced diet

Hyperosmolar hyperglycemic nonketotic syndrome

Description

- Acute complication of hyperglycemic crisis in patient with diabetes; characterized by severe hyperglycemia, profound dehydration, undetectable ketonuria, and absence of acidosis
- If not treated properly; may result in coma or death
- Also called *HHNS*

Causes

- Acute insulin deficiency; causes include illness, stress, and infection
- Hemodialysis, peritoneal dialysis, total parenteral nutrition, or enteral feedings
- Type 2 diabetes mellitus (most commonly in these patients)

Signs and symptoms

- Rapid onset of drowsiness, stupor, and coma
- Polyuria
- Hypotension, tachycardia, and diaphoresis
- Poor skin turgor, dry mucous membranes, decreased peripheral pulses, cool skin temperature, decreased reflexes, and orthostatic hypotension

Management

- Treatment of underlying cause
- Oxygen therapy with airway support and mechanical ventilation if indicated
- I.V. insulin therapy and fluid and electrolyte replacements
- Blood glucose and electrolyte monitoring
- Monitoring of cardiac status, vital signs, and intake and output
- Testing urine for glucose and ketones

ALERT If untreated, the patient with HHNS is at risk for shock, coma, and death. In addition, the patient is at risk for acute and long-term complications associated with diabetes mellitus.

Hypertensive crisis

Description

• Abrupt, acute, and marked increase in blood pressure from the patient's baseline, ultimately leading to acute and rapidly progressing end-organ damage (see *What happens in hypertensive crisis,* page 82)
• Typically, diastolic blood pressure greater than 120 mm Hg

Causes

• Chronic, poorly controlled or untreated primary hypertension
• Conditions responsible for secondary hypertension (pheochromocytoma, Cushing's syndrome, chronic renal failure, eclampsia)
• Disturbance in one of the intrinsic mechanisms: renin-angiotensin-aldosterone system, autoregulation, sympathetic nervous system, or antidiuretic hormone

Signs and symptoms

• Severe, throbbing headache in the back of the head (most common complaint)
• Blood pressure measurement, obtained several times at an interval of at least 2 minutes, reveals an elevated diastolic pressure above 120 mm Hg
• Nausea, vomiting, or anorexia
• Irritability, dizziness, confusion, somnolence, stupor
• Vision loss, blurred vision, or diplopia
• Dyspnea on exertion, orthopnea, paroxysmal nocturnal dyspnea, and edema secondary to heart failure
• With hypertensive encephalopathy: decreased level of consciousness; disorientation; seizures; focal neurologic deficits, such as hemiparesis; and unilateral sensory deficits
• Fourth heart sound (with left ventricular hypertrophy)
• Acute retinopathy and hemorrhage, retinal exudates, papilledema, and arterial-venous nicking

Management

• Medications: I.V. nitroprusside (Nipride), labetalol (Normodyne), nitroglycerin (Nitro-Bid IV), or hydralazine (Apresoline)

ALERT Know that nitroprusside is metabolized to thiocyanate, which is excreted by the kidneys. Be alert for signs and symptoms of thiocyanate toxicity, such as fatigue, nausea, tinnitus, blurred vision, and delirium.

• Lifestyle changes, such as weight reduction, smoking cessation, exercise, and dietary changes

Disorders

SNAPSHOT

What happens in hypertensive crisis

Hypertensive crisis is a severe rise in arterial blood pressure caused by a disturbance in one or more of the regulating mechanisms. If untreated, hypertensive crisis may result in renal, cardiac, or cerebral complications and, possibly, death.

Causes of hypertensive crisis

- Abnormal renal function
- Eclampsia
- Hypertensive encephalopathy
- Intracerebral hemorrhage
- Monoamine oxidase inhibitor interactions with food containing tyramine (beer, aged cheese)
- Myocardial ischemia
- Pheochromocytoma
- Untreated hypertension
- Withdrawal of antihypertensive drugs (abrupt)

↓

Prolonged hypertension

↓

Inflammation and necrosis of arterioles

↓

Narrowing of blood vessels

↓

Restriction of blood flow to major organs

↓

Organ damage

↓

Renal

- Decreased renal perfusion
- Progressive deterioration of nephrons
- Decreased ability to concentrate urine
- Increased serum creatinine and blood urea nitrogen
- Increased renal tubule permeability with protein leakage into tubules
- Renal insufficiency
- Uremia
- Renal failure

Cardiac

- Decreased cardiac perfusion
- Coronary artery disease
- Angina or myocardial infarction
- Increased cardiac workload
- Left ventricular hypertrophy
- Heart failure

Cerebral

- Decreased cerebral perfusion
- Increased stress on vessel wall
- Arterial spasm
- Ischemia
- Transient ischemic attacks
- Weakening of vessel intima
- Aneurysm formation
- Intracranial hemorrhage

- Blood pressure monitoring
- Monitoring of neurologic status

Hyperthermia

Description

- Elevation in body temperature over 99° F (37.2° C) that results from environmental and internal factors that increase heat production or decrease heat loss beyond the body's ability to compensate
- Three categories: heat cramps, heat exhaustion, and heatstroke
- Also called *heat syndrome*

Causes

- Conditions increasing heat production, such as drugs (for example, amphetamines), excessive exercise, and infection
- Factors impairing heat dissipation include cardiovascular disease; dehydration; drugs, such as phenothiazines and anticholinergics; excess clothing; high temperatures or humidity; lack of acclimatization; obesity; and sweat gland dysfunction

Signs and symptoms

Mild hyperthermia (heat cramps)

- Temperature ranging from 99° to 102° F (37.2° to 38.9° C)
- Mild agitation, muscle twitching and spasms
- Mild hypertension, tachycardia
- Moist, cool skin and muscle tenderness; involved muscle groups may be hard and lumpy
- Nausea, abdominal cramps

Moderate hyperthermia (heat exhaustion)

- Temperature elevated up to 104° F (40° C)
- Dizziness, syncope, confusion, weakness
- Headache, nausea, vomiting
- Hypotension; rapid, thready pulse
- Muscle cramping
- Oliguria; pale, moist skin; thirst

Critical hyperthermia (heat stroke)

- Temperature greater than 106° F (41.1° C)
- Confusion, combativeness, delirium, loss of consciousness, seizures
- Hypertension followed by hypotension, atrial or ventricular tachycardia, tachypnea
- Fixed, dilated pupils
- Hot, dry, reddened skin

ALERT Heat stroke, a medical emergency, can lead to hypovolemic or cardiogenic shock, cardiac arrhythmias, and renal failure caused by rhabdomyolysis, disseminated intravascular coagulation, and hepatic failure.

Management

- For mild hyperthermia (heat cramps): cool environment, rest, and oral or I.V. fluid and electrolyte replacement
- For moderate hyperthermia (heat exhaustion): cool environment, rest, and oral fluid and electrolyte replacement; if I.V. fluid replacement is necessary, laboratory test results determine the choice of I.V. solution—usually normal saline or isotonic glucose solution
- For critical hyperthermia (heat stroke): hypothermia blankets and ice packs to the groin and axillae, I.V. normal saline solution; supportive measures
- Monitoring of vital signs, oxygenation, and cardiac rhythm

ALERT Too rapid a reduction of temperature can lead to vasoconstriction, which can cause shivering. Shivering increases metabolic demand and oxygen consumption.

- Monitoring of neurologic status for changes

Hypothermia

Description

- Core body temperature below 95° F (35° C), affecting chemical changes in the body
- May be classified as mild (89.6° to 95° F [32° to 35° C]), moderate (86° to 89.6° F [30° to 32° C]), or severe (77° to 86° F [25° to 30° C]); severe hypothermia can be fatal
- Risk increases with youth, old age, lack of insulating body fat, wet or inadequate clothing, drug abuse, cardiac disease, smoking, fatigue, malnutrition and depletion of caloric reserves, and excessive alcohol intake

Causes

- Administration of large amounts of cold blood or blood products
- Cold water near drowning
- Possibly occurring in normal temperatures if disease or debility alters the patient's homeostasis
- Prolonged exposure to cold temperatures

Signs and symptoms

- With mild hypothermia: severe shivering, slurred speech, and amnesia
- With moderate hypothermia: unresponsive, with peripheral cyanosis and muscle rigidity
- With severe hypothermia: patient appears dead, with no palpable pulse and no audible heart sounds; dilated pupils; appears to be in a state of rigor mortis; ventricular fibrillation and a loss of deep tendon reflexes commonly occur and patient is at risk for cardiopulmonary arrest

Management

- Passive rewarming: warm blankets and a warm room
- Active external rewarming: hyperthermia blanket, warm water immersion, and radiant heat lamps
- Active core rewarming: heated I.V. fluids, genitourinary tract irrigation, extracorporeal rewarming, hemodialysis or peritoneal dialysis, gastric and mediastinal lavage, and heated, humidified oxygen

ALERT Be sure to rewarm the patient internally and externally at the same time; rewarming the surface first could cause rewarming shock with potentially fatal ventricular fibrillation. Rewarm slowly—if warmed blood is returned to a cold heart too fast, ventricular fibrillation and cardiovascular collapse can occur.

ALERT Arrhythmias that develop usually convert to normal sinus rhythm with rewarming. If the patient has no pulse or respirations, cardiopulmonary resuscitation is needed until rewarming raises the core temperature to at least 89.6° F (32° C).

- Oxygen therapy and mechanical ventilation, if indicated
- Monitoring of electrolyte levels

Meningitis

Description

• Inflammation of brain and spinal cord meninges that may affect all three meningeal membranes (dura mater, arachnoid membrane, and pia mater) (see *Inflammation in meningitis*)
• Usually follows onset of respiratory symptoms
• Sudden onset, causing serious illness within 24 hours
• Bacterial meningitis: acute infection that occurs in the subarachnoid space

Causes

• Bacterial infection, usually from *Neisseria meningitidis* and *Streptococcus pneumoniae*
• Fungi
• Possibly follows lumbar puncture, penetrating head wound, skull fracture, or ventricular shunting procedures
• Protozoa
• Secondary to another bacterial infection such as pneumonia
• Viruses

Signs and symptoms

• History of headache, fever, nausea, vomiting, weakness, myalgia, photophobia, confusion, delirium, and seizures
• Meningismus, rigors

ALERT Meningismus and fever are commonly absent in neonates and the only clinical clues may be nonspecific, such as refusal to feed, high-pitched cry, and irritability.

Elderly patients may exhibit an insidious onset, exhibiting lethargy and variable signs of meningismus and no fever.

• Profuse sweating, rash (with meningococcemia)
• Kernig's and Brudzinski's signs (elicited in only 50% of adults)
• Declining level of consciousness
• Cranial nerve palsies; focal neurologic deficits such as visual field defects
• Signs of increased intracranial pressure (in later stages)

Management

• Hypothermia measures and fluid therapy
• Medication: I.V. antibiotics, antiarrhythmics, osmotic diuretics, anticonvulsants, aspirin or acetaminophen
• Respiratory isolation for the first 24 hours (with meningococcal meningitis)
• Oxygen therapy
• Monitoring of neurologic status

SNAPSHOT
Inflammation in meningitis

In meningitis, pathogens trigger an inflammatory response in the brain and spinal cord. Often, inflammation begins in the pia-arachnoid (pia mater and arachnoid space) and progresses to congestion of adjacent tissues, where exudates cause nerve cell destruction and increased intracranial pressure. This results in engorged blood vessels, disrupted blood supply, thrombosis or rupture, and possibly cerebral infarction.

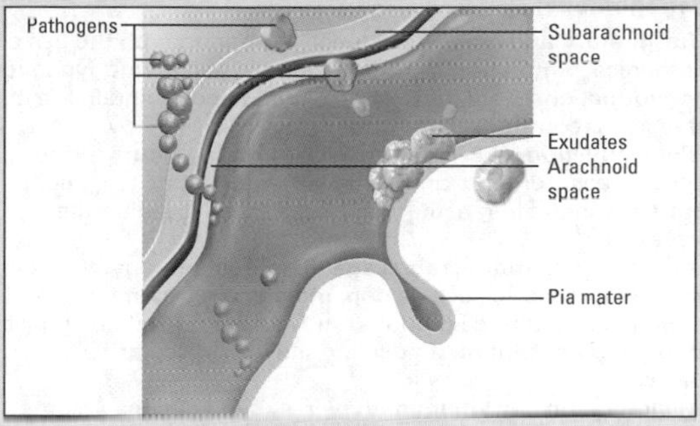

Multisystem organ dysfunction syndrome

Description

- Occurs when two or more organs or organ systems become affected and are unable to function in their role of maintaining homeostasis; intervention necessary to support and maintain organ function
- Not an illness by itself; occurs as a manifestation of another progressive underlying condition
- Also called *MODS*

Causes

- Infection
- Ischemia
- Multisystem injury
- Reperfusion injury
- Trauma

Signs and symptoms

- Fever, usually greater than 101° F (38.3° C)
- Tachycardia; narrowed pulse pressure
- Tachypnea
- Decreased pulmonary artery pressure, pulmonary artery wedge pressure, and central venous pressure and increased cardiac output (due to tachycardia)
- Signs of impaired perfusion of specific tissues and organs, such as decreasing level of consciousness, respiratory depression, diminished bowel sounds, jaundice, oliguria, or anuria

Management

- Respiratory and circulatory function support with the use of mechanical ventilation, supplemental oxygen, hemodynamic monitoring, and fluid infusion to expand and maintain the intravascular compartment
- Renal function closely monitored, including hourly urine output measurements and serial laboratory tests to evaluate for trends indicating acute renal failure; dialysis ultimately necessary
- Medications: antimicrobial agents to treat underlying infection; vasopressors, such as dopamine and norepinephrine
- Isotonic crystalloid solutions, such as normal saline and lactated Ringer's solution, to expand the intravascular fluid spaces
- Colloids, such as albumin, to help expand plasma volume without the added risk of causing fluid overload
- Some agents are being used with varying success, such as antitumor necrosis factor, endotoxin, and anti-interleukin-1 antibodies

Myocardial infarction

Description

- Reduced blood flow through one or more coronary arteries, causing myocardial ischemia and necrosis (see *Viewing the coronary vessels*)
- Infarction site dependent on the vessels involved
- Also called *MI* and *heart attack*

Causes

- Atherosclerosis
- Coronary artery stenosis or spasm
- Platelet aggregation
- Thrombosis

ALERT Risk factors include increased age (40 to 70); diabetes mellitus; elevated serum triglyceride, low-

SNAPSHOT

Viewing the coronary vessels

If an occlusion in a coronary artery causes a myocardial infarction (MI), the amount of damage to the myocardium depends on several factors. The area of the heart supplied by the affected vessel is a concern as well as the demand for oxygen in the affected area of the heart. In addition, the collateral circulation in the affected area of the heart affects the outcome. Collateral circulation is an alternate circulation that develops when blood flow to a tissue is blocked. The illustration here shows the major coronary vessels that may be involved in an MI.

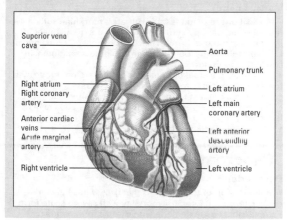

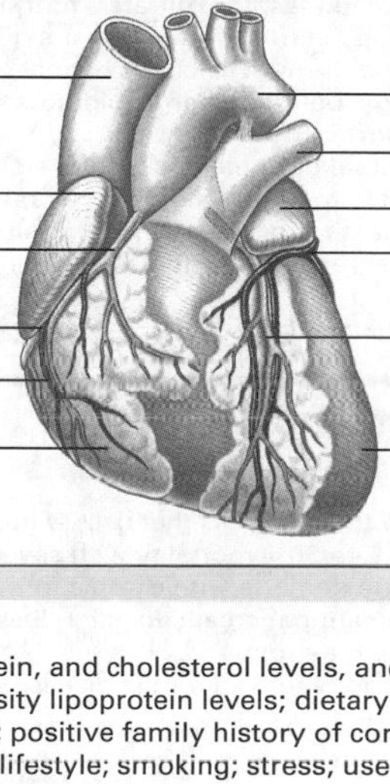

density lipoprotein, and cholesterol levels, and decreased serum high-density lipoprotein levels; dietary factors; hypertension; obesity; positive family history of coronary artery disease; sedentary lifestyle; smoking; stress; use of drugs, such as amphetamines or cocaine

Signs and symptoms

- Increasing frequency, severity, or duration of angina
- Cardinal symptom of MI: persistent, crushing substernal pain or pressure possibly radiating to the left arm, jaw, neck, and shoulder blades; for women: fatigue and back pain
- In elderly patients or those with diabetes, pain possibly absent; in others, pain possibly mild and confused with indigestion

- Feeling of impending doom, fatigue, nausea, vomiting, and shortness of breath
- Sudden death (may be the first and only indication of MI)
- Extreme anxiety and restlessness
- Dyspnea, diaphoresis
- Tachycardia, hypertension; bradycardia and hypotension, in inferior MI
- Third and fourth heart sounds and paradoxical splitting of the second heart sound with ventricular dysfunction; systolic murmur of mitral insufficiency; pericardial friction rub with transmural MI or pericarditis
- Low-grade fever during the next few days

Management

- Medications: oxygen, aspirin, nitrates, morphine sulfate, I.V. thrombolytic therapy started within 3 hours of the onset of symptoms, antiarrhythmics, calcium channel blockers, heparin I.V., inotropic drugs, beta-adrenergic blockers, angiotensin-converting inhibitors, stool softeners
- Temporary pacemaker or electric cardioversion (for arrhythmias not responsive to pharmacologic therapy)
- Intra-aortic balloon pump for cardiogenic shock
- Surgery: surgical revascularization, percutaneous revascularization
- Cardiac rehabilitation

Pancreatitis

Description

- Inflammation of the pancreas that occurs in acute and chronic forms; 10% to 30% mortality with severe acute form
- Irreversible tissue damage with chronic form; tends to progress to significant pancreatic function loss (see *Understanding acute pancreatitis*)
- May be associated with biliary tract disease, alcoholism, trauma, and certain drugs

Causes

- Abnormal organ structure (heredity)
- Alcoholism
- Ampullary stenosis
- Biliary tract disease
- Metabolic or endocrine disorders
- Pancreatic cysts or tumors
- Penetrating peptic ulcers
- Penetrating trauma
- Risk factors: use of drugs, such as glucocorticoids, hormonal contraceptives, sulfonamides, and thiazides; renal failure and

SNAPSHOT

Understanding acute pancreatitis

Inflammation of the pancreas may be acute or chronic. Acute pancreatitis, which is life-threatening, may be classified as edematous (interstitial) or necrotizing. In both types, inappropriate activation of enzymes causes tissue damage.

The mechanism that triggers this activation is unknown; however, several conditions are associated with it. The most common include biliary tract obstruction by gallstones and alcohol abuse (alcohol increases stimulation of pancreatic secretions).

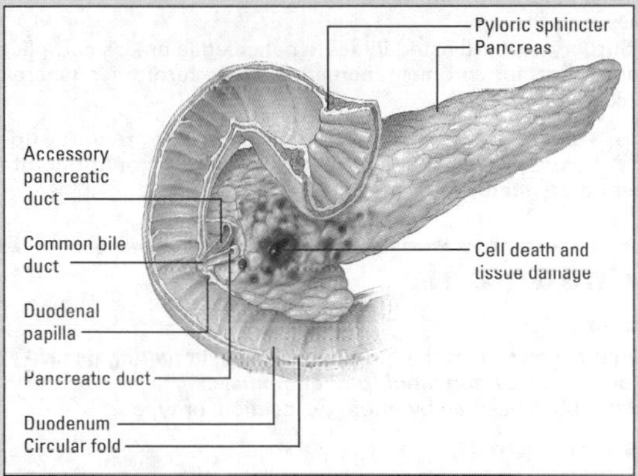

kidney transplantation; endoscopic retrograde cholangiopancreatography; heredity; and emotional or neurogenic factors
- Vascular insufficiency
- Viral or bacterial infection

Signs and symptoms

- Intense epigastric pain centered close to the umbilicus and radiating to the back, between the 10th thoracic and 6th lumbar vertebrae; usually aggravated by fatty foods, alcohol consumption, or recumbent position
- Weight loss with nausea and vomiting
- Hypotension, tachycardia
- Fever
- Dyspnea, orthopnea, pleural effusion
- Generalized jaundice

- Cullen's sign (bluish periumbilical discoloration), Turner's sign (bluish flank discoloration)
- Steatorrhea (with chronic pancreatitis)
- Abdominal tenderness, rigidity, and guarding

Management

- Emergency treatment of shock, as needed; vigorous I.V. replacement of fluid, electrolytes, and proteins; blood transfusions (for hemorrhage) and albumin as indicated
- Nasogastric suctioning
- Medications: analgesics, antacids, histamine antagonists, antibiotics, anticholinergics, pancreatic enzymes, insulin
- Total parenteral nutrition
- Oxygen therapy
- Surgery: not indicated in acute pancreatitis unless complications occur; for chronic pancreatitis, sphincterotomy; pancreaticojejunostomy

ALERT Respiratory complications may require support with mechanical ventilation. Close monitoring of respiratory status is vital.

Pneumonia

Description

- Acute infection of the lung parenchyma impairing gas exchange (see *Understanding pneumonia*)
- Possibly classified by etiology, location, or type

Causes

Aspiration pneumonia

- Caustic substance entering airway

Bacterial and viral pneumonia

- Abdominal and thoracic surgery
- Alcoholism
- Aspiration
- Atelectasis
- Bacterial or viral respiratory infections
- Chronic illness (such as cancer) and debilitation
- Endotracheal intubation or mechanical ventilation
- Exposure to noxious gases
- Immunosuppressive therapy
- Influenza
- Malnutrition
- Sickle cell disease
- Smoking
- Tracheostomy

SNAPSHOT
Understanding pneumonia

In bacterial pneumonia, an infection triggers alveolar inflammation and edema. This produces an area of low ventilation with normal perfusion. Capillaries become engorged with blood, causing stasis. As the alveolocapillary membrane breaks down, alveoli fill with blood and exudates, resulting in atelectasis.

In viral pneumonia, the virus attacks bronchial epithelial cells, causing inflammation and desquamation. The virus also invades mucus glands and goblet cells, spreading to the alveoli, which fill with blood and fluid.

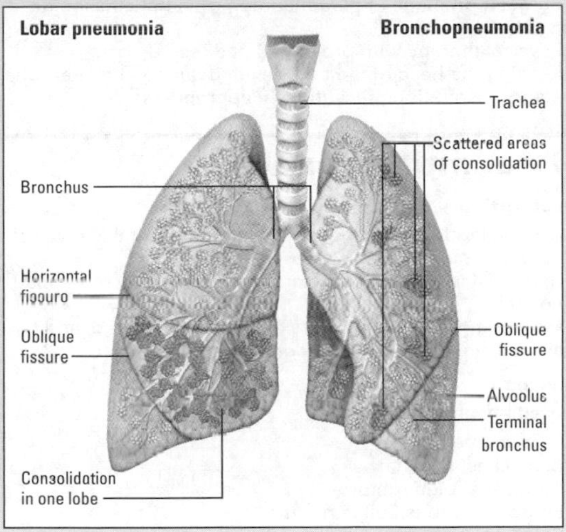

Signs and symptoms

- Bacterial pneumonia: sudden onset of pleuritic chest pain that worsens during inspiration, cough, purulent sputum production, and chills
- Viral pneumonia: nonproductive cough, constitutional symptoms, and fever
- Aspiration pneumonia: fever, weight loss, and malaise
- Fatigue
- Fever

- Sputum production
- Dullness over the affected area
- Crackles, wheezing, or rhonchi; decreased breath sounds; decreased fremitus (with emphysema or pleural effusion); increased fremitus in presence of consolidation
- Tachypnea, use of accessory muscles, shallow breathing

Management

- Mechanical ventilation (positive end-expiratory pressure) for respiratory failure; chest physiotherapy
- High-calorie, high-protein diet; adequate fluids; bed rest
- Medications: antibiotics, humidified oxygen, analgesics, bronchodilators
- Surgery: drainage of parapneumonic pleural effusion or lung abscess
- Physical therapy with prolonged bed rest
- Keeping the head of the bed elevated during and after tube feedings; aspiration precautions if appropriate

Pneumothorax

Description

- Accumulation of air or gas between the parietal and visceral pleurae, leading to lung collapse
- Degree of lung collapse determined by amount of trapped air or gas
- Most common pneumothorax types: open, closed, and tension (see *Understanding tension pneumothorax*)

Causes

Closed pneumothorax

- Barotrauma
- Blunt chest trauma
- Congenital bleb rupture
- Emphysematous bullae rupture
- Erosive tubercular or cancerous lesions
- Interstitial lung disease
- Rib or clavicle fracture
- Smoking

Open pneumothorax

- Central venous catheter insertion
- Chest surgery
- Penetrating chest injury
- Thoracentesis
- Transbronchial biopsy or percutaneous lung biopsy

SNAPSHOT

Understanding tension pneumothorax

In tension pneumothorax, air accumulates intrapleurally and can't escape.

On inspiration, increasing intrathoracic pressures cause the mediastinum to shift toward the unaffected lung, impairing ventilation.

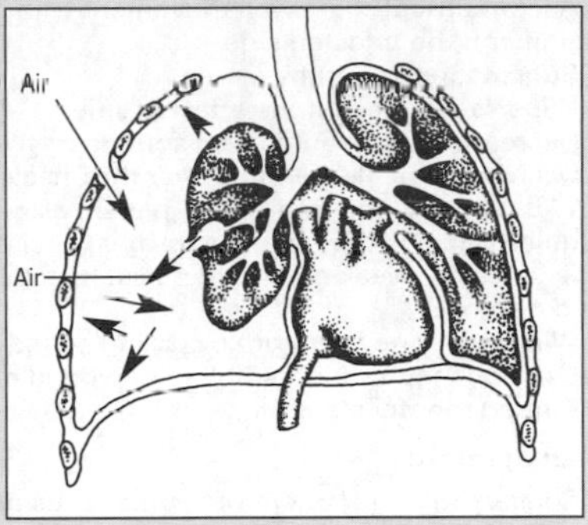

On expiration, the mediastinal shift distorts the vena cava and reduces venous return, producing hypotension and shock.

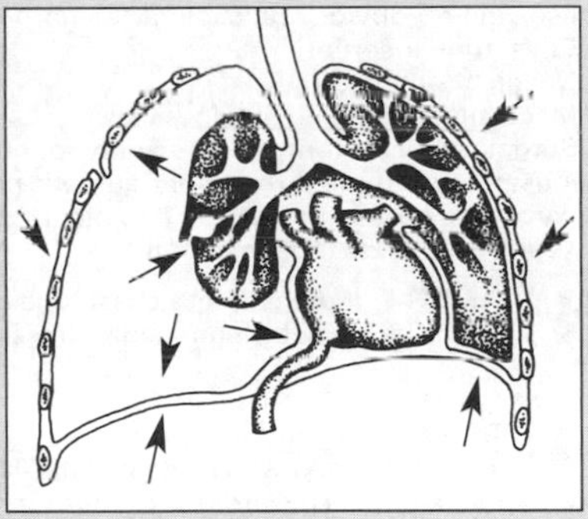

Tension pneumothorax

- Chest tube occlusion or malfunction
- High positive end-expiratory pressures, causing rupture of alveolar blebs
- Lung or airway puncture from positive-pressure ventilation
- Mechanical ventilation after chest injury
- Penetrating chest wound

Disorders

Signs and symptoms

- May be asymptomatic (with small pneumothorax)
- Sudden, sharp, pleuritic pain that worsens with chest movement, breathing, and coughing
- Shortness of breath, possible cyanosis (with tension pneumothorax)
- Asymmetrical chest wall movement with overexpansion and rigidity on the affected side
- Subcutaneous emphysema
- Hyperresonance on the affected side
- Decreased or absent breath sounds on the affected side
- Decreased tactile fremitus over the affected side
- With tension pneumothorax, patient also exhibits distended jugular veins, pallor, anxiety, tracheal deviation away from the affected side, weak and rapid pulse, hypotension, tachypnea, and cyanosis
- With open pneumothorax, sucking sound occurs from wound on inspiration; bubbling of wound on expiration
- Altered mental status

Management

- Conservative treatment of spontaneous pneumothorax with no signs of increased pleural pressure, less than 30% lung collapse, and no obvious physiologic compromise
- Chest tube insertion
- Needle thoracostomy
- Medications: oxygen, analgesics
- Surgery: thoracotomy, pleurectomy for recurring spontaneous pneumothorax; repair of traumatic pneumothorax; doxycycline or talc installation into pleural space
- Assist with chest tube insertion

ALERT If the patient's chest tube dislodges, immediately place a petroleum gauze dressing over the opening.

ALERT Watch for signs and symptoms of tension pneumothorax, which can be fatal. These include anxiety, hypotension, tachycardia, tachypnea, and cyanosis.

Pulmonary edema

Description

- Accumulation of fluid in the extravascular spaces of the lung that results from either increased pulmonary capillary hydrostatic pressure or decreased colloid osmotic pressure (see *Understanding pulmonary edema*)

SNAPSHOT

Understanding pulmonary edema

In pulmonary edema, diminished function of the left ventricle causes blood to back up into pulmonary veins and capillaries. The increasing capillary hydrostatic pressure pushes fluid into the interstitial spaces and alveoli. These illustrations show a normal alveolus and an alveolus affected by pulmonary edema.

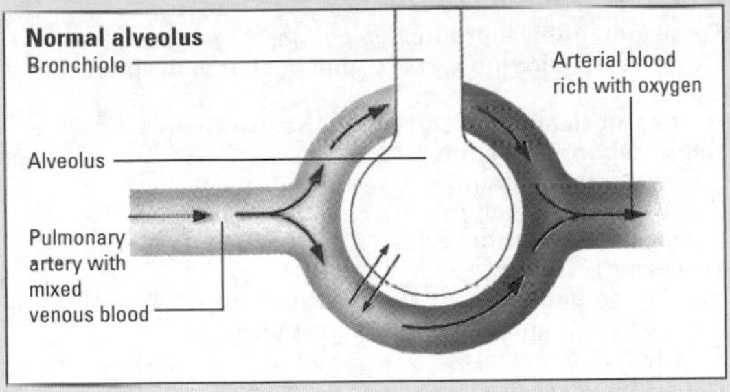

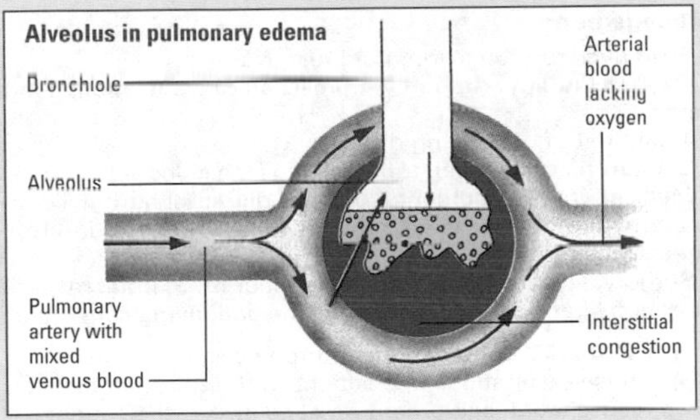

- Common complication of cardiovascular disorders
- May be chronic or acute, possibly becoming fatal rapidly

Causes

- Acute myocardial ischemia and infarction
- Arrhythmias
- Barbiturate or opiate poisoning
- Fluid overload

• Impaired pulmonary lymphatic drainage
• Inhalation of irritating gases
• Left atrial myxoma
• Left-sided heart failure or diastolic dysfunction
• Pneumonia
• Pulmonary veno-occlusive disease
• Thoracentesis
• Valvular heart disease

Signs and symptoms

• Persistent, intense productive cough
• Dyspnea on exertion, paroxysmal nocturnal dyspnea, orthopnea
• Restlessness and anxiety; mental status changes
• Rapid, labored breathing
• Frothy, bloody sputum
• Jugular vein distention
• Sweaty, cold, clammy skin
• Wheezing, crackles
• Third heart sound audible on auscultation
• Tachycardia, hypotension, thready pulse
• Peripheral edema
• Hepatomegaly

Management

• Fluid overload reduction, fluid restriction
• Oxygen therapy: support with mechanical ventilation, if indicated
• Treatment of underlying disease
• Sodium-restricted diet; tube feedings if needed
• Medications: supplemental oxygen, diuretics, nitroglycerin, antiarrhythmics, morphine, bronchodilators, positive inotropic agents, vasopressors
• Surgery: valve repair or replacement or myocardial revascularization, if appropriate, to correct the underlying cause

ALERT Be aware that morphine can further compromise respirations in a patient with respiratory distress. Keep resuscitation equipment on hand in case the patient stops breathing.

Pulmonary embolism

Description

• Obstruction of the pulmonary arterial bed from a thrombus lodged in the main pulmonary artery or branch, partially or completely obstructing it, resulting in ventilation-perfusion mismatch and hypoxemia

SNAPSHOT

How pulmonary embolism happens

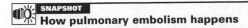

Blood clot forms in the deep venous system.

↓

Clot dislodges and travels through systemic venous system, right chambers of heart, and into pulmonary circulation.

↓

Clot lodges in branch of circulatory system.

↓

Blood flow distal to obstruction is blocked.

↓

Embolus prevents alveoli from producing enough surfactant to maintain alveolar integrity; alveoli collapse and atelectasis develops.

↓

Large clot can cause tissue death.

- Usually originates in deep veins of the leg (see *How pulmonary embolism happens*)
- May be asymptomatic, but sometimes causing rapid death from pulmonary infarction

Causes

- Atrial fibrillation
- Deep vein thrombosis
- Pelvic, renal, and hepatic vein thrombosis
- Rarely, other types of emboli, such as bone, air, fat, amniotic fluid, tumor cells, or a foreign body
- Right heart thrombus
- Upper extremity thrombosis
- Valvular heart disease

Signs and symptoms

- Shortness of breath for no apparent reason
- Pleuritic pain or angina
- Tachycardia, weak and rapid pulse, hypotension
- Low-grade fever
- Productive cough, possibly with blood-tinged sputum
- Warmth, tenderness, and edema of the lower leg
- Restlessness

• Transient pleural friction rub, crackles
• Third and fourth heart sounds with increased intensity of the pulmonic component of the second heart sound
• With a large embolus: cyanosis, syncope, distended jugular veins

Management

• Mechanical ventilation, if indicated; oxygen therapy
• Possible fluid restriction
• Medications: thrombolytics, anticoagulation, corticosteroids (controversial), diuretics, antiarrhythmics, vasopressors (for hypotension), antibiotics (for septic embolus)
• Surgery: vena caval interruption, vena caval filter placement, pulmonary embolectomy
• Avoid massaging the lower legs; encourage early postoperative ambulation

Renal failure, acute

Description

• Sudden interruption of renal function that results from obstruction, reduced circulation, or renal parenchymal disease
• Classified as prerenal failure, intrarenal failure (also called *intrinsic* or *parenchymal failure*), or postrenal failure
• Usually reversible with medical treatment; if not treated, may progress to end-stage renal disease, uremia, and death
• Normally occurs in three distinct phases: oliguric, diuretic, and recovery
• Oliguric phase: may last a few days or several weeks where urine output drops below 400 ml/day; fluid volume excess, azotemia, and electrolyte imbalance occurs; local mediators are released, causing intrarenal vasoconstriction; medullary hypoxia causes cellular swelling and adherence of neutrophils to capillaries and venules; hypoperfusion, cellular injury, and necrosis occurs; reperfusion causes reactive oxygen species to form, leading to further cellular injury
• Diuretic phase: renal function recovers and urine output gradually increases; glomerular filtration rate improves, although tubular transport systems remain abnormal
• Recovery phase: may last 3 to 12 months, or longer with gradual return to normal or near normal renal function (see *What happens in acute renal failure*)

Causes

Prerenal failure

• Hemorrhagic blood loss
• Hypotension or hypoperfusion

SNAPSHOT

What happens in acute renal failure

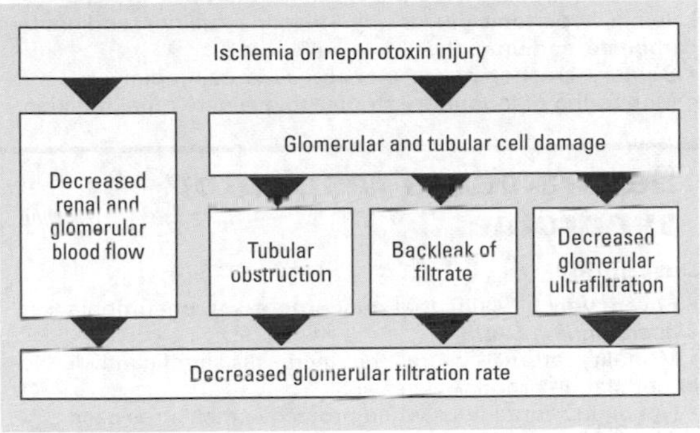

- Hypovolemia
- Loss of plasma volume
- Water and electrolyte losses

Intrarenal failure

- Acute tubular necrosis
- Coagulation defects
- Glomerulopathies
- Malignant hypertension

Postrenal failure

- Bladder neck obstruction
- Obstructive uropathies, usually bilateral
- Ureteral destruction

Signs and symptoms

- Oliguria or anuria, depending on renal failure phase
- Hypervolemia, edema
- Tachycardia
- Bibasilar crackles
- Irritability, drowsiness, confusion, altered level of consciousness
- Bleeding abnormalities
- Dry, pruritic skin; dry mucous membranes
- Uremic breath odor

Management

- Hemodialysis or continuous renal replacement therapy

- High-calorie, low-protein, low-sodium, and low-potassium diet; fluid restriction
- Medications: supplemental vitamins, diuretics; in hyperkalemia, hypertonic glucose-and-insulin infusions, sodium bicarbonate, sodium polystyrene sulfonate
- Surgery: creation of vascular access for hemodialysis
- Monitoring of laboratory studies to evaluate renal function

Disorders

Severe acute respiratory syndrome

Description

- Severe viral infection that may progress to pneumonia (see *Understanding SARS*)
- Mortality rate 10% overall, but increases significantly in older population groups
- Not highly contagious when protective measures used
- Also known as *SARS*

Causes

- Type of coronavirus known as SARS-associated coronavirus (SARS-CoV)
- Risk factors: close contact with an infected person, contact with aerosolized (exhaled) droplets and bodily secretions from an infected person, or travel to endemic areas

Signs and symptoms

- Headache, body aches
- Nonproductive cough
- Rash
- High fever
- Diarrhea
- Respiratory distress in later stages

Management

- Symptomatic treatment; may require mechanical ventilation
- Isolation for hospitalized patients; strict respiratory and mucosal barrier precautions
- Quarantine of exposed people to prevent spread; instruction on proper hand hygiene to prevent spread
- Global surveillance and reporting of suspected cases to national health authorities
- Medications: antipyretics, antivirals, steroids, oxygen
- Monitoring of respiratory status

SNAPSHOT

Understanding SARS

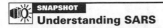

Although the exact origin of severe acute respiratory syndrome (SARS) is unknown, close contact with civet cats may have transmitted a mutated form of the coronavirus to humans. Viral infection of a human host cell could occur as follows:

The SARS virion (A) attaches to receptors on the host-cell membrane and releases enzymes (called *absorption*) (B) that weaken the membrane and enable the SARS virion to penetrate the cell. The SARS virion removes the protein coat that protects its genetic material (C), replicates (D), and matures, and then escapes from the cell by budding from the plasma membrane (E). The infection then can spread to other host cells.

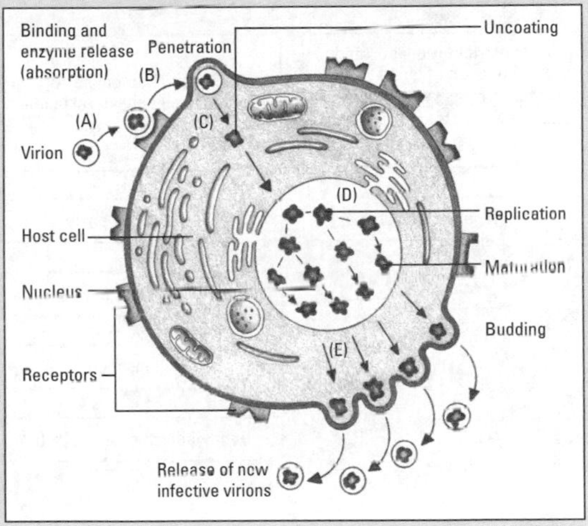

Shock, cardiogenic

Description

- Diminished cardiac output that severely impairs tissue perfusion
- Most lethal form of shock; sometimes called *pump failure* (see *What happens in cardiogenic shock,* page 104)

SNAPSHOT

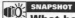

What happens in cardiogenic shock

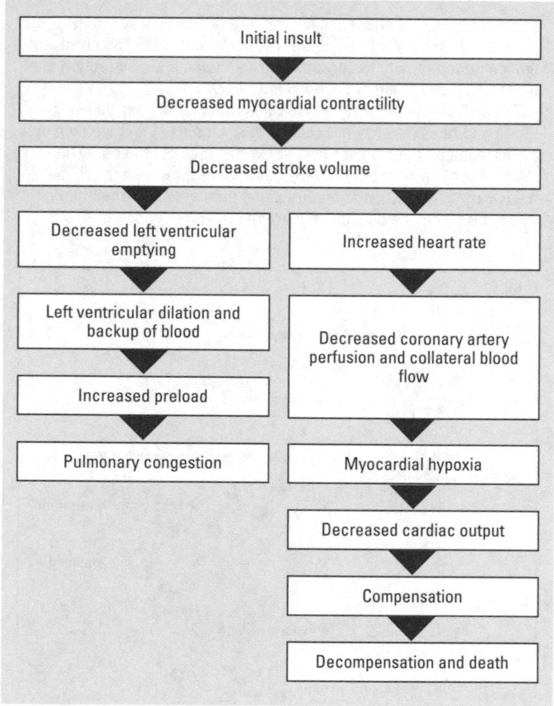

Causes

- Acute mitral or aortic insufficiency
- End-stage cardiomyopathy
- Myocardial infarction (most common)
- Myocardial ischemia
- Myocarditis
- Papillary muscle dysfunction
- Ventricular aneurysm
- Ventricular septal defect

Signs and symptoms
- Anginal pain
- Urine output less than 20 ml/hour
- Pale, cold, clammy skin
- Decreased sensorium and level of consciousness; severe anxiety
- Rapid, shallow respirations; pulmonary crackles
- Rapid, thready pulse; mean arterial pressure of less than 60 mm Hg in adults
- Gallop rhythm, faint heart sounds and, possibly, a holosystolic murmur
- Jugular vein distention

Management
- Medications: antiarrhythmics, analgesics, osmotic diuretics, inotropics, oxygen, sedatives, vasoconstrictors, vasodilators, and vasopressors
- Intra-aortic balloon pump
- Hemodynamic monitoring
- Possible parenteral nutrition or tube feedings
- Surgery: ventricular assist device, heart transplantation, or revascularization

Shock, hypovolemic

Description
- Reduced intravascular blood volume that causes circulatory dysfunction and inadequate tissue perfusion, resulting from loss of blood, plasma, or fluids (see *What happens in hypovolemic shock,* page 106)
- Potentially life-threatening

Causes
- Acute blood loss (about one-fifth of total volume)
- Burns
- Dehydration, as from excessive perspiration, severe diarrhea, protracted vomiting, diabetes insipidus, diuresis, or inadequate fluid intake
- Diuretic abuse
- Internal extravascular fluid loss caused by acute pancreatitis, ascites, intestinal obstruction, or peritonitis (third spacing)

Signs and symptoms
- Pale, cool, clammy skin
- Decreased sensorium, anxiety, irritability
- Rapid, shallow respirations
- Urine output usually less than 20 ml/hour

SNAPSHOT

What happens in hypovolemic shock

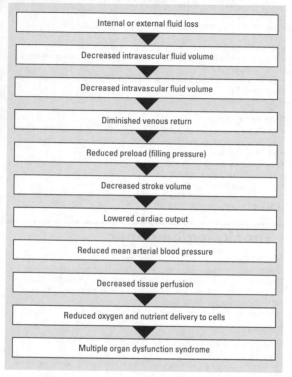

Internal or external fluid loss

↓

Decreased intravascular fluid volume

↓

Decreased intravascular fluid volume

↓

Diminished venous return

↓

Reduced preload (filling pressure)

↓

Decreased stroke volume

↓

Lowered cardiac output

↓

Reduced mean arterial blood pressure

↓

Decreased tissue perfusion

↓

Reduced oxygen and nutrient delivery to cells

↓

Multiple organ dysfunction syndrome

- Rapid, thready pulse; mean arterial pressure (MAP) less than 60 mm Hg in adults (with chronic hypotension, MAP may fall below 50 mm Hg before signs of shock)

Management

- Oxygen administration
- Bleeding control by direct application of pressure and related measures
- Medications: positive inotropes, vasopressors
- Prompt and vigorous blood and fluid replacement

- Hemodynamic monitoring
- Surgery to correct underlying problem
- Intra-aortic balloon pump, ventricular assist device, or pneumatic antishock garment

Shock, septic

Description

- Inflammatory response to infection that releases microbes or an immune mediator
- Characterized by low systemic vascular resistance and an elevated cardiac output in early stages; late stages, decreased cardiac output and progression to multiple organ dysfunction syndrome (MODS) (see *What happens in septic shock,* page 108)

Causes

- Any pathogenic organism that invades the bloodstream

Signs and symptoms

Hyperdynamic or warm phase

- Peripheral vasodilation; skin possibly pink, flushed or warm and dry
- Altered level of consciousness (LOC) reflected in agitation, anxiety, irritability, and shortened attention span
- Respirations rapid and shallow
- Urine output below normal
- Rapid, full, bounding pulse; blood pressure normal or slightly elevated
- Fever

Hypodynamic or cold phase

- Peripheral vasoconstriction and inadequate tissue perfusion; pale, cold, clammy skin and possible cyanosis
- Decreased LOC; possible obtundation and coma
- Respirations possibly rapid and shallow; crackles or rhonchi if pulmonary congestion present
- Urine output possibly less than 25 ml/hour or absent
- Rapid, weak, thready pulse; irregular pulse if arrhythmias present; hypotension

Management

- Remove and replace I.V., intra-arterial or urinary drainage catheters whenever possible
- In patients immunosuppressed from drug therapy, discontinue or reduce drugs, if possible
- Mechanical ventilation
- Fluid volume replacement

SNAPSHOT
What happens in septic shock

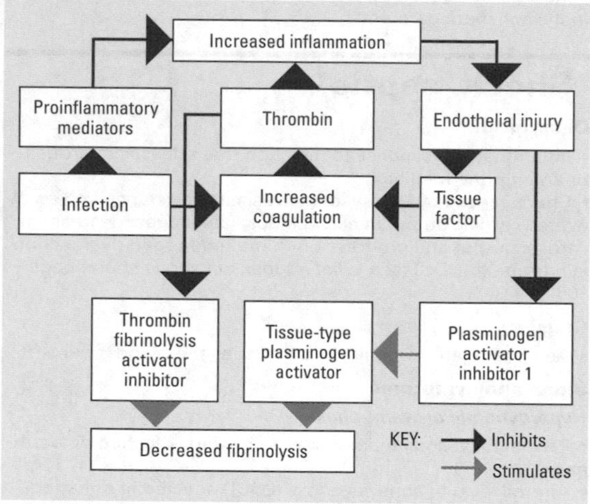

• Hemodynamic monitoring
• Medications: antimicrobial, antipyretics, colloid or crystalloid infusions, diuretics, granulocyte transfusions, oxygen, vasopressors
• Recombinant human-activated protein C (Xigris) infusion may be used
• Monitoring for multisystem organ dysfunction syndrome

Stroke

Description

• Sudden impairment of blood circulation to the brain resulting from thrombus, emboli, or hemorrhage (see *Understanding stroke*)
• Recurrences possible within weeks, months, or years
• Also known as *cerebrovascular accident* or *brain attack*

Causes

Cerebral embolism

• Cardiac arrhythmias

SNAPSHOT
Understanding stroke

Strokes are typically classified as ischemic or hemorrhagic, depending on the underlying cause. In either type of stroke, the patient is deprived of oxygen and nutrients.

Ischemic stroke

An ischemic stroke results from a blockage or reduction of blood flow to an area of the brain. The blockage may result from atherosclerosis or blood clot formation.

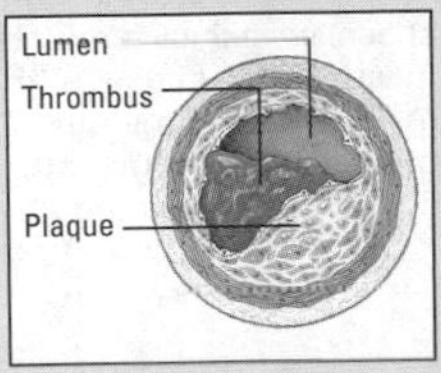

Common sites of plaque formation

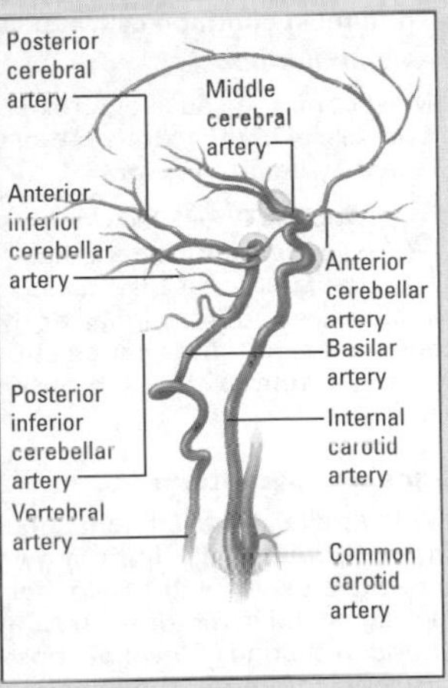

Hemorrhagic stroke

A hemorrhagic stroke is caused by bleeding within and around the brain. Bleeding that fills the spaces between the brain and the skull (called *subarachnoid hemorrhage*) is caused by ruptured aneurysms, arteriovenous malformation, and head trauma. Bleeding within the brain tissue itself (known as *intracerebral hemorrhage*) is primarily caused by hypertension.

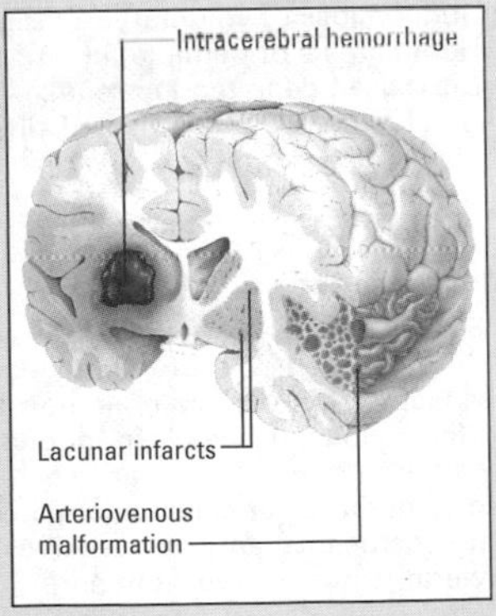

- Endocarditis
- History of rheumatic heart disease
- Post-open-heart surgery
- Posttraumatic valvular disease
- Second most common cause of stroke

Cerebral hemorrhage

- Arteriovenous malformation
- Cerebral aneurysms
- Chronic hypertension
- Third most common cause of stroke

Cerebral thrombosis

- Most common cause of stroke results from obstruction of a blood vessel in the extracerebral vessels
- Site may be intracerebral

Disorders

ALERT Risk factors for stroke include history of transient ischemic attack, heart disease, smoking, familial history of cerebrovascular disease, obesity, alcohol use, high red blood cell count, cardiac arrhythmias, diabetes mellitus, gout, high serum triglyceride and cholesterol levels, use of hormonal contraceptives in conjunction with smoking and hypertension.

Signs and symptoms

- With stroke in the left hemisphere, signs and symptoms on right side; with stroke in right hemisphere, signs and symptoms on left side; with stroke that causes cranial nerve damage, signs and symptoms on same side
- Sudden change in level of consciousness
- Sudden communication and mobility difficulties
- Sudden loss of voluntary muscle control
- Hemiparesis or hemiplegia on one side of the body
- Decreased deep tendon reflexes
- Hemianopsia on the affected side of the body
- Vision disturbances
- Headache
- Sensory losses

Management

- Secure patent airway
- Careful blood pressure management; titration of fluids and vasoactive drugs to maintain normotension
- Medications: tissue plasminogen activator when the cause isn't hemorrhagic (emergency care within 3 hours of onset of the symptoms); analgesics, anticoagulants, anticonvulsants, antidepressants, antihypertensives, antiplatelets, lipid-lowering agents, stool softeners

- Surgery: craniotomy, endarterectomy, extracranial-intracranial bypass, ventricular shunts
- Aspiration precautions: pureed dysphagia diet or tube feedings if indicated
- Physical, speech, and occupational rehabilitation; helping the patient adapt to specific deficits
- Monitoring of neurologic status

Syndrome of inappropriate antidiuretic hormone

Disorders

Description

- Disease of the posterior pituitary marked by excessive release of an antidiuretic hormone (vasopressin) from the posterior lobe of the pituitary gland (see *What happens in syndrome of inappropriate antidiuretic hormone,* page 112)
- Potentially life-threatening; prognosis dependent on underlying disorder and response to treatment
- Also known as *SIADH*

Causes

- Central nervous system disorders, such as tumor, trauma, infection, stroke, subarachnoid hemorrhage
- Drugs, such as exogenous vasopressin, nonsteroidal anti-inflammatory drugs, diuretics
- Miscellaneous conditions (myxedema and psychosis)
- Oat cell carcinoma of the lung or other neoplastic diseases
- Pulmonary disorders, such as tumors, chronic obstructive pulmonary disease, tuberculosis
- Surgery

Signs and symptoms

- Nausea, vomiting
- Headaches, blurred vision
- Agitation, irritability
- Tachycardia
- Disorientation, seizures, and coma
- Sluggish deep tendon reflexes, muscle cramps and weakness

Management

- Correction of the underlying cause
- Restricted water intake (500 to 1,000 ml/day)
- High-sodium, high-protein diet or urea supplements to enhance water excretion

SNAPSHOT

What happens in syndrome of inappropriate antidiuretic hormone

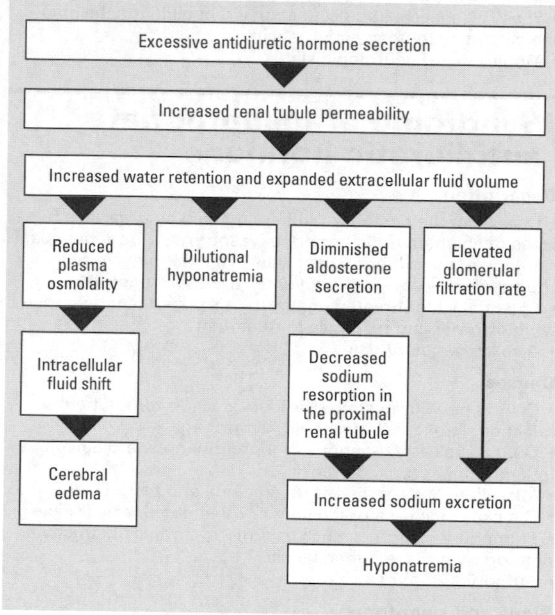

- Medications: corticosteroids, antidiuretic hormone antagonists, arginine and vasopressin receptor antagonist, vasopressin, loop and osmotic diuretics
- Careful administration of 3% sodium chloride solution if serum sodium level less than 120 or if the patient is having seizures
- Surgery to treat underlying cause such as cancer

ALERT Watch the patient closely for signs and symptoms of heart failure, which may occur because of fluid overload.

Diagnostic tests

Crisis values of laboratory tests

The abnormal laboratory test values listed here have immediate life-or-death significance to the patient. Report such values to the patient's physician immediately.

Test	Low value	Common causes and effects
Ammonia	< 15 mcg/dl	Renal failure
Calcium, serum	< 7 mg/dl	Vitamin D or parathyroid hormone deficiency: tetany, seizures
Carbon dioxide and bicarbonate, blood	< 10 mEq/L	Complex pattern of metabolic and respiratory factors
Creatine kinase isoenzymes		
Creatinine, serum		
D-dimer, serum or cerebrospinal fluid (CSF)		
Glucose, blood	< 40 mg/dl	Excessive insulin administration: brain damage
Gram stain, CSF		
Hemoglobin	< 8 g/dl	Hemorrhage or vitamin B_{12} or iron deficiency: heart failure
International Normalized Ratio		
Partial pressure of carbon dioxide, in arterial blood	< 20 mm Hg	Complex pattern of metabolic and respiratory factors
Partial pressure of oxygen, in arterial blood	< 50 mm Hg	Complex pattern of metabolic and respiratory factors

High value	Common causes and effects
> 50 mcg/dl	Severe hepatic disease: hepatic coma, Reye's syndrome, GI hemorrhage, heart failure
> 12 mg/dl	Hyperparathyroidism: coma
> 40 mEq/L	Complex pattern of metabolic and respiratory factors
> 5%	Acute myocardial infarction (MI)
> 4 mg/dl	Renal failure: coma
> 250 mcg/ml	Disseminated intravascular coagulation (DIC), pulmonary embolism, arterial or venous thrombosis, subarachnoid hemorrhage (CSF only), secondary fibrinolysis
> 300 mg/dl (with ketonemia and electrolyte imbalance)	Diabetes: diabetic coma
Gram-positive or gram-negative	Bacterial meningitis
> 18 g/dl	Chronic obstructive pulmonary disease: thrombosis, polycythemia vera
> 3.0	DIC, uncontrolled oral anticoagulation
> 70 mm Hg	Complex pattern of metabolic and respiratory factors

(continued)

Diagnostic tests

Crisis values of laboratory tests *(continued)*

Test	Low value	Common causes and effects
Partial thromboplastin time		
pH, arterial blood	< 7.2	Complex pattern of metabolic and respiratory factors
Platelet count	< 50,000/µl	Bone marrow suppression: hemorrhage
Potassium, serum	< 3 mEq/L	Vomiting and diarrhea, diuretic therapy: cardiotoxicity, arrhythmia, cardiac arrest
Prothrombin time		
Sodium, serum	< 120 mEq/L	Diuretic therapy: cardiac failure
Troponin I		
White blood cell (WBC) count	< 2,000/µl	Bone marrow suppression: infection
WBC count, CSF		

Arterial blood gas analysis

Purpose

- To evaluate the efficiency of pulmonary gas exchange and the integrity of the ventilatory control system and to determine the acid base level of the blood
- To measure the partial pressure of arterial oxygen (Pao_2), the partial pressure of arterial carbon dioxide ($Paco_2$), pH, oxygen content (O_2CT), arterial oxygen saturation (Sao_2), and bicarbonate (HCO_3^-) values

High value	Common causes and effects
> 40 seconds (> 70 seconds for patient on heparin)	Anticoagulation factor deficiency: hemorrhage
> 7.0	Chronic obstructive pulmonary disease. Thrombosis, polycythemia vera
> 500,000/μl	Leukemia, reaction to acute bleeding: hemorrhage
> 6 mEq/L	Renal disease, diuretic therapy: cardiotoxicity, arrhythmia
> 14 seconds (> 20 seconds for patient on warfarin)	Anticoagulant therapy, anticoagulation factor deficiency: hemorrhage
> 160 mEq/L	Dehydration: vascular collapse
> 2 mcg/ml	Acute MI
> 20,000/μl	Leukemia: infection
> 10/μl	Meningitis, encephalitis: infection

Patient preparation

- Explain the purpose and tell the patient that the arterial blood gas analysis requires a blood sample. Explain who will perform the arterial puncture, when it will occur, and where the puncture site will be: radial, brachial, or femoral artery.
- Tell the patient he need not restrict food and fluids and that he can breathe normally during the test.
- Tell him he may experience brief cramping or throbbing pain at the site.

Procedure

ALERT Wait at least 20 minutes before drawing arterial blood when starting, changing, or discontinuing oxygen therapy; after initiating or changing settings of mechanical ventilation; or after extubation.

- Use a heparinized blood gas syringe to draw the sample.
- Confirm the patient's identity using two patient identifiers.
- Perform an arterial puncture or draw blood from an arterial line after discarding the appropriate amount of the sample.
- Eliminate air from the sample, place it on ice immediately, and prepare to transport it for analysis.
- Note on the laboratory request when the sample was collected, patient's temperature, the flow rate of oxygen therapy and method of delivery. If the patient is on a ventilator, note the fraction of inspired oxygen, and positive and expiratory pressure.

Postprocedure care

- Apply pressure to the puncture site for 3 to 5 minutes or until bleeding stops, then tape a gauze pad firmly over it. If receiving anticoagulants or if the patient has a coagulopathy, apply pressure longer than 5 minutes if necessary.

ALERT If the puncture site is on the arm, don't tape the entire circumference; this may restrict circulation.

- Monitor vital signs and observe for signs of circulatory impairment, such as swelling, discoloration, pain, numbness, and tingling in the bandaged arm or leg.

Normal results

- Pao_2: 80 to 100 mm Hg (SI, 10.6 to 13.3 kPa)
- $Paco_2$: 35 to 45 mm Hg (SI, 4.7 to 5.3 kPa)
- pH: 7.35 to 7.45 (SI, 7.35 to 7.45)
- O_2CT: 15% to 23% (SI, 0.15 to 0.23)
- Sao_2: 94% to 100% (SI, 0.94 to 1)
- HCO_3^-: 22 to 25 mEq/L (SI, 22 to 25 mmol/L)

Abnormal results

- Low Pao_2, O_2CT, and Sao_2 levels and a high $Paco_2$ resulting from conditions that impair respiratory function, such as respiratory muscle weakness or paralysis, respiratory center inhibition (from head injury, brain tumor, or drug abuse), and airway obstruction (from mucus plugs or tumor)
- Low readings possibly resulting from bronchiole obstruction caused by asthma or emphysema, an abnormal ventilation-perfusion ratio caused by partially blocked alveoli or pulmonary capillaries, or from alveoli that are damaged or filled with fluid because of disease, hemorrhage, or near-drowning (see *Understanding arterial blood gas values*)
- Inspired air possibly containing insufficient oxygen, Pao_2, O_2CT, and Sao_2 decrease but $Paco_2$ may be normal in pneu-

Understanding arterial blood gas values

This chart compares abnormal arterial blood gas values and their significance for patient care.

Disorder	pH	$Paco_2$ (mm Hg)	HCO_3^- (mEq/L)	Compensation
Normal	7.35 to 7.45	35 to 45	22 to 26	
Respiratory acidosis	< 7.35	> 45	• Acute: may be normal • Chronic: > 26	• Renal: increased secretion and excretion of acid; compensation taking 24 hours to begin • Respiratory: rate increasing to expel CO_2
Respiratory alkalosis	> 7.45	< 35	• Acute: normal • Chronic: < 22	• Renal: decreased H+ secretion and active secretion of HCO_3^- into urine • Respiratory: lungs expelling more CO_2 by increasing rate and depth of respirations
Metabolic acidosis	< 7.35	< 35	< 22	• Respiratory: hypoventilation occurring immediately but limited due to ensuing hypoxemia
Metabolic alkalosis	> 7.45	> 45	> 26	• Renal: more effective but slow to excrete less acid and more base

mothorax, impaired diffusion between alveoli and blood (caused by interstitial fibrosis, for example), or an arteriovenous shunt that permits blood to bypass the lungs

• Low O_2CT—with normal Pao_2, Sao_2 and, possibly, $Paco_2$ values—possibly resulting from severe anemia, decreased blood volume, and reduced hemoglobin oxygen-carrying capacity

ALERT Results may be altered by failure to heparinize the syringe, send it to the laboratory immediately; exposing the sample to air (increase or decrease in Pao_2 and $Paco_2$); venous blood in the sample (possible decrease in Pao_2 and increase in $Paco_2$); medications the patient may be taking (acetazolamide, methicillin, nitrofurantoin, and tetracycline cause possible decrease in $Paco_2$; HCO_3^-, ethacrynic acid, hydrocortisone, metolazone, prednisone, and thiazides cause possible increase in Paco2); and fever (possible false-high Pao_2 and $Paco_2$).

Bronchoscopy

Purpose

• To allow direct visualization of the larynx, trachea, and bronchi using a rigid or fiber-optic bronchoscope
• To allow visual examination of tumors, obstructions, secretions, or foreign bodies in the tracheobronchial tree
• To diagnose bronchogenic carcinoma, tuberculosis, interstitial pulmonary disease, and fungal or parasitic pulmonary infections
• To obtain specimens for microbiological and cytologic examination
• To locate bleeding sites in the tracheobronchial tree
• To remove foreign bodies, malignant or benign tumors, mucus plugs, and excessive secretions from the tracheobronchial tree

Patient preparation

• Make sure an appropriate consent form has been signed and report any allergies.
• Instruct the patient to fast for 6 to 12 hours before the test.
• Obtain vital signs and results of preprocedure studies; report any abnormal findings.
• An I.V. sedative may be given.
• If appropriate, remove the patient's dentures.
• Tell the patient the test takes 45 to 60 minutes.
• Inform the patient that blocking of the airway won't occur, but that hoarseness, loss of voice, hemoptysis, and sore throat may occur.

Procedure

• Position the patient properly and give supplemental oxygen if ordered.

• Monitor pulse oximetry, vital signs, and cardiac rhythm.
• Local anesthetic is sprayed into the mouth and throat.
• The bronchoscope is inserted through the mouth or nose; a bite block is placed in the mouth if using the oral approach.
• When the bronchoscope is just above the vocal cords, about 3 to 4 ml of 2% to 4% lidocaine is flushed through the inner channel to the vocal cords.
• A fiber-optic camera is used to take photographs for documentation.
• Tissue specimens are obtained from suspect areas.
• A suction apparatus may remove foreign bodies or mucus plugs.
• Bronchoalveolar lavage may remove thickened secretions or may diagnose infectious causes of infiltrates.
• Specimens are prepared properly and immediately sent to the laboratory.

Postprocedure care

• Position a conscious patient in semi-Fowler's position; position an unconscious patient on one side, with the head of the bed slightly elevated.
• Instruct the patient to spit out saliva rather than swallow it.
• Observe the patient for bleeding.
• Resume the patient's usual diet, beginning with sips of clear liquid or ice chips, when the gag reflex returns.
• Provide lozenges or a soothing liquid gargle to ease discomfort when the gag reflex returns.
• Check the follow-up chest X-ray for pneumothorax.
• Monitor vital signs, characteristics of sputum, and respiratory status.

ALERT Complications include subcutaneous crepitus, which may indicate tracheal or bronchial perforation or pneumothorax; laryngeal edema or laryngospasm causing stridor and dyspnea; hypoxemia, cardiac arrhythmias, bleeding, infection, and bronchospasm.

Normal results

• Bronchi structurally similar to the trachea
• Right bronchus slightly larger and more vertical than the left
• Smaller segmental bronchi branching off from the main bronchi

Abnormal results

• Structural abnormalities of the bronchial wall: indicate inflammation, ulceration, tumors, and enlargement of submucosal lymph nodes
• Structural abnormalities of endotracheal origin: suggest stenosis, compression, ectasia, and diverticula

• Structural abnormalities of the trachea or bronchi: suggest calculi, foreign bodies, masses, and paralyzed vocal cords
• Tissue and cell study abnormalities: suggest interstitial pulmonary disease, infection, carcinoma, and tuberculosis

Cardiac blood pool imaging

Purpose

• To evaluate regional and global ventricular performance after I.V. injection of human serum albumin or red blood cells (RBCs) tagged with the isotope technetium 99m (^{99m}Tc) pertechnetate
• In first-pass imaging, to record (by a scintillation camera) the radioactivity emitted by the isotope in its initial pass through the left ventricle
• To record higher counts of radioactivity that occur during diastole because there's more blood in the ventricle; to record lower counts that occur during systole as the blood is ejected
• To evaluate left ventricular function
• To detect aneurysms of the left ventricle, abnormalities of the myocardial wall (areas of akinesia or dyskinesia), or intracardiac shunting

Patient preparation

• Make sure an informed consent form has been signed.
• Explain that cardiac blood pooling imaging permits assessment of the heart's left ventricle. Describe the test, who will perform it, where it will take place, and its expected duration.
• Tell the patient that he need not restrict food and fluids.
• Explain that he'll receive an I.V. injection of a radioactive tracer and that a detector positioned above his chest will record circulation through his heart.
• Reassure the patient that the tracer poses no radiation hazard and rarely produces adverse effects.
• Inform the patient that he may experience slight discomfort from the needle puncture but that the imaging itself is painless.
• Instruct the patient to remain silent and motionless during imaging, unless otherwise instructed.

Procedure

• The patient is placed in a supine position beneath the detector of a scintillation camera and 15 to 20 millicuries of albumin or RBCs tagged with ^{99m}Tc pertechnetate is injected I.V.
• For the next minute, the scintillation camera records the first pass of the isotope through the heart to locate the aortic and mitral valves.

• Using an electrocardiogram, the camera is gated for 60-millisecond intervals, representing end-systole and end-diastole, and 500 to 1,000 cardiac cycles are recorded.
• To observe septal and posterior wall motion, a modified left or right anterior oblique position may be used and the patient given 0.4 mg of nitroglycerin sublingually. The scintillation camera then records additional gated images to evaluate abnormal contraction in the left ventricle.
• The patient may be asked to exercise as the scintillation camera records gated images.

Postprocedure care

• Monitor vital signs and response to the testing.

Normal results

• Left ventricle contracts symmetrically; isotope evenly distributed in the scans
• Normal ejection fraction: 55% to 65%

Abnormal results

• In coronary artery disease: usually asymmetrical blood distribution to the myocardium, producing segmental abnormalities of ventricular wall motion; may also result from preexisting conditions (myocarditis)
• In cardiomyopathy: globally reduced ejection fractions
• In left-to-right shunt: recirculating radioisotope prolongs the down slope of the curve of scintigraphic data; early arrival of activity in left ventricle or aorta signifies a right-to-left shunt

Cardiac catheterization

Purpose

• To measure pressure in the heart chambers; record films of the ventricles (contrast ventriculography) and arteries (coronary arteriography) involving passage of a catheter into the right, left, or both sides of the heart
• To assess patency of the coronary arteries and function of left ventricle in left-sided heart catheterization; or, in right-sided catheterization, to assess pulmonary artery pressures
• To evaluate valvular insufficiency or stenosis, septal defects, congenital anomalies, myocardial function, myocardial blood supply, and cardiac wall motion
• To aid in diagnosing left ventricular enlargement, aortic root enlargement, ventricular aneurysms, and intracardiac shunts

Patient preparation

- Make sure an informed consent form has been signed, and notify the physician of hypersensitivity to shellfish, iodine, or contrast media.
- Stop anticoagulant as ordered to reduce complications of bleeding.
- Restrict food and fluids for at least 6 hours before the test.
- Explain that a mild sedative may be given.
- Warn the patient that a transient hot, flushing sensation or nausea may occur.
- Tell the patient that the test will take 1 to 2 hours.

Procedure

- The patient is placed in a supine position on a padded table and heart rate and rhythm, respiratory status, and blood pressure are monitored throughout the procedure.
- An I.V. line is started and a local anesthetic is injected.
- A small incision is made into the artery or vein, depending on whether the test is for the left or right.
- The catheter is passed through the sheath into the vessel and guided using fluoroscopy.
- In right-sided heart catheterization, the catheter is inserted into the antecubital or femoral vein and advanced through the vena cavae into the right side of the heart and into the pulmonary artery.
- In left-sided heart catheterization, the catheter is inserted into the brachial or femoral artery and advanced retrograde through the aorta into the coronary artery ostium and left ventricle.
- When the catheter is in place, contrast medium is injected.
- Nitroglycerin is given to eliminate catheter-induced spasm or watch its effect on the coronary arteries.
- After the catheter is removed, direct pressure is applied to the incision site until bleeding stops, and a sterile dressing is applied.

Postprocedure care

- Reinforce the dressing as needed.
- Enforce bed rest for 6 to 8 hours.
- If the femoral route was used for catheter insertion, keep the affected leg straight at the hip for 6 to 8 hours.
- If the antecubital fossa route was used, keep the affected arm straight at the elbow for at least 3 hours.
- Resume medications and give analgesics as ordered.
- Encourage fluid intake unless contraindicated.
- Monitor vital signs, intake and output, cardiac rhythm, neurologic and respiratory status, and peripheral vascular status distal to the puncture site.

• Check the catheter insertion site and dressings for signs and symptoms of infection.

ALERT Complications include infective endocarditis; left- or right-sided heart catheterization: myocardial infarction, arrhythmias, cardiac tamponade, infection, hypovolemia, pulmonary edema, hematoma, blood loss, adverse reaction to contrast media, and vasovagal response; left-sided heart catheterization: arterial thrombus or embolism, and stroke; right-sided heart catheterization: thrombophlebitis and pulmonary embolism.

Normal results

- No abnormalities of heart valves, chamber size, pressures, configuration, wall motion or thickness, and blood flow present
- Coronary arteries showing smooth and regular outline

Abnormal results

- Coronary artery narrowing greater than 70% suggests significant coronary artery disease
- Narrowing of the left main coronary artery and occlusion or narrowing high in the left anterior descending artery suggests the need for revascularization surgery
- Impaired wall motion suggests myocardial incompetence
- Pressure gradient indicates valvular heart disease
- Retrograde flow of the contrast medium across a valve during systole indicating valvular incompetence

Cerebral angiography

Purpose

- To radiographically examine the cerebral vasculature after injection of intra-arterial contrast medium
- To detect cerebrovascular abnormalities, such as aneurysm or arteriovenous malformation, thrombosis, narrowing, or occlusion
- To evaluate vascular displacement caused by tumor, hematoma, edema, herniation, vasospasm, increased intracranial pressure, or hydrocephalus
- To locate clips applied to blood vessels during surgery and to evaluate the postoperative status of such vessels
- To evaluate the presence and degree of carotid artery disease

Patient preparation

- Make sure a consent form has been signed and report any allergies.

- Have the patient fast for 8 to 10 hours before the test.
- Tell the patient that his head will be immobilized, he'll need to lie still, and that he'll receive a local anesthetic.
- Warn that nausea, warmth, or burning may occur with contrast injection.
- Initiate an I.V. access and give I.V. fluids and a sedative as ordered.
- Explain to the patient that the test takes 2 to 4 hours.

Procedure

- The patient is placed in a supine position on a radiographic table.
- The access site is prepared and draped and a local anesthetic is injected.
- The artery is punctured with the appropriate needle and catheterized under fluoroscopic guidance.
- Catheter placement is verified by fluoroscopy and a contrast medium is injected.
- A series of radiographs is taken and reviewed.
- Arterial catheter patency is maintained by continuous or periodic flushing.
- Vital signs and neurologic status are monitored continuously.
- The catheter is removed, firm pressure is applied to the access site until bleeding stops, and a pressure dressing is applied.

Postprocedure care

- Enforce bed rest and apply an ice bag.
- If active bleeding or expanding hematoma occurs, apply firm pressure to the puncture site and inform the physician immediately.
- Ensure adequate hydration.
- Provide analgesia as ordered.
- Monitor vital signs, along with intake and output.
- Monitor the neurovascular status of the extremity distal to the access site.
- If the femoral approach was used, keep the involved leg straight at the hip and check pulses distal to the site (dorsalis pedis, posterior tibial and popliteal).
- If the carotid artery was used as the access site, watch for dysphagia or respiratory distress, which can result from hematoma or edema. Also watch for disorientation, weakness, or numbness in the extremities (signs of neurovascular compromise) and for arterial spasms, which produce symptoms of transient ischemic attacks (TIAs). Notify the physician immediately if abnormal signs develop.
- If the brachial artery was used, keep the arm straight at the elbow and assess distal pulses (radial and ulnar). Avoid

venipuncture and blood pressures in the affected arm. Observe the extremity for changes in color, temperature, or sensation. If it becomes pale, cool, or numb, notify the physician immediately.

ALERT Complications include adverse reaction to contrast media, embolism, bleeding, hematoma, infection, vasospasm, thrombosis, TIA, or stroke.

Normal results

- Normal cerebral vasculature
- During arterial phase of perfusion: contrast medium fills and opacifies superficial and deep arteries and arterioles
- During venous phase: contrast medium opacifies superficial and deep veins

Abnormal results

- Changes in the caliber of vessel lumina: suggest vascular disease
- Vessel displacement: suggests possible tumor

Computed tomography

Purpose

- To produce cross-sectional images of various layers of tissue not readily seen on standard X-rays

Patient preparation

- Make sure a consent form has been signed and report any allergies.
- The specific type of CT scan dictates the need for an oral or I.V. contrast medium.
- Warn the patient about transient discomfort from the needle puncture and a warm or flushed feeling from an I.V. contrast medium, if used.
- Instruct the patient to remain still during the test and to immediately report feelings of nausea, vomiting, dizziness, headache, itching, or hives.
- Tell the patient that the study takes from 5 minutes to 1 hour depending on the type of CT and his ability to remain still.

Procedure

- The patient is positioned on an adjustable table inside a scanning gantry.
- A series of transverse radiographs is taken and recorded.
- The information is reconstructed by a computer and selected images are photographed.

• After the images are reviewed, an I.V. contrast enhancement may be ordered and additional images are obtained.
• The patient is observed carefully for adverse reactions to the contrast medium.

Postprocedure care

• The patient's normal diet and activities may resume, unless otherwise ordered.

Normal results

• Specific type of CT scan dictating normal findings
• Tissue densities appearing as black, white, or shades of gray on the CT image
• Bone (has the densest tissue) appearing white
• Cerebrospinal fluid (has no tissue) appearing black

Abnormal results

• Specific type of CT dependent on the area of study (see *Types of CT scans*, pages 129 to 133)

ALERT Interfering factors include oral or I.V. contrast media use in previous diagnostic tests, which may obscure the images.

Digital subtraction angiography, cerebral

Purpose

• To provide a high-contrast view of blood vessels
• To show extracranial and intracranial cerebral blood flow
• To detect and evaluate cerebrovascular abnormalities
• To aid postoperative evaluation of cerebrovascular surgery

Patient preparation

• Make sure an appropriate consent form has been signed.
• Check history for any allergies, including hypersensitivity to iodine, iodine-containing substances such as shellfish, and contrast media; if allergies are present, notify the physician.
• Notify the physician of any abnormal laboratory studies, such as elevated blood urea nitrogen or creatinine.
• Instruct the patient to fast for 4 hours before test; he need not restrict fluids.
• Stress the importance of lying still during the procedure; even swallowing can interfere with imaging. The patient will need to hold his breath for 10-second intervals at various times during the test.

(Text continues on page 133.)

Types of CT scans

Area	Purpose	Abnormal findings
Abdominal and pelvic	• Evaluate soft tissue and organs of the abdomen, pelvis, and retroperitoneal space • Evaluate inflammatory disease • Aid staging of neoplasms • Evaluate trauma • Detect tumors, cysts, hemorrhage, and edema • Evaluate response to chemotherapy	• Primary and metastatic neoplasms • Abscesses • Cysts • Obstructive disease from a tumor or calculi
Bone and skeletal	• Determine the existence and extent of primary bone tumors, skeletal metastases, soft-tissue tumors, ligament or tendon injuries, and fractures • Diagnose joint abnormalities	• Primary bone tumors • Soft-tissue tumors • Skeletal metastasis • Bone fractures • Joint abnormalities
Brain	• Diagnose intracranial lesions and abnormalities • Monitor the effects of surgery, radiotherapy, or chemotherapy in treatment of intracranial tumors • Guide cranial surgery • Assess focal neurologic abnormalities • Evaluate suspected head injury such as subdural hematoma	• Cerebral atrophy • Hydrocephalus • Cerebral edema • Arteriovenous malformation • Intracranial tumors • Intracranial hematoma • Cerebral atrophy • Infarction • Edema • Congenital anomalies
Cardiac scoring	• Diagnose coronary artery calcium content • Screen for coronary artery calcium content in high-risk patients and patients with pain of unknown origin	• Score between 101 and 400: indicates significant calcified plaque in the arteries (an increased risk of MI) • Score > 400: signifies extensive calcification and critical narrowing of the arteries due to plaque

(continued)

Types of CT scans *(continued)*

Area	Purpose	Abnormal findings
Ear	• Investigate the cause of bilateral hearing loss • Confirm cochlear abnormalities • Differentiate chronic inflammation from cholesteatoma • Evaluate ossification of the cochlea coils before cochlear implantation • Depict osseous changes in the temporal and petrous bone • Define appropriate surgical and therapeutic approaches for patients with middle and inner ear disorders • Assess postsurgical management of patients with middle and inner ear disorders	• Tympanosclerosis • Osseous changes of the external auditory canal and middle and inner ear structures • Cochlear abnormalities
Intracranial	• Diagnose intracranial lesions and abnormalities • Monitor the effects of surgery, radiation therapy, or chemotherapy on intracranial tumors • Guide cranial surgery	• Congenital anomalies • Intracranial tumors • Astrocytomas • Subdural and epidural hematomas • Hemorrhage • Cerebral atrophy • Cerebral infarction • Cerebral edema
Renal	• Detect and evaluate renal abnormalities, such as tumor, obstruction, calculi, polycystic disease, congenital anomalies, and abnormal fluid accumulation • Evaluate the retroperitoneum	• Renal masses or cysts • Renal cell carcinoma • Vascular or adrenal tumors • Obstructions • Calculi • Polycystic kidney disease • Congenital anomalies • Hematomas • Lymphoceles • Abscesses • Kidney damage or infection

Types of CT scans *(continued)*

Area	Purpose	Abnormal findings
Liver and biliary tract	• Distinguish between obstructive and nonobstructive jaundice • Detect intrahepatic tumors and abscesses, subphrenic and subhepatic abscesses, cysts, and hematomas	• Focal hepatic defects • Small lesions • Neoplasms • Hepatic abscesses • Hepatic cysts • Hematomas • Biliary duct dilation • Calculi • Pancreatic carcinoma
Orbital	• Evaluate pathologic conditions of the orbit and eye • Evaluate fractures of the orbit and adjoining structures • Determine the cause of unilateral exophthalmos	• Space-occupying lesions • Lymphomas and metastatic carcinomas • Encapsulated tumors (benign hemangiomas and meningiomas) • Intracranial tumors (gliomas, meningiomas, and secondary tumors) • Early erosion or expansion of the medial orbital wall • Space-occupying lesions in the orbit or paranasal sinuses • Thickening of the medial and lateral rectus muscles
Pancreatic	• Detect pancreatic carcinoma or pseudocysts • Detect or evaluate pancreatitis • Distinguish between pancreatic disorders and disorders of the retroperitoneum	• Pancreatic carcinoma • Pseudocysts • Metastases • Adenocarcinoma • Islet cell tumors • Cystadenomas • Cystadenocarcinomas • Acute and chronic pancreatitis • Abscesses • Ascites • Pleural effusion • Biliary obstruction

(continued)

Types of CT scans *(continued)*

Area	Purpose	Abnormal findings
Spinal	• Diagnose spinal lesions and abnormalities • Monitor the effects of spinal surgery or therapy	• Spinal lesions and abnormalities • Neurinoma (schwannoma) • Meningioma • Degenerative processes and structural changes • Herniated nucleus pulposus • Spinal cord compression • Cervical spondylosis • Cervical cord compression • Lumbar stenosis • Facet disorders • Spurring of the vertebrae • Fluid-filled arachnoidal and other paraspinal cysts • Vascular malformations • Congenital spinal malformations (meningocele, myelocele, and spina bifida)
Thoracic	• Locate suspected neoplasms (as in Hodgkin's disease), especially with mediastinal involvement • Differentiate calcified lesions (indicating tuberculosis) from tumors • Differentiate emphysema or bronchopleural fistula from lung abscess • Distinguish tumors adjacent to the aorta from aortic aneurysms	• Tumors • Nodules • Cysts • Aortic aneurysms • Enlarged lymph nodes

Types of CT scans *(continued)*

Area	Purpose	Abnormal findings
Thoracic *(continued)*	• Detect the invasion of a neck mass in the thorax • Evaluate primary malignancy that may metastasize to the lungs, especially in the patient with a primary bone tumor, soft-tissue sarcoma, or melanoma • Evaluate the mediastinal lymph nodes • Evaluate the severity of lung disease such as emphysema • Detect a dissection or leak of an aortic aneurysm or aortic arch aneurysm • Plan radiation treatment	• Pleural effusion • Accumulations of blood, fluid, or fat

Diagnostic tests

- Warn that he may experience warmth, headache, metallic taste, nausea, or vomiting after injection of the contrast medium.
- Explain that the test may take 1 to 2 hours.

Procedure

- The patient is placed in a supine position on a radiography table with his arms at his sides.
- An initial series of fluoroscopic pictures (mask images) is taken.
- The access site is shaved and prepared (a vein or artery may be used).
- The patient is given a local anesthetic and an I.V. sedative.
- The vessel is cannulated; a catheter inserted and advanced to the area to be studied.
- The contrast medium is injected and films are taken in various views.
- Vital signs and neurologic status are monitored. The patient is observed for signs of a hypersensitivity reaction.

Postprocedure care

- The patient should drink at least 1 qt (1 L) of fluid on the day of the procedure. Instruct him to resume a normal diet.
- Monitor vital signs, intake and output, puncture site, neurologic status, infection, delayed hypersensitivity reaction, and thrombotic events.

• If bleeding occurs, apply firm pressure to the puncture site, and tell the physician immediately.

Normal results

• Contrast medium: fills and opacifies all superficial and deep arteries, arterioles, and veins

Abnormal results

• Vascular filling defects: may indicate arteriovenous occlusion or stenosis
• Outpouchings in vessel lumina: may reflect aneurysms
• Vessel displacement or vascular masses: may indicate a tumor

Doppler ultrasound

Purpose

• To noninvasively evaluate blood flow in the major veins and arteries of the arms and legs and in the extracranial cerebrovascular system
• To permit direct listening and graphic recording of blood flow with a handheld transducer that directs high-frequency sound waves to an artery or vein (see *How to detect thrombi with a Doppler probe*)
• To aid the diagnosis of venous insufficiency, superficial and deep vein thromboses, and peripheral artery disease and arterial occlusion
• To monitor patients with arterial reconstruction and bypass grafts
• To detect abnormalities of carotid artery blood
• To evaluate arterial trauma

Patient preparation

• Make sure a consent form has been signed; report any allergies.
• Explain to the patient that the procedure takes about 20 minutes and doesn't involve risk or discomfort.

Procedure

• Doppler ultrasonography is performed bilaterally.
• The patient is assisted into a supine position on the examination table with his arms at his sides.

Peripheral arterial evaluation

• For peripheral arterial evaluation in the leg, the usual test sites are the common and superficial femoral, popliteal, posterior tibial, and dorsalis pedis arteries.
• For peripheral arterial evaluation in the arm, the usual test sites are the subclavian, brachial, radial, and ulnar arteries.

How to detect thrombi with a Doppler probe

The Doppler probe is typically used to detect venous thrombi by first positioning the transducer and then occluding the blood vessel by compression (as illustrated in the normal leg at right). Water-soluble conductive gel is applied to the tip of the transducer to provide coupling between the skin and the transducer.

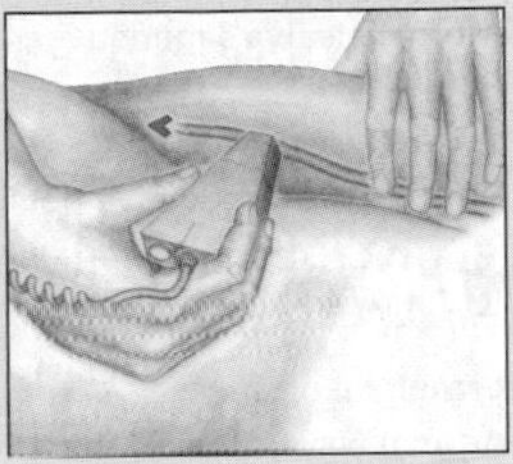

When pressure is released, allowing blood flow to resume, the transducer picks up the sudden augmentation of the flow sound and permits graphic recording of blood flow. If a thrombus is present, a compression maneuver fails to produce the augmented flow sound because the blood flow (as shown at right in the femoral vein) is significantly impaired.

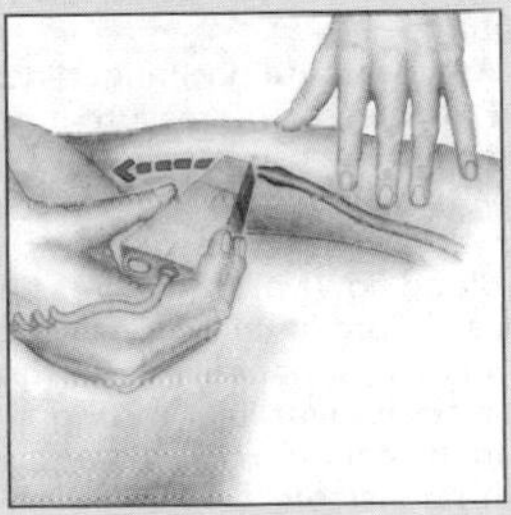

- Brachial blood pressure is measured, and the transducer is placed at various points along the test arteries.
- The signals are monitored, and the waveforms are recorded for analysis.
- The blood flow velocity is monitored and recorded over the test artery.
- Segmental limb blood pressures are obtained to localize arterial occlusive disease.

Peripheral venous evaluation

- For peripheral venous evaluation in the leg, the usual test sites are the popliteal, superficial and common femoral veins, and posterior tibial vein.
- For extracranial cerebrovascular evaluation, usual test sites are the supraorbital artery; the common, external, and internal carotid arteries; the vertebral arteries; and the brachial, axillary, subclavian, and jugular veins.
- The transducer is placed over the appropriate vessel, waveforms are recorded, and respiratory modulations are noted.
- Proximal limb compression maneuvers are performed.

• Augmentation after release of compression is noted to evaluate venous valve competency.
• For tests involving the legs and feet, the patient is asked to perform Valsalva's maneuver, and venous blood flow is recorded.

Postprocedure care

• Remove the conductive gel from the patient's skin.

ALERT Bradyarrhythmias may occur if the probe is placed near the carotid sinus.

Normal results

• Arterial waveforms of the arms and legs multiphasic, with a prominent systolic component and one or more diastolic sounds
• Arm pressure unchanged despite postural changes
• Proximal thigh pressure normally 20 to 30 mm Hg greater than arm pressure
• Venous blood flow velocity phasic with respiration, with a lower pitch than arterial flow
• Blood flow velocity increasing with distal compression or release of proximal limb compression
• Valsalva's maneuver interrupting venous flow velocity
• In cerebrovascular testing, a strong velocity signal present
• In the common carotid artery, blood flow velocity increasing during diastole
• Periorbital arterial flow normally anterograde out of the orbit
• Ankle-brachial index (ABI): 0.9

Abnormal results

• Diminished blood flow velocity signal: suggests arterial stenosis or occlusion
• Absent velocity signals: suggest complete occlusion and lack of collateral circulation
• ABI, 0.5 to 0.9, claudication; ABI, 0.5, resting ischemic pain; ABI, 0.2, gangrenous foot or leg
• Venous blood flow velocity unchanged by respirations, not increased with compression or Valsalva's maneuver, or absent: indicates venous thrombosis
• Reversed flow velocity signal: may indicate chronic venous insufficiency and varicose veins
• Absent Doppler signals during cerebrovascular examination: suggests total arterial occlusion

Echocardiography

Purpose

- To noninvasively examine size, shape, and motion of cardiac structures, using sound waves
- To diagnose and evaluate valvular abnormalities
- To measure and evaluate the size of the heart's chambers and valves
- To help diagnose cardiomyopathies and atrial tumors
- To evaluate cardiac function or wall motion after myocardial infarction
- To detect pericardial effusion or mural thrombi

Patient preparation

- Tell the patient that he may be asked to breathe in and out slowly, to hold his breath, or to inhale a gas with a slightly sweet odor (amyl nitrite) while changes in heart function are recorded.
- Warn about possible adverse effects of amyl nitrite (dizziness, flushing, and tachycardia), but reassure him that such effects quickly subside.
- Stress the need to remain still because movement may distort results.
- Explain that the test takes 15 to 30 minutes.

Procedure

- The patient is placed in a supine position and conductive gel is applied to the third or fourth intercostal space to the left of the sternum. The transducer is placed directly over it.
- The transducer directs ultra-high-frequency sound waves toward cardiac structures, which reflect these waves; the transducer picks up the echoes, converts them to electrical impulses, and relays them to an echocardiography machine for display.
- In M-mode (motion mode), a single, pencil-like ultrasound beam strikes the heart and produces a vertical view, which is useful for recording the motion and dimensions of intracardiac structures.
- In two-dimensional echocardiography, a cross-sectional view of the cardiac structures is used for recording the lateral motion and spatial relationship between structures.
- The transducer is systematically angled to direct ultrasonic waves at specific parts of the patient's heart.
- During the test, the screen is observed; significant findings are recorded on a strip chart recorder or on a videotape recorder.
- For a left lateral view, the patient is placed on his left side.

• Doppler echocardiography also may be used where color flow simulates red blood cell flow through the heart valves. The sound of blood flow also may be used to assess heart sounds and murmurs as they relate to cardiac hemodynamics.

Postprocedure care

• Remove the conductive gel from the patient's skin.

Normal results

• For mitral valve: anterior and posterior mitral valve leaflets separating in early diastole and attaining maximum excursion rapidly, then moving toward each other during ventricular diastole; after atrial contraction, mitral valve leaflets coming together and remaining together during ventricular systole
• For aortic valve: aortic valve cusps moving anteriorly during systole and posteriorly during diastole
• For tricuspid valve: motion of the valve resembling that of the mitral valve
• For pulmonic valve: movement occurring posterior during atrial systole and during ventricular systole; in right ventricular ejection, cusp moving anteriorly, attaining its most anterior position during diastole
• For ventricular cavities: left ventricular cavity normally an echo-free space between the interventricular septum and the posterior left ventricular wall
• Right ventricular cavity normally an echo-free space between the anterior chest wall and the interventricular septum

Abnormal results

• In mitral stenosis: valve narrowing abnormally because of the leaflets' thickening and disordered motion; during diastole, both mitral valve leaflets moving anteriorly instead of posteriorly
• In mitral valve prolapse: one or both leaflets ballooning into the left atrium during systole
• In aortic insufficiency: aortic valve leaflet fluttering during diastole
• In stenosis: aortic valve thickening and generating more echoes
• In bacterial endocarditis: disrupted valve motion and fuzzy echoes usually on or near the valve
• Large chamber size: may indicate cardiomyopathy, valvular disorders, or heart failure; small chamber size: may indicate restrictive pericarditis
• Hypertrophic cardiomyopathy: identified by systolic anterior motion of the mitral valve and asymmetrical septal hypertrophy
• Myocardial ischemia or infarction: may cause absent or paradoxical motion in ventricular walls

- Pericardial effusion: fluid accumulates in the pericardial space, causing an abnormal echo-free space
- In large effusions: pressure exerted by excess fluid restricting pericardial motion

Electrocardiography

Purpose

- To measure the electrical potential from 12 different leads: the standard limb leads (I, II, III), the augmented limb leads (aV_F, aV_L, and aV_R), and the precordial, or chest, leads (V_1 through V_6)
- To identify conduction abnormalities, cardiac arrhythmias, myocardial ischemia or infarction (MI)
- To monitor recovery from MI
- To document pacemaker performance

Patient preparation

- Explain the need for the patient to lie still, relax, and breathe normally.
- Note current cardiac drug therapy on the test request form and pertinent information, such as chest pain or pacemaker presence.
- Explain that the test is painless and takes 5 to 10 minutes.

Procedure

- Confirm the patient's identity using two patient identifiers.
- Place the patient in a supine or semi-Fowler's position and provide privacy. Expose the chest, ankles, and wrists.
- Place electrodes on the inner aspect of the wrists, on the medial aspect of the lower legs, and on the chest, then connect the leadwires.
- Press the START button and input any required information.
- Make sure that all leads are represented in the tracing. If not, determine which electrode has come loose, reattach it, and restart the tracing.

ALERT All recording and other nearby electrical equipment should be properly grounded. Make sure that the electrodes are firmly attached.

Postprocedure care

- Disconnect the equipment, remove the electrodes, and remove the gel with a moist cloth towel.
- If the patient is having recurrent chest pain or if serial electrocardiograms are ordered, leave the electrode patches in place.

Normal results

- Cardiac rate, 60 to 100 beats/minute; normal sinus rhythm
- P wave: precedes each QRS complex
- PR interval: lasts 0.12 to 0.20 second
- QRS complex: lasts 0.06 to 0.10 second
- ST segment: not more than 0.1 mV
- T wave: appears rounded and smooth and positive in leads I, II, V_3, V_4, V_5, and V_6
- QT-interval duration: varies but usually lasts 0.36 to 0.44 second

Abnormal results

- Heart rate less than 60 beats/minute: reveals bradycardia
- Heart rate greater than 100 beats/minute: reveals tachycardia (See *Cardiac rhythms*)
- Missing P waves: may indicate atrioventricular (AV) block, atrial arrhythmia, or junctional rhythm
- Short PR interval: may indicate a junctional arrhythmia; a prolonged PR interval may indicate an AV block (see *Comparing heart blocks,* pages 146 and 147)
- Prolonged QRS complex: may suggest intraventricular conduction defects; missing QRS complexes: may suggest an AV block or ventricular asystole
- ST-segment elevation of 0.2 mV or more above baseline: may indicate myocardial injury; ST-segment depression: may indicate myocardial ischemia or injury
- T-wave inversion in leads I, II, and V_3 to V_6, myocardial ischemia; peaked T waves, hyperkalemia or myocardial ischemia; variations in T-wave amplitude, electrolyte imbalances
- Prolonged QT interval: may suggest life-threatening ventricular arrhythmias

(Text continues on page 148.)

Cardiac rhythms

Normal sinus rhythm

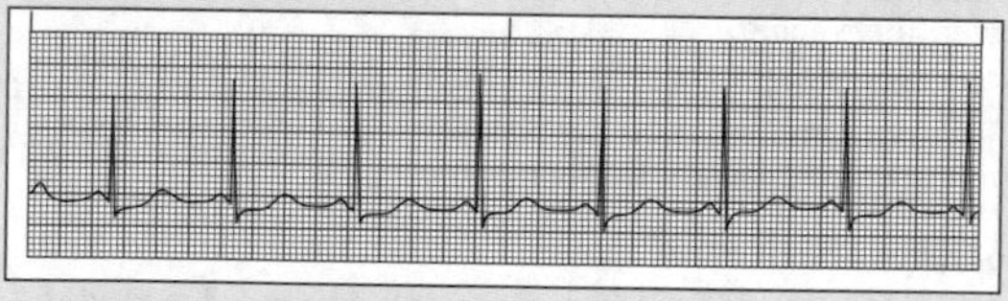

Rhythm .... regular
Rate .... 60 to 100 beats/minute
P wave .... normal, upright
PR interval .... 0.12 to 0.20 second
QRS complex .... 0.06 to 0.10 second

Sinus bradycardia

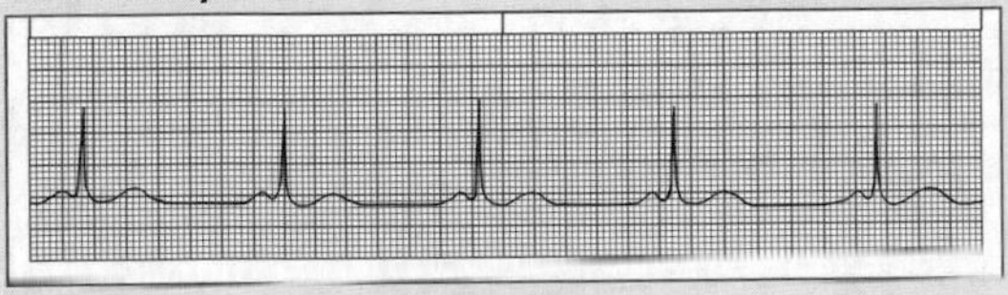

Rhythm ....regular
Rate ....< 60 beats/minute
P wave ....normal
PR interval ....0.12 to 0.20 second
QRS complex ....0.06 to 0.10 second

Sinus tachycardia

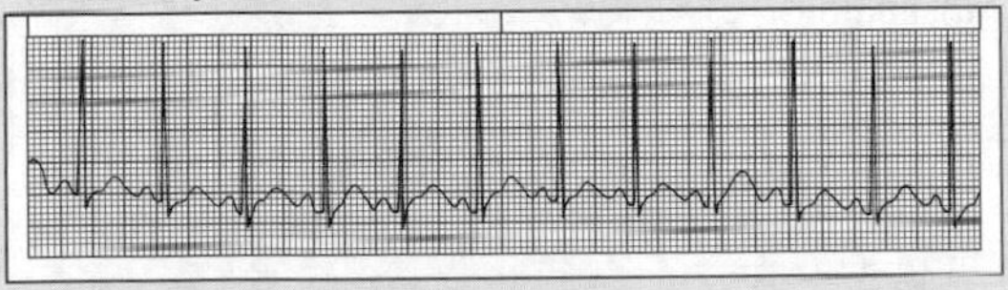

Rhythm ....regular
Rate ....100 to 160 beats/minute
P wave ....normal
PR interval ....0.12 to 0.20 second
QRS complex ....0.06 to 0.10 second

Premature atrial contractions

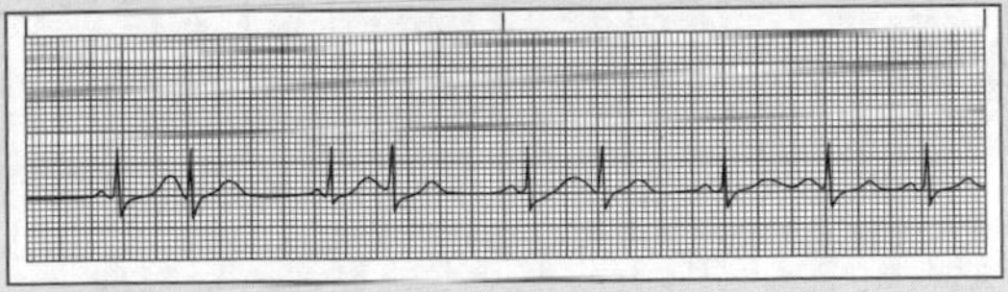

Rhythm ....irregular
Rate ....varies with underlying rhythm
P wave ....premature and abnormally shaped with premature atrial contractions
PR interval ....usually within normal limits, but varies depending on ectopic focus
QRS complex ..0.06 to 0.10 second

(continued)

Atrial tachycardia

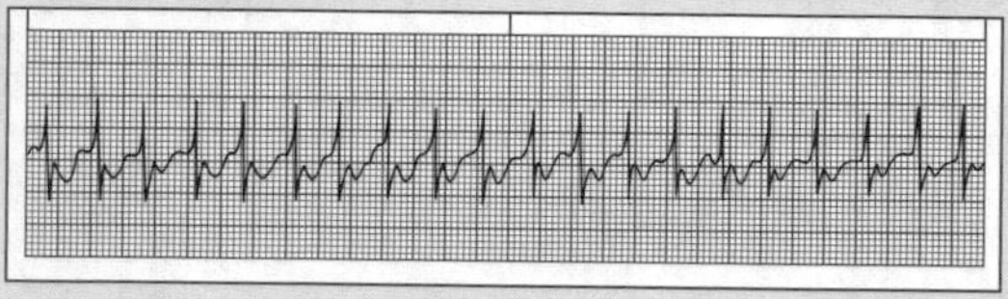

Rhythm ....regular
Rate ....150 to 250 beats/minute; ventricular rate depends on atrioventricular conduction rates
P wave ....hidden in the preceding T wave
PR interval ....not visible
QRS complex . .0.06 to 0.10 second

Atrial flutter

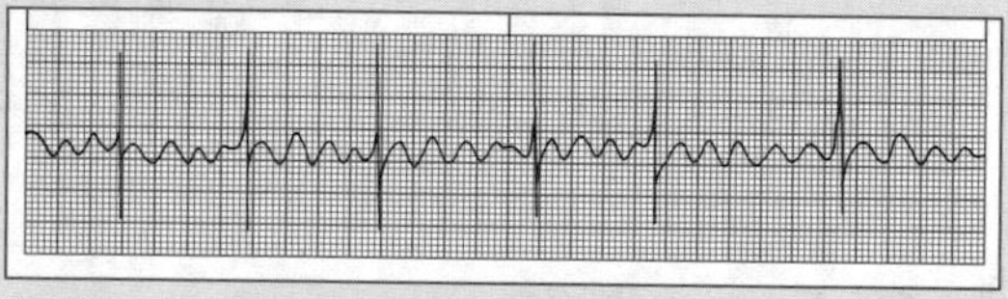

Rhythm ....atrial—regular; ventricular—typically irregular
Rate ....beats/minute; ventricular rate depends on degree of atrioventricular block
P wave ....classic sawtooth appearance
PR interval ....unmeasurable
QRS complex . .0.06 to 0.10 second

Atrial fibrillation

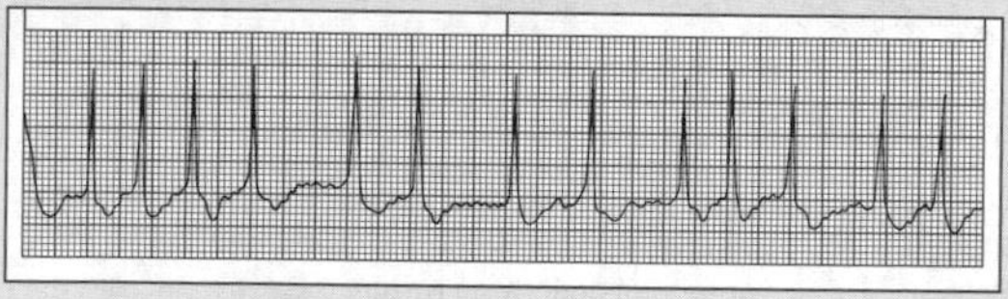

Rhythm ....irregularly irregular
Rate ....atrial—usually > 400 beats/minute; ventricular—varies
P wave ....absent; replaced by fine fibrillatory waves, or f waves
PR interval ....indiscernible
QRS complex . .0.06 to 0.10 second

Premature junctional contractions (PJCs)

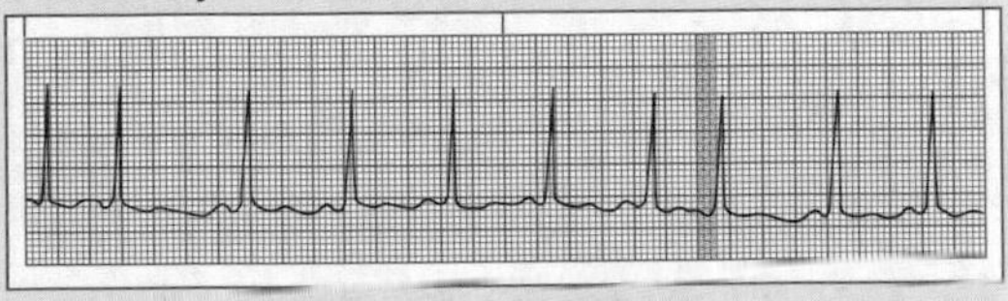

Rhythm . . . . .irregular atrial and ventricular rhythms during PJCs
Rate . . . . .reflects the underlying rhythm
P wave . . . . . . .usually inverted and may occur before or after or be hiddenwithin the QRS complex (see shaded area)
PR interval . . . .< 0.12 second if P wave precedes QRS complex; otherwise unmeasurable
QRS complex . .0.06 to 0.10 second

Junctional escape rhythm

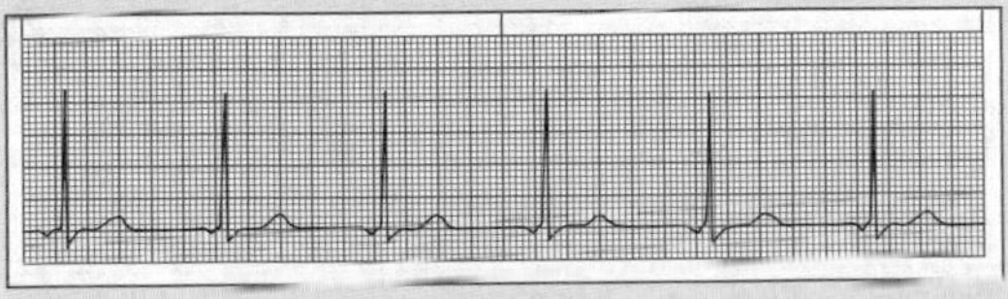

Rhythm . . . . . . .regular
Rate . . . . .40 to 60 beats/minute
P wave . . . . . . .usually inverted and may occur before or after or be hidden within the QRS complex
PR interval . . . .< 0.12 second if P wave precedes QRS complex; otherwise unmeasurable
QRS complex . .0.10 second

(continued)

Accelerated junctional rhythm

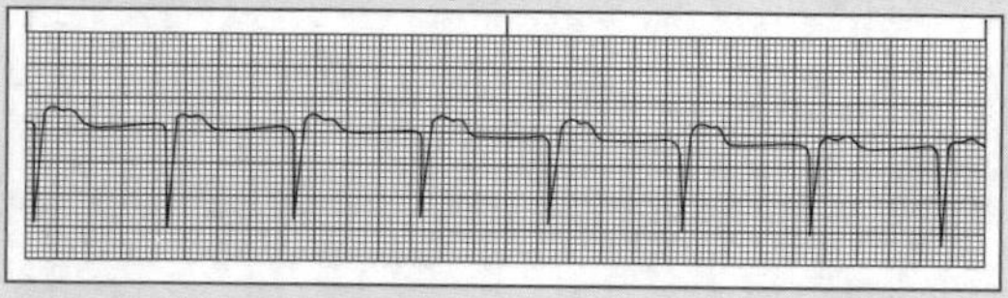

Rhythm . . . . . . .regular
Rate . . . . .60 to 100 beats/minute
P wave . . . . . . .usually inverted and may occur before or after or be hidden within the QRS complex
PR interval . . . .< 0.12 second if P wave precedes QRS complex; otherwise unmeasurable
QRS complex . .0.06 to 0.10 second

Premature ventricular contractions (PVCs)

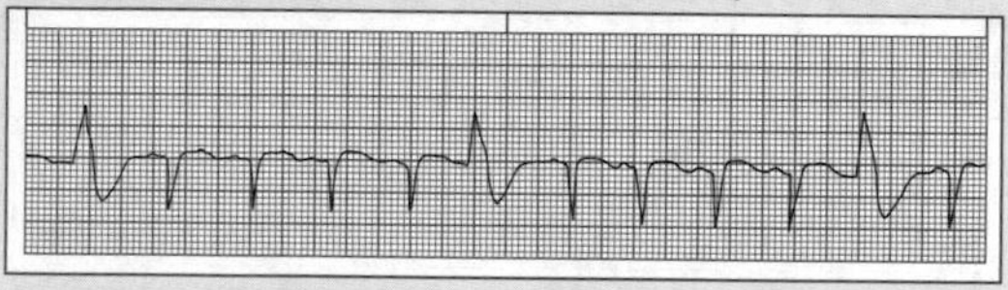

Rhythm . . . . irregular
Rate . . . . .reflects the underlying rhythm
P wave . . . . . . .none with PVC, but P wave present with other QRS complexes
PR interval . . . .unmeasurable except in underlying rhythm
QRS complex . .early, with bizarre configuration and duration of > 0.12 second; QRS complexes are normal in underlying rhythm

Ventricular tachycardia

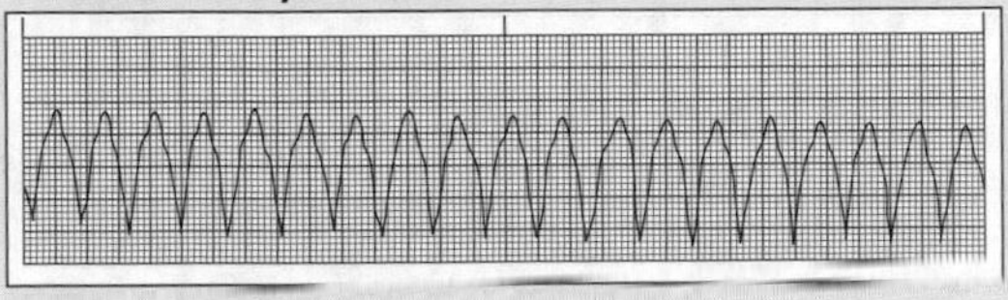

Rhythm . . . . regular
Rate . . . . atrial—can't be determined; ventricular—100 to 250 beats/minute
P wave . . . . absent
PR interval . . . . unmeasurable
QRS complex . . > 0.12 second; wide and bizarre

Ventricular fibrillation

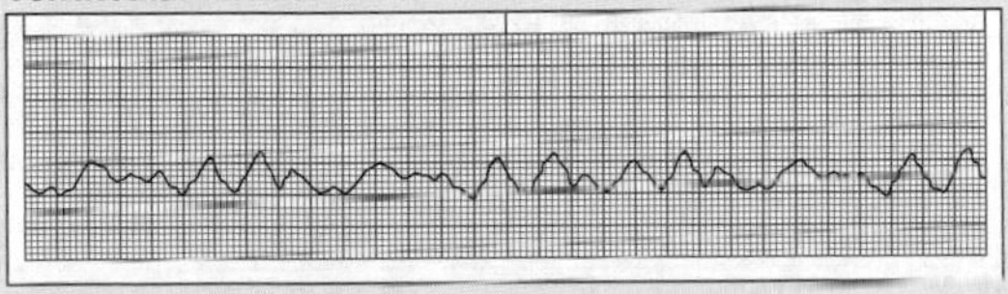

Rhythm . . . . chaotic
Rate . . . . can't be determined
P wave . . . . absent
PR interval . . . . unmeasurable
QRS complex . . indiscernible

Asystole

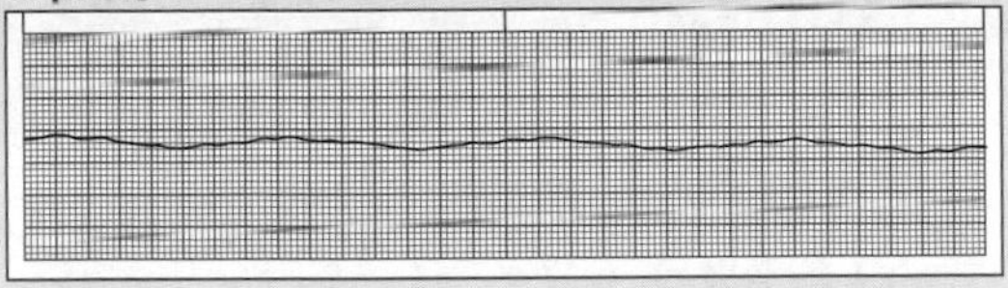

Rhythm . . . . atrial—usually indiscernible; ventricular—absent
Rate . . . . atrial—usually indiscernible; ventricular—absent
P wave . . . . may be present
PR interval . . . . unmeasurable
QRS complex . . absent or occasional escape beats

Comparing heart blocks

First-degree atrioventricular block

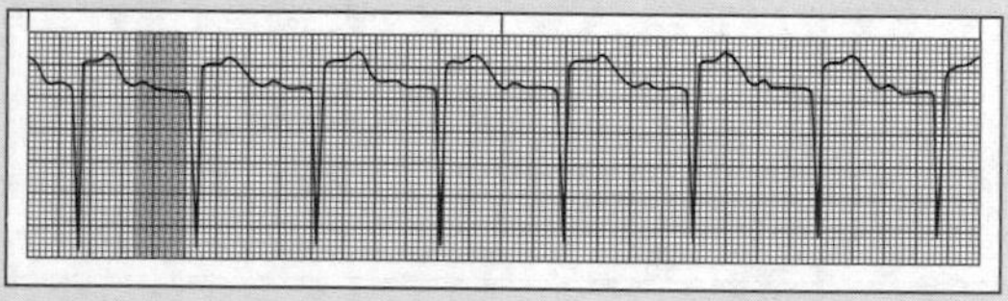

Rhythm . . . . . . .regular
Rate . . . . .within normal limits
P wave . . . . . . .normal
PR interval . . . .> 0.20 second (see shaded area) but constant
QRS complex . .0.06 to 0.10 second

Type I second-degree atrioventricular block

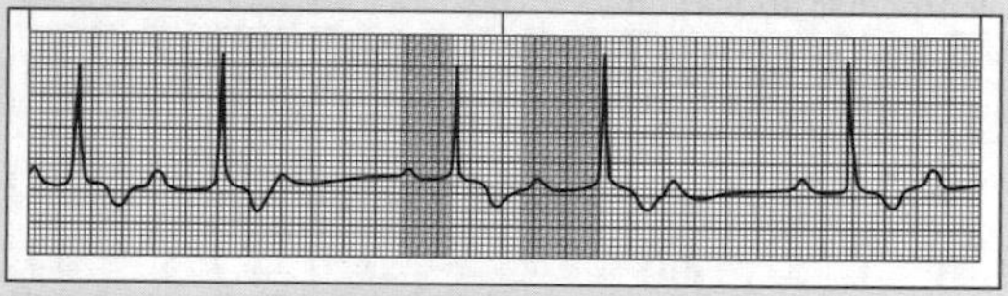

Rhythm . . . . . . .atrial—regular; ventricular—irregular
Rate . . . . .atrial—exceeds ventricular rate; both remain within normal limits
P wave . . . . . . .normal
PR interval . . . .progressively prolonged (see shaded areas) until a P wave appears without a QRS complex
QRS complex . .0.06 to 0.10 second

Comparing heart blocks *(continued)*

Type II second-degree atrioventricular block

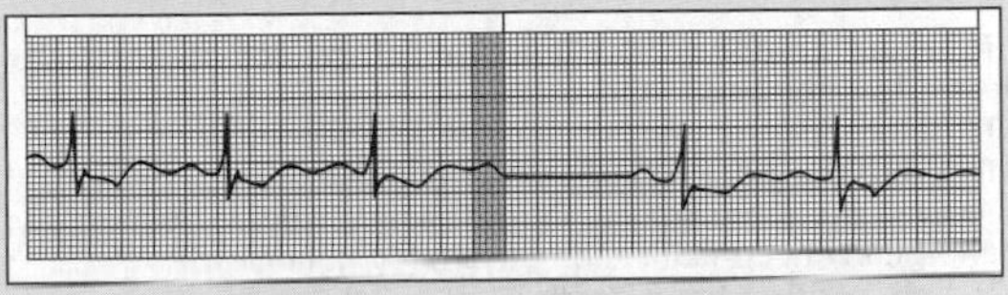

Rhythm ....atrial—regular; ventricular—irregular
Rate ....atrial—within normal limits; ventricular—slower than atrial but may be within normal limits
P wave ....normal
PR interval ....constant for the conducted beats
QRS complex ..within normal limits; absent for dropped beat

Third-degree atrioventricular block

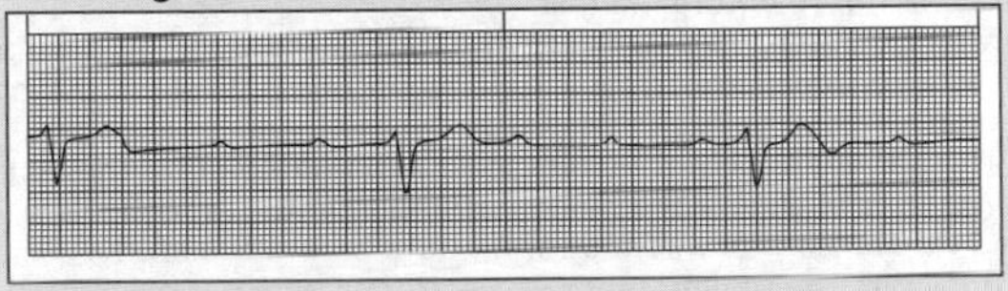

Rhythm ....regular
Rate ....atria and ventricles beat independently; atrial—60 to 100 beats/minute; ventricular—40 to 60 intranodal block, < 40 infranodal block
P wave ....normal
PR interval ....varied; not applicable or measurable
QRS complex ..normal or widened

Electroencephalography

Purpose

- To record portions of the brain's electrical activity through electrodes attached to the scalp
- To determine the presence and type of epilepsy
- To aid in the diagnosis of intracranial lesions
- To evaluate brain activity in metabolic disease, head injury, meningitis, encephalitis, and psychological disorders
- To help confirm brain death

Patient preparation

- Make sure a consent form has been signed; report any allergies.
- Wash and dry the patient's hair to remove hair sprays, creams, or oils.
- Withhold tranquilizers, barbiturates, and other sedatives for 24 to 48 hours before the test.
- Minimize sleep (4 to 5 hours) the night before the study. If a sleep EEG is ordered, give a sedative to promote sleep during the test.
- The patient need not restrict food and fluids before the test; stimulants such as caffeine-containing beverages, chocolate, and tobacco are prohibited for 8 hours before the study.
- Reassure the patient that the electrodes won't shock him. If the test will involve needle electrodes, warn that he might feel pricking sensations during insertion.
- Explain that the test takes about 1 hour.

Procedure

- The patient is positioned and electrodes are attached to the scalp.
- During recording, the patient is carefully observed and any movements, such as blinking, swallowing, or talking are noted.
- The patient may undergo testing in various stress situations including hyperventilation and photic stimulation.

Postprocedure care

- Tell the patient he may resume drug therapy.
- Provide a safe environment.
- Monitor the patient for seizures and maintain seizure precautions.
- Help the patient remove electrode paste from his hair.
- If brain death is confirmed, provide emotional support for the family.

Normal results

• Alpha waves: occur at frequencies of 8 to 13 cycles/second in regular rhythm; present only in the waking state when the patient's eyes are closed but he's mentally alert; usually disappear with visual activity or mental concentration and decrease with apprehension or anxiety, appearing most prominently in the occipital leads
• Beta waves (13 to 30 cycles/second): indicate normal activity when the patient appears alert with eyes open; appear mostly in the frontal and central regions of the brain
• Theta waves (4 to 7 cycles/second): occur most commonly in children and young adults and appear primarily in the parietal and temporal regions, indicating drowsiness or emotional stress in adults
• Delta waves (fewer than 4 cycles/second): visible in deep sleep stages and in serious brain dysfunction

Abnormal results

• Spikes and waves at frequency of 3 cycles/second: suggest absence seizures
• Multiple, high-voltage, spiked waves in both hemispheres: suggest generalized tonic-clonic seizures
• Spiked waves in affected temporal region: suggest temporal lobe epilepsy
• Localized, spiked discharges: suggest focal seizures
• Slow waves (usually delta waves but possibly unilateral beta waves): suggest intracranial lesions
• Focal abnormalities in injured area: suggest vascular lesions
• Generalized, diffuse, and slow brain waves: suggest metabolic or inflammatory disorders or increased intracranial pressure
• Absent EEG pattern or a flat tracing (except for artifacts): may indicate brain death

ALERT Skipping a meal before the test can cause hypoglycemia and alter brain wave patterns. Anticonvulsants, tranquilizers, barbiturates, and other sedatives may alter wave patterns as well.

Electrophysiology studies

Purpose

• To measure discrete conduction intervals during the slow withdrawal of an electrode catheter from the right ventricle through the bundle of His to the sinoatrial node
• To diagnose arrhythmias and conduction anomalies

- To determine the need for an implanted pacemaker, internal cardioverter-defibrillator, and cardioactive drugs
- To locate the site of a bundle-branch block, especially in asymptomatic patients with conduction disturbances
- To determine the presence and location of accessory-conducting pathways

Patient preparation

- Make sure a consent form has been signed; report any allergies.
- Instruct the patient to restrict food and fluids for at least 6 hours before the test.
- Provide reassurance to the patient that he'll remain conscious during the test, which takes 1 to 3 hours. Instruct him to report any discomfort or pain.

Procedure

- The patient is placed in a supine position on a special table and electrocardiogram (ECG) monitoring starts.
- The insertion site (usually the groin or antecubital fossa) is shaved and prepared. A local anesthetic is injected.
- A catheter is inserted intravenously, using fluoroscopic guidance and advanced into the right ventricle, then slowly withdrawn.
- Recordings of conduction intervals are taken from each pole of the catheter, either simultaneously or sequentially.
- After recordings and measurements are complete, the catheter is removed.
- The insertion site is cleaned and a sterile dressing applied.

ALERT Emergency resuscitation equipment should be immediately available in case of arrhythmias during the test.

Postprocedure care

- Monitor vital signs and obtain a 12-lead resting ECG; monitor for cardiac arrhythmias, anginal or embolism symptoms, and ECG changes.
- Enforce bed rest; have the patient resume his usual diet.
- Monitor the insertion site for bleeding and signs of infection.

ALERT Complications include arrhythmias, pulmonary emboli and thromboemboli, hemorrhage, and infection.

Normal results

- Intra-atrial conduction time (PA interval): 20 to 40 msec
- Conduction time from the bundle of His to the Purkinje fibers (HV interval): 35 to 55 msec

• Conduction time from the atrioventricular node to the bundle of His (AH interval): 45 to 150 msec

Abnormal results

• Prolonged HV interval: suggests possible acute or chronic disease
• AH-interval delay: suggests atrial pacing, chronic conduction system disease, carotid sinus pressure, recent myocardial infarction, and use of certain drugs
• PA-interval delay: suggests possible acquired, surgically induced, or congenital atrial disease and atrial pacing

Endoscopy

Purpose

• To diagnose inflammatory, ulcerative, and infectious diseases, using a flexible scope.
• To diagnose benign and malignant tumors and other lesions of the mucosa

Patient preparation

• Make sure a consent form has been signed; report any allergies.
• Give the patient an I.V. sedative before the endoscope insertion.
• Explain that the test takes about 1 hour.

ALERT For a patient taking an anticoagulant, it may be necessary to adjust his drug regimen. For high-risk procedures, the patient should stop taking warfarin 3 to 5 days before the procedure; an appropriate drug such as low molecular-weight heparin should be ordered. Stop aspirin or nonsteroidal anti-inflammatory drugs 3 to 7 days before the test.

Procedure

• I.V. access is started, if indicated.
• Vital signs, pulse oximetry, and cardiac rhythm are monitored throughout the procedure.
• Follow the procedure for the specific endoscopy to be performed (arthroscopy, bronchoscopy, colonoscopy, colposcopy, cystourethroscopy, endoscopic retrograde cholangiopancreatography, esophagogastroduodenoscopy, hysteroscopy, laparoscopy, laryngoscopy, mediastinoscopy, proctosigmoidoscopy, sigmoidoscopy, thoracoscopy).

Postprocedure care

• Provide a safe environment.

- Withhold food and fluids until the gag reflex returns.
- Monitor vital signs, respiratory and neurologic status, and cardiac rhythm.

ALERT Complications include adverse reaction to sedation, cardiac arrhythmias, respiratory depression, and bleeding.

Normal results

- See specific endoscopy procedure
- Structure and function of the studied organ within normal parameters for the patient's age

Abnormal results

- See specific endoscopy procedure (see *Types of endoscopy*)
- Abnormalities specific to the studied organ

(Text continues on page 156.)

Types of endoscopy

Type and area	Purpose	Abnormal findings
ARTHROSCOPY • Joint	• Detect and diagnose meniscal, patellar, condylar, extrasynovial, and synovial diseases • Monitor disease progression • Guide joint surgery • Monitor the effectiveness of therapy	• Meniscal disease • Patellar disease • Condylar disease • Extrasynovial disease • Synovial disease • Foreign bodies associated with gout, pseudogout, and osteochondromatosis
BRONCHOSCOPY • Trachea • Bronchial trees	• Visually examine a tumor, an obstruction, secretions, bleeding, or a foreign body in the tracheobronchial tree • Help diagnose bronchogenic carcinoma, tuberculosis, interstitial pulmonary disease, and fungal or parasitic pulmonary infection	• Bronchial wall abnormalities • Endotracheal abnormalities • Blood • Secretions • Calculi • Foreign bodies • Interstitial pulmonary disease

Types of endoscopy *(continued)*

Type and area	Purpose	Abnormal findings
BRONCHOSCOPY *(continued)*	• Remove foreign bodies, malignant or benign tumors, mucus plugs, and excessive secretions from the tracheobronchial tree	• Bronchogenic carcinoma • Tuberculosis • Other pulmonary infections
CAPSULE ENDOSCOPY (CAMERA PILL) • Stomach walls • Small intestine	• Detect polyps or cancer • Detect causes of bleeding and anemia	• Bleeding sites • Erosions • Crohn's disease • Celiac disease • Benign and malignant small intestine tumors • Vascular disorders • Small-bowel injuries or disorders
COLONOSCOPY • Colon • Large intestine	• Detect or evaluate inflammatory and ulcerative bowel disease • Locate the origin of lower GI bleeding • Help diagnose colonic strictures and benign or malignant lesions • Evaluate the colon postoperatively for recurrence of polyps and malignant lesions	• Proctitis • Granulomatous or ulcerative colitis • Crohn's disease • Malignant or benign lesions • Diverticular disease • Lower GI bleeding
COLPOSCOPY • Vagina	• Help confirm cervical intraepithelial neoplasia or invasive carcinoma after a positive Pap test • Evaluate vaginal or cervical lesions • Monitor conservatively treated cervical intraepithelial neoplasia	• Cervical intraepithelial neoplasia or invasive carcinoma • Inflammatory changes (usually from infection), atrophic changes (usually from aging or, less com-

(continued)

Diagnostic tests

Types of endoscopy *(continued)*

Type and area	Purpose	Abnormal findings
COLPOSCOPY *(continued)*	• Monitor the patient whose mother received diethylstilbestrol during pregnancy	monly, hormonal contraceptives), erosion (probably from increased pathogenicity of vaginal flora due to changes in vaginal pH), and papilloma and condyloma (possibly from viruses)
CYSTOURETHROSCOPY		
• Cervix • Bladder • Urethra • Urinary tract • Uretal orifices • Prostate	• Diagnose and evaluate urinary tract disorders • Perform a biopsy, lesion resection, calculi removal, dilatation of a constricted urethra, and catheterization of the ureteral orifices for retrograde pyelography	• Enlarged prostate gland • Urethral stricture • Calculi • Tumors • Diverticula • Ulcers • Polyps • Bladder wall trabeculation • Congenital anomalies
ENDOSCOPIC RETROGRADE CHOLANGIOPANCREATOGRAPHY		
• Liver's biliary tree • Gallbladder • Pancreatic duct	• Evaluate obstructive jaundice • Diagnose cancer of the duodenal papilla, pancreas, and biliary ducts • Locate calculi and stenosis in the pancreatic ducts and hepatobiliary tree • Identify leaks from trauma or surgery • Evaluate abdominal pain of unknown etiology • Perform stent placement or papillotomy	• Biliary cirrhosis • Carcinoma of the bile ducts, duodenal papilla, or pancreas head • Chronic pancreatitis • Obstructive jaundice • Pancreatic cyst or tumor • Pancreatic fibrosis • Papillary stenosis • Primary sclerosing cholangitis

Types of endoscopy *(continued)*

Type and area	Purpose	Abnormal findings
ESOPHAGOGASTRODUODENOSCOPY		
• Upper GI system	• Diagnose inflammatory disease, malignant and benign tumors, ulcers, Mallory-Weiss syndrome, and structural abnormalities • Evaluate the stomach and duodenum postoperatively • Obtain emergency diagnosis of duodenal ulcer or esophageal injury	• Acute or chronic ulcers • Benign or malignant tumors • Diverticula • Duodenitis • Esophageal and pyloric stenoses • Esophageal hiatal hernia • Esophageal rings • Esophagitis • Gastritis • Mallory-Weiss syndrome • Varices
LARYNGOSCOPY		
• Larynx	• Detect lesions, strictures, or foreign bodies • Remove benign lesions or foreign bodies from the larynx • Help diagnose laryngeal or upper airway abnormalities • Examine the larynx when indirect laryngoscopy is inadequate	• Laryngeal carcinoma • Benign lesions • Strictures • Foreign bodies • Laryngeal edema • Radiation reaction or tumor • Vocal cord dysfunction
PROCTOSCOPY, SIGMOIDOSCOPY, PROCTOSIGMOIDOSCOPY		
• Rectum and sigmoid colon	• Help diagnose inflammatory, infectious, and ulcerative bowel disease • Detect hemorrhoids, hypertrophic anal papilla, polyps, fissures, fistulas, and abscesses in the rectum and anal canal	• Internal and external hemorrhoids • Hypertrophic anal papilla • Anal fissures and fistulas • Anorectal abscesses • Inflammatory bowel diseases • Polyps, cancer, and other tumors

(continued)

Diagnostic tests

Types of endoscopy *(continued)*

Type and area	Purpose	Abnormal findings
THORACOSCOPY • Pleura, pleural spaces, mediastinum, and pericardium	• Diagnose pleural disease • Obtain biopsy specimens • Treat pleural conditions, such as cysts, blebs, and effusions • Perform wedge resections	• Lesions (tumors, ulcers, and bleeding sites) • Carcinoma • Empyema • Pleural effusion • Tuberculosis • Inflammatory process

Laparoscopy, peritoneal cavity

Purpose

- To allow many types of abdominal surgery, such as tubal ligation and cholecystectomy, to be performed simultaneously
- To identify the cause of pelvic pain
- To detect endometriosis, ectopic pregnancy, or pelvic inflammatory disease (PID)
- To evaluate pelvic masses
- To evaluate infertility
- To stage a carcinoma

Patient preparation

- Make sure a consent form has been signed; report any allergies.
- Inform the physician if the patient takes aspirin, nonsteroidal anti-inflammatory drugs, or other drugs that affect clotting.
- Tell the patient to fast after midnight before the test or for at least 8 hours before surgery.
- Explain the use of a local or general anesthetic.
- Warn the patient that she may experience pain at the puncture site and in the shoulder.
- Instruct the patient to empty her bladder just before the test.
- Explain that the test takes 15 to 30 minutes.

Procedure

- The patient is anesthetized and helped into the lithotomy position.
- The bladder is catheterized.
- A bimanual examination of the pelvic area may be performed to detect abnormalities.

• An incision is made at the inferior rim of the umbilicus.
• The peritoneal cavity is insufflated with carbon dioxide or nitrous oxide.
• A laparoscope is inserted to examine the pelvis and abdomen.
• A second incision may be made just above the pubic hair line for some procedures.
• After the examination, minor surgical procedures, such as ovarian biopsy, may be performed.

Postprocedure care

• Instruct the patient to resume her usual diet.
• Instruct the patient to restrict activity for 2 to 7 days.
• Explain that abdominal and shoulder pain should disappear within 24 to 36 hours.
• Provide analgesics.
• Monitor vital signs, adverse reactions to anesthetic, intake and output, bleeding, and signs and symptoms of infection.

ALERT Complications include punctured visceral organ and peritonitis.

Normal results

• Uterus and fallopian tubes normal in size and shape, free from adhesions, and mobile
• Ovaries normal in size and shape
• No cysts and no endometriosis

Abnormal results

• Bubble on surface of the ovary: suggests a possible ovarian cyst
• Sheets or strands of tissue: suggest possible adhesions
• Small, blue powder burns on peritoneum or serosa: suggest endometriosis
• Growths on the uterus: suggest fibroids
• Enlarged fallopian tube: suggests possible hydrosalpinx
• Enlarged or ruptured fallopian tube: suggests a possible ectopic pregnancy
• Infection or abscess: suggests possible PID

Laryngoscopy, direct

Purpose

• To detect lesions, strictures, or foreign bodies in the larynx
• To aid the diagnosis of laryngeal cancer or vocal cord impairment
• To remove benign lesions or foreign bodies from the larynx

• To examine the larynx when the view by indirect laryngoscopy is inadequate
• To evaluate symptoms of pharyngeal or laryngeal disease (stridor or hemoptysis)

Patient preparation

• Make sure a consent form has been signed; report any allergies.
• Instruct the patient to fast for 6 to 8 hours before the test.
• Give the patient a sedative to help him relax and a drug to reduce secretions.
• Give a general or local anesthetic to numb the gag reflex.
• Explain that the test takes about 30 minutes; it takes longer if minor surgery is performed as part of the procedure.

Procedure

• The patient is assisted into a supine position.
• A general anesthetic is given, or the mouth or nose and throat are sprayed with local anesthetic.
• The laryngoscope is inserted through the mouth.
• The larynx is examined for abnormalities; specimens may be collected.
• Minor surgery (polyp removal) may occur at this time.

Postprocedure care

• Assist the patient onto his side with his head slightly elevated.
• Restrict food and fluids until the gag reflex returns (usually 2 hours).
• Reassure that voice loss, hoarseness, and sore throat are most likely temporary.
• Provide throat lozenges or a soothing liquid gargle after the gag reflex returns.
• Monitor the patient and immediately report to the physician any adverse reaction to the anesthetic or sedative.
• Apply an ice collar to prevent or minimize laryngeal edema.

ALERT Observe sputum for blood, and notify the physician immediately if excessive bleeding or respiratory compromise occurs.

• After a biopsy, instruct the patient to refrain from clearing his throat and coughing, and to avoid smoking.
• Monitor vital signs, respiratory status, sputum, and voice quality.

ALERT Immediately report signs of respiratory difficulty, such as laryngeal stridor or dyspnea. Keep emergency resuscitation equipment and a tracheotomy tray readily available for 24 hours.

• Watch for edema and subcutaneous emphysema.

ALERT Complications include subcutaneous crepitus around the patient's face and neck—a sign of tracheal perforation, airway obstruction (in the patient with epiglottiditis), adverse reaction to anesthetic, or bleeding.

Normal results

• No inflammation, lesions, strictures, or foreign bodies

Abnormal results

• Abnormal lesions (combined with the results of a biopsy): suggest possible laryngeal cancer or benign lesions
• Narrowing: suggests stricture
• Inflammation: suggests possible laryngeal edema secondary to radiation or tumor
• Asynchronous vocal cords: suggest possible vocal cord dysfunction

Collaboration

Specialists may be consulted to assist with patient care, depending on the results of the test. An oncologist may be consulted if the patient has cancer; a thoracic surgeon may be consulted if surgery is required.

Lung perfusion scan

Purpose

• To produce a visual image of pulmonary blood flow after I.V. injection of a radiopharmaceutical
• To assess arterial perfusion of the lungs
• To detect pulmonary emboli
• To evaluate pulmonary function

Patient preparation

• Make sure a consent form has been signed; report any allergies.
• Tell the patient that he need not restrict food and fluids before the test.
• Stress the importance of lying still during imaging.
• Explain that the test takes about 30 minutes and the amount of radioactivity is minimal.

Procedure

• The patient is assisted into a supine position on a nuclear medicine table.
• The radiopharmaceutical is injected I.V.
• A gamma camera takes a series of images in various views.

• Images projected on an oscilloscope screen show the distribution of radioactive particles.

Postprocedure care

• Monitor the injection site for hematoma; apply pressure if one develops.

Normal results

• Hot spots (areas of high uptake): indicate normal blood perfusion
• Uptake pattern uniform

Abnormal results

• Cold spots (areas of low uptake): indicate poor perfusion, suggesting an embolism
• Decreased regional blood flow (without vessel obstruction): suggests possible pneumonitis

Lung ventilation scan

Purpose

• To differentiate areas of ventilated lung from areas of underventilated lung
• To diagnose pulmonary emboli when used in combination with a lung perfusion scan
• To identify areas of the lung that are capable of ventilation
• To evaluate regional respiratory function
• To locate regional hypoventilation

Patient preparation

• Make sure a consent form has been signed; report any allergies.
• Tell the patient that he need not restrict food or fluids.
• Stress the importance of lying still during imaging.
• Tell the patient that he will wear a tight-fitting mask during the test.
• Explain that the test takes 15 to 30 minutes.

Procedure

• The patient is assisted into a supine position on a nuclear medicine table.
• A tight-fitting mask is applied, covering the patient's nose and mouth.
• The patient inhales air mixed with a small amount of radioactive gas through the tightly fitted mask.
• Distribution of the gas in the lungs is monitored on a nuclear scanner.
• The patient's chest is scanned as the gas is exhaled.

Postprocedure care

- Reinstate oxygen therapy as appropriate.
- Monitor the patient's vital signs and respiratory status.

ALERT Panic attacks may occur from wearing the tight-fitting mask.

Normal results

- Gas equally distributed in both lungs

Abnormal results

- Gas distributed unequally in both lungs: suggests poor ventilation or airway obstruction in areas with low radioactivity
- Vascular obstruction with normal ventilation (when performed with a lung perfusion scan): suggests decreased perfusion as in pulmonary embolism
- Both ventilation and perfusion abnormalities: suggest possible parenchymal disease

Magnetic resonance imaging

Purpose

- To produce computerized images of internal organs and tissues using powerful magnetic field and radiofrequency waves
- To obtain images of internal organs and tissues not readily visible on standard X-rays

Patient preparation

- Patients requiring life-support equipment, including ventilators, require special preparation; contact the magnetic resonance imaging (MRI) staff ahead of time.
- Tell the patient that he need not restrict food or fluids.
- Make sure a consent form has been signed; report any allergies.
- A claustrophobic patient may require sedation or an open MRI to reduce anxiety.
- Instruct the patient to remove any metal objects.

ALERT Be aware that any metal or tattoos located on or within the patient's body may cause burns.

- Advise patient that he'll be asked to remain still during the procedure.
- Warn the patient that the machine makes loud clacking sounds.
- Explain that the test takes about 30 to 90 minutes.

Procedure

• If the patient is to receive a contrast medium, an I.V. line is started and the medium is administered before the procedure.
• The patient is checked for metal objects at the scanner room door.
• The patient is placed in a supine position on a padded scanning table; the table is positioned in the opening of the scanning gantry.
• A call bell or intercom is used to maintain verbal contact.
• The patient may wear earplugs if needed.
• Varying radiofrequency waves are directed at the area being scanned.
• A computer reconstructs information as images on a television screen.

Postprocedure care

• Tell the patient to resume his normal diet and activities unless otherwise indicated.
• Monitor vital signs and watch for orthostatic hypotension.

Normal results

• Results dependent on specific type of MRI
• Structure and function of the studied organ within normal parameters for the patient

Abnormal results

• Results dependent on specific type of MRI (see *Types of MRI*)
• Abnormalities dependent on the particular organ studied

ALERT Metal objects, such as I.V. pumps, ventilators, other metallic equipment, or computer-based equipment, in the MRI area may cause interference.

(Text continues on page 165.)

Types of MRI

Area	Purpose	Abnormal findings
Abdominal and pelvic	• Visualize the liver, pancreas, adrenals, spleen, kidneys, blood vessels, and reproductive organs • Stage uterine, vulvar, and cervical carcinoma and prostate cancer	• Neoplasms • Renal implant abnormalities • Retroperitoneal structural abnormalities

Types of MRI *(continued)*

Area	Purpose	Abnormal findings
Blood vessels (magnetic resonance angiography)	• Detect, diagnose, and assist in the treatment of heart disorders, stroke, and blood vessel diseases • Screen for familial tendency for arterial aneurysms	• Atherosclerosis • Disease in the aorta and in blood vessels supplying the kidneys, lungs, and legs • Graft patency • Aneurysms • Stenosis • Occlusions
Intracranial	• Help diagnose intracranial and spinal lesions and soft-tissue abnormalities	• Cerebral edema • Aneurysms • Demyelinating disease • Edematous fluid • Multiple sclerosis (MS) lesions • Pontine and cerebellar tumors • Tumors • Stroke • Hydrocephalus • Ischemia • Arnold-Chiari malformation
Breast	• Visualize complex breast lesions • Differentiate between benign and malignant breast tumors • Detect breast tumors in women with implants • Stage breast cancer	• Complex breast lesion • Benign and malignant breast tumors

(continued)

Types of MRI *(continued)*

Area	Purpose	Abnormal findings
Cardiac	• Evaluate cardiac wall motion • Visualize cardiac structures, valves, and coronary arteries	• Abnormal heart chamber size • Pericarditis • Congenital heart disorders • Thrombic clotting disorders • Aortic dissection • Aortic aneurysm • Cardiac ischemia
Musculoskeletal	• Identify primary and metastatic bone tumors • Delineate muscles, ligaments, and bones • Contrast body tissues and sharply define healthy, benign, and malignant tissues	• Bony and soft-tissue tumors • Changes in bone marrow composition • Spinal disorders
Spinal	• Visualize diseases of the spinal canal and cord • Detect a bulging, degenerated, or herniated intervertebral disk • Assess for spinal infection or tumors that arise in, or have spread to, the spine • Help visualize needle placement for steroids to relieve spinal pain	• Disk herniation • Primary and metastatic neoplasms • Inflammatory disease • Demyelinating disease (MS) • Congenital abnormalities • Disk degeneration
Urinary tract	• Evaluate genitourinary tumors and abdominal or pelvic masses • Detect prostate stones and cysts • Detect cancer invasion into seminal vesicles and pelvic lymph nodes	• Tumors • Strictures • Stenosis • Thrombosis • Malformations • Abscess • Inflammation • Edema • Fluid collection • Bleeding • Hemorrhage • Organ atrophy

Myocardial perfusion imaging, radiopharmaceutical

Purpose

- To assess coronary arteries in patients who can't tolerate exercise stress tests; it's also known as *chemical stress test imaging*
- To assess the presence and degree of coronary artery disease
- To evaluate a patient's response after therapeutic procedures (such as bypass surgery and coronary angioplasty)

Patient preparation

- Confirm that the patient isn't pregnant.
- Adenosine, dobutamine, or dipyridamole are used to chemically stress the patient, simulating effects of exercise by increasing blood flow in coronary arteries or by increasing heart rate and contractility.
- A radiopharmaceutical is injected; resting and stress images are obtained and compared to evaluate coronary perfusion.
- For dobutamine administration, withhold beta-adrenergic blockers for 48 hours before the test. Give drugs such as antihypertensives.
- Withhold theophylline for 24 to 36 hours and nitrates 6 hours before the test.
- Instruct the patient to avoid caffeine for 12 hours before testing.
- Tell the patient that he must fast—but may drink water—for 3 to 4 hours before the test.
- Make sure a consent form has been signed; report any allergies.
- Screen for bronchospastic lung disease or asthma (adenosine and dipyridamole are contraindicated). Screen for presence of a pacemaker; dobutamine may be contraindicated.
- Weigh the patient to determine the appropriate drug dosage.
- Warn the patient that he may experience flushing, shortness of breath, dizziness, headache, chest pain, increased heart rate, or palpitations during the infusion, depending on the drug in use. Explain that signs and symptoms generally stop as soon as the infusion ends.
- Explain that the study takes 1 to 2 hours but may take longer, depending on the type of nuclear medicine equipment.
- Give adenosine or dipyridamole as ordered.

Procedure

- The patient is placed in a supine position on the examination table; I.V. access is obtained.
- Baseline electrocardiogram (ECG) and vital signs are obtained.
- The chemical stress medication is infused. Vital signs and cardiac rhythm are monitored continuously.
- At the appropriate time, the radiopharmaceutical is injected.
- Rest imaging may be done before stress imaging or 3 to 4 hours after stress imaging, depending on the radiopharmaceutical used.
- After the images are completed, the I.V. access is removed.

Postprocedure care

- Tell the patient to resume his regular diet and activity.
- Monitor vital signs, ECG, cardiac rhythm, and respiratory status.
- Monitor anginal symptoms, heart and breath sounds.
- Reversal drugs that should be readily available include I.V. aminophylline for adenosine and dipyridamole and I.V. beta-adrenergic blocker for dobutamine.

ALERT Complications include serious arrhythmias and myocardial ischemia or infarction.

Normal results

- No perfusion defects on imaging
- No ischemic changes on ECG

Abnormal results

- Cold spots: indicate areas of decreased uptake, possibly suggesting coronary artery disease (most common); myocardial fibrosis, attenuation caused by soft tissue (breast and diaphragm), or coronary spasm

Nuclear medicine scans

Purpose

- To produce imaging of specific body organs or systems by a scintillating scanning camera after I.V. injection, inhalation, or oral ingestion of a radioactive tracer compound
- To produce tissue analysis and images not readily seen on standard X-rays
- To detect or rule out malignant lesions when X-ray findings are normal or questionable

Patient preparation

- Make sure a consent form has been signed; report any allergies.
- Note any prior nuclear medicine procedures. Make sure the patient isn't scheduled for more than one radionuclide scan on the same day.
- Advise the patient that he'll be asked to take various positions on a scanner table.
- Stress how important it is for the patient to remain still during the procedure.
- Explain that the study takes about 1 to 2 hours, but the time varies depending on the specific nuclear medicine scan.

Procedure

- If the patient will receive an I.V. tracer isotope, an I.V. line is started.
- The detector of a scintillation camera is directed at the area being scanned and displays the image on a monitor.
- Scintigraphs are obtained and reviewed for clarity; if necessary, additional views are obtained.

Postprocedure care

- Tell the patient to resume his normal diet and activities.
- Monitor vital signs; watch for infection and orthostatic hypotension.

Normal results

- Results dependent on specific type of nuclear medicine scan
- Structure and function of studied organ normal

Abnormal results

- Results dependent on specific type of nuclear medicine scan
- Abnormalities dependent on studied structure or organ

Pulmonary angiography

Purpose

- To radiographically examine the pulmonary circulation after injection of a radiopaque contrast medium into the pulmonary artery or one of its branches
- To detect pulmonary embolism in a symptomatic patient with an equivocal lung scan
- To evaluate pulmonary circulation abnormalities
- To provide accurate preoperative evaluation of patients with shunt physiology caused by congenital heart disease
- To treat identified pulmonary embolism with thrombolysis

Patient preparation

• Make sure a consent form has been signed; report any allergies.
• Check for and report history of anticoagulation or renal insufficiency.
• Note and inform the physician of any abnormal laboratory results.
• Instruct the patient to fast for 8 hours before the test.
• Stop heparin infusion 3 to 4 hours before the test.
• Explain the need to use a local anesthetic.
• Warn the patient that he may have a possible urge to cough, a flushed feeling, or a salty taste for 3 to 5 minutes after the injection.
• Explain that the test takes about 1 to 2 hours and that he'll be monitored during the test.

Procedure

• The patient is placed in a supine position.
• The access site is cleaned and prepared, which is usually the right groin.
• A local anesthetic is injected.
• The vein is accessed; a catheter is introduced under image-guidance and advanced through the right atrium, the right ventricle, and into the pulmonary artery.
• Pulmonary artery pressures are measured and blood samples may be drawn from various regions of the pulmonary circulation.
• The contrast medium is injected and images are obtained.
• Thrombolysis is initiated, if indicated.
• After the catheter is removed, hemostasis is obtained.
• The access site is cleaned and dressed.

Postprocedure care

• Maintain bed rest.
• Have the patient resume his usual diet.
• Restart anticoagulation.
• Encourage the patient to drink fluids, or give I.V. fluids to help eliminate the contrast medium.
• Monitor vital signs, intake and output, renal function studies, and adverse reaction to the contrast medium.

ALERT Observe the site for bleeding and swelling. If these occur, maintain pressure at the insertion site for at least 10 minutes, and notify the radiologist.

ALERT Complications include myocardial perforation or rupture, ventricular arrhythmias and conduction defects, acute renal failure, bleeding and hematoma formation, infection, adverse reaction to the contrast medium, cardiac valve damage, and right-sided heart failure.

Normal results

- Contrast medium flowing symmetrically and without interruption through the pulmonary circulation

Abnormal results

- Interruption of blood flow and filling defects: suggest possible acute pulmonary embolism
- Arterial webs, stenoses, irregular occlusions, wall-scalloping, and "pouching" defects (a concave edge of thrombus facing the opacified lumen): suggest chronic pulmonary embolism

Pulmonary function tests

Purpose

- To evaluate pulmonary function through a series of spirometric measurements
- To assess effectiveness of a specific therapeutic regimen
- To evaluate pulmonary status

Patient preparation

- Make sure a consent form has been signed; report any allergies.
- Stress the need for the patient to avoid smoking for 12 hours before the tests. Stress the need to avoid a heavy meal before the tests.
- Withhold bronchodilators for 8 hours.

Procedure

- For tidal volume (V_T), the patient breathes normally into the mouthpiece 10 times.
- For expiratory reserve volume (ERV), the patient breathes normally for several breaths and then exhales as completely as possible.
- For vital capacity (VC), the patient inhales as deeply as possible and exhales into the mouthpiece as completely as possible. This is repeated three times, and the largest volume is recorded.
- For inspiratory capacity (IC), the patient breathes normally for several breaths and inhales as deeply as possible.
- For functional residual capacity (FRC), the patient breathes normally into a spirometer. After a few breaths, the levels of gas in the spirometer and in the lungs reach equilibrium. FRC is calculated by subtracting the spirometer volume from the original volume.

- For forced vital capacity (FVC) and forced expiratory volume (FEV), the patient inhales as slowly and deeply as possible and then exhales into the mouthpiece as quickly and completely as possible. This is repeated three times, and the largest volume is recorded. The volume of air expired at 1 second (FEV_1), at 2 seconds (FEV_2), and at 3 seconds (FEV_3) during all three repetitions is recorded.
- For maximal voluntary ventilation, the patient breathes into the mouthpiece as quickly and deeply as possible for 15 seconds.
- For diffusing capacity for carbon monoxide, the patient inhales a gas mixture with a low level of carbon monoxide and holds his breath for 10 to 15 seconds before exhaling.

Postprocedure care

- Pulmonary function tests may be contraindicated in patients with acute coronary insufficiency, angina, or recent myocardial infarction. Watch for respiratory distress, changes in pulse rate and blood pressure, coughing, and bronchospasm in these patients.

ALERT Complications include respiratory distress, bronchospasm, and physical exhaustion.

Normal results

- Results dependent on age, height, weight, and sex (values expressed as a percentage)
- V_T: 5 to 7 mg/kg of body weight
- ERV: 25% of VC
- IC: 75% of VC
- FEV_1: 83% of VC after 1 second
- FEV_2: 94% of VC after 2 seconds
- FEV_3: 97% of VC after 3 seconds

Abnormal results

- FEV_1 less than 80%: suggests obstructed pulmonary disease
- FEV_1-to-FVC ratio greater than 80%: suggests restrictive pulmonary disease
- Decreased VT: suggests possible restrictive disease
- Decreased minute volume (MV): may suggest disorders such as pulmonary edema
- Increased MV: may suggest acidosis, exercise, or low compliance states
- Reduced CO_2 response: may suggest emphysema, myxedema, obesity, hypoventilation syndrome, or sleep apnea
- Residual volume greater than 35% of total lung capacity after maximal expiratory effort: suggests obstructive disease
- Decreased IC: suggests restrictive disease
- Increased FRC: may suggest obstructive pulmonary disease

- Low total lung capacity (TLC): suggests restrictive disease
- High TLC: suggests obstructive disease
- Decreased FVC: suggests flow resistance from obstructive disease or from restrictive disease
- Low forced expiratory flow: suggests obstructive disease of the small and medium-sized airways
- Decreased peak expiratory flow rate: suggests upper airway obstruction
- Decreased diffusing capacity for carbon monoxide: suggests possible interstitial pulmonary disease

Technetium-99m pyrophosphate scanning

Purpose

- To detect a hot spot on a scan made with a scintillation camera via I.V. tracer isotope (technetium-99m pyrophosphate) that accumulates in damaged myocardial tissue (possibly by combining with calcium in the damaged myocardial cells)
- To be used when serum cardiac enzyme tests are unreliable or when patients have equivocal electrocardiograms (ECGs) such as in left bundle-branch block
- To confirm a recent myocardial infarction (MI)
- To define the size and location of a recent MI
- To assess prognosis after an acute MI

Patient preparation

- Make sure a consent form has been signed; report any allergies.
- Tell the patient that he need not restrict food and fluids.
- Reassure the patient that he'll feel only transient discomfort during isotope injection and that the scan itself is painless.
- Stress the need to remain quiet and motionless during scanning.

Procedure

- Technetium-99m pyrophosphate is injected into the antecubital vein.
- After 2 to 3 hours, assist the patient into a supine position.
- Attach ECG electrodes for continuous monitoring during the test.
- Scans are usually taken in several positions; anterior, left anterior oblique, right anterior oblique, and left lateral. Each scan takes about 10 minutes.

Postprocedure care

- Answer the patient's questions about the test.

Normal results

- No isotope in the myocardium

Abnormal results

- Isotope taken up by the sternum and ribs and their activity compared with that of the heart; 2+, 3+, and 4+ activity (equal to or greater than bone): suggest a positive myocardial scan
- Areas of isotope accumulation, or hot spots: suggest damaged myocardium

Thallium imaging

Purpose

- To evaluate blood flow after I.V. injection of the radioisotope thallium-201 or Cardiolite
- To assess myocardial perfusion
- To demonstrate the location and extent of an myocardial infarction (MI)
- To diagnose coronary artery disease (CAD) (stress imaging)
- To evaluate coronary artery patency following surgical revascularization
- To evaluate effectiveness of antianginal therapy or percutaneous revascularization interventions (stress imaging)

Patient preparation

- Make sure a consent form has been signed; report any allergies.
- For stress imaging, instruct the patient to wear comfortable walking shoes during the treadmill exercise.
- Tell the patient he must restrict his use of alcohol, tobacco, and nonprescription medications for 24 hours before the test.
- Have the patient fast after midnight the night before the test.
- Urge the patient to report fatigue, pain, shortness of breath, or other anginal symptoms immediately.

Procedure

- For stress imaging, the patient walks on a treadmill at a regulated pace that's gradually increased while his electrocardiogram (ECG), blood pressure, and heart rate are monitored.
- When the patient reaches peak stress, give 1.5 to 3 mCi of thallium.
- The patient exercises an additional 45 to 60 seconds to permit circulation and uptake of the isotope.

ALERT Stop the stress imaging immediately if the patient develops chest pain, dyspnea, fatigue, syncope, hypotension, ischemic ECG changes, significant arrhythmias, or other critical signs or symptoms (confusion, staggering, or pale, clammy skin).

- Disconnect the patient from monitoring equipment if he's stable, and position him on his back under the nuclear medicine camera.
- Additional scans may be taken after the patient rests and occasionally after 24 hours.
- Scanning after rest is helpful in differentiating between an ischemic area and an infarcted or scarred area of the myocardium.
- For resting imaging, give the patient an injection of thallium I.V. or Cardiolite. Scanning is performed as in stress imaging.

Postprocedure care

- If further scanning is required, have the patient rest and restrict foods and beverages other than water.
- Monitor vital signs and ECGs; watch for cardiac arrhythmias and anginal symptoms.

ALERT Complications include cardiac arrhythmias, myocardial ischemia, MI, respiratory distress, cardiac arrest, hypotension, or hypertension.

Normal results

- Normal distribution of the isotope throughout left ventricle without defects (cold spots)
- Improved regional perfusion after coronary artery bypass surgery: suggests graft patency
- Improved perfusion after nonsurgical revascularization interventions: suggests increased coronary flow

Abnormal results

- Persistent defects: suggests MI
- Transient defects (those that disappear after a 3- to 6-hour rest): suggest myocardial ischemia caused by CAD

Transesophageal echocardiography

Purpose

- To provide a better view of the heart's structures combining ultrasonography with endoscopy
- To allow images to be taken from the posterior aspect of the heart involving a small transducer attached to the end of a gastroscope and inserted into the esophagus

- To visualize and evaluate thoracic and aortic disorders, such as dissection and aneurysm; valvular disease (especially of the mitral valve); endocarditis; and congenital heart disease
- To visualize and evaluate intracardiac thrombi, cardiac tumors, cardiac tamponade, and ventricular dysfunction

Patient preparation

- Make sure a consent form has been signed; report any allergies.
- Review the patient's medical history and report possible contraindications to the test, such as esophageal obstruction or varices, GI bleeding, previous mediastinal radiation therapy, or severe cervical arthritis.
- Note and report any loose teeth.
- Tell the patient that he must fast for 6 hours before the procedure.
- Instruct the patient to remove dentures or oral prostheses.
- Explain the use of a topical anesthetic throat spray.
- Warn the patient that he may gag when the tube is inserted.
- Explain the need for I.V. sedation and continuous monitoring.
- Explain the study takes about 2 hours, including preparation and recovery.

Procedure

- Connect the patient to monitors for continual blood pressure, heart rate, and pulse oximetry assessment.
- Assist the patient into a supine position on his left side and give him a sedative.
- The back of his throat is sprayed with a topical anesthetic.
- A bite block is placed in the patient's mouth and he's instructed to close his lips around it.
- The endoscope is inserted and advanced 12" to 14" (30 to 36 cm) to the level of the right atrium.
- To visualize the left ventricle, the scope is advanced 16" to 18" (41 to 46 cm).
- Ultrasound images are obtained and reviewed.

Postprocedure care

- Ensure patient safety and a patent airway until the sedative wears off.
- Withhold food and water until his gag reflex returns.
- If the procedure is done on an outpatient basis, advise the patient to have someone drive him home.
- Monitor level of consciousness, vital signs, respiratory status, and cardiac arrhythmias.
- Watch for bleeding and observe for gag reflex; observe closely for a vasovagal response, which may occur with gagging.

• Keep resuscitation and suction equipment immediately available.
• Use pulse oximetry to detect hypoxia.
• If bleeding occurs, stop the procedure immediately.

ALERT Complications include laryngospasm, cardiac arrhythmias, bleeding, and adverse reactions to sedation.

Normal results

• Heart without structural abnormalities
• No visible vegetations or thrombi
• No visible tumors

Abnormal results

• Structural thoracic and aortic abnormalities: suggest possible endocarditis, congenital heart disease, intracardiac thrombi, or tumors
• Congenital defects: suggest possible patent ductus arteriosus

ALERT Laryngospasm, arrhythmias, or bleeding increase the risk of complications. If any of these occur, postpone the test.

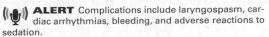

Ultrasonography

Purpose

• To measure organ size and evaluate structure
• To detect foreign bodies and differentiate between a cyst and solid tumor
• To monitor tissue response to radiation or chemotherapy

Patient preparation

• Make sure a consent form has been signed; report any allergies.
• Explain that the procedure is painless and safe and that no radiation exposure is involved.
• Stress the importance of remaining still during scanning.

Procedure

• Assist the patient into a supine position; use pillows to support the area to be examined.
• The target area is coated with a water-soluble jelly. The transducer is used to scan the area, projecting the images on the oscilloscope screen. The image on the screen is photographed for subsequent examination.

• It may be necessary to assist the patient into right or left lateral positions for subsequent views.

Postprocedure care

• After the procedure, remove the conductive gel from the patient's skin.

Normal results

• Results dependent on specific type of ultrasonography (abdominal aorta, gallbladder and biliary system, kidney and perirenal, liver, pancreas, pelvis, spleen, and thyroid)
• Structure and function of the studied organ within normal parameters for the patient's age

Abnormal results

• Results dependent on specific type of ultrasonography (abdominal aorta, gallbladder and biliary system, kidney and perirenal, liver, pancreas, pelvis, spleen, and thyroid) (see *Types of ultrasonography*)
• Abnormalities specific to the studied organ

Types of ultrasonography

Area	Purpose	Abnormal findings
Abdominal aorta	• Detect and measure a suspected abdominal aortic aneurysm • Detect and measure the expansion of a known abdominal aortic aneurysm	• Aneurysm • Aneurysm with high risk of rupture
Carotid	• Detect cerebral blood flow • Evaluate ischemia, headache, dizziness, paresthesia, hemiparesis, and speech and visual disturbances	• Plaque • Stenosis • Obstruction • Dissection • Aneurysm • Carotid body tumor • Arteritis
Gallbladder and biliary system	• Confirm cholelithiasis • Diagnose acute cholecystitis • Distinguish between obstructive and nonobstructive jaundice	• Acute cholecystitis • Biliary obstruction • Biliary sludge • Gallstones within the gallbladder lumen or the biliary system • Polyps and carcinoma

Types of ultrasonography *(continued)*

Area	Purpose	Abnormal findings
Leg	• Confirm deep vein thrombosis • Distinguish clot formation from venous obstruction • Evaluate congenital venous abnormalities • Assess deep vein valvular competence • Locate a suitable vein for arterial bypass grafting • Evaluate chronic venous disease	• Deep vein thrombosis • Congenital venous malformations • Venous obstruction • Clot formation • Valve incompetencies
Liver	• Distinguish between obstructive and nonobstructive jaundice • Screen for hepatocellular disease • Detect hepatic metast[illegible] and hem[illegible]	• Abscesses • Ascitic fluid • Benign tumors • Cysts • He[illegible]

Types of ultrasonography *(continued)*

Area	Purpose	Abnormal findings
Pelvic area	• Demonstrate splenomegaly • Monitor the progression of primary and secondary splenic disease • Evaluate the effectiveness of therapy • Evaluate the spleen after abdominal trauma • Help detect splenic cysts and subphrenic abscesses	• Splenomegaly (but not the cause) • Splenic rupture • Subcapsular hematoma • Subphrenic abscess • Cystic or solid lesions
Thyroid	• Estimate thyroid weight • Determine the size, depth, and dimension of thyroid goiters and masses • Evaluate a neck mass	• Goiter • Parathyroid lesions • Congenital deformities (brachial cleft cyst, cystic hygroma, thyroglossal duct cyst) • Benign adenomas • Malignant tumors
Vaginal	• Establish early pregnancy (fifth to sixth week of gestation) with fetal heart motion • Identify ectopic pregnancy • Monitor follicular growth during infertility treatm... • Evaluate abno... cy (such a... mis...	• Peritonitis • Ectopic pregnancy • Cancer of the uterus, ovaries, vagin... oth...

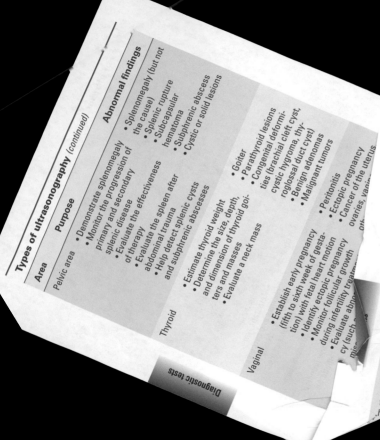

In... sopharyngeal airway

Fir... y beside the patient's face to make sure it's the pro... wn below left). It should be slightly smaller than the ... l diameter and slightly longer than the distance fro... nose to his earlobe.

T... rway, hyperex-ten... s neck (unless co...). Lubricate the air... ter-soluble gel. Th... he tip of his nose an... irway into his nos-tril ... below right). Avoid

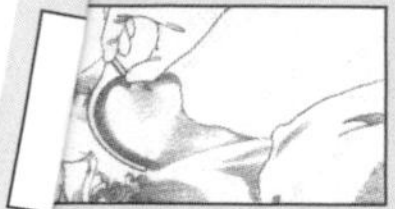

pu... ainst any resistance to ... tissue trauma and air-wa... g. Be sure to have the bevel facing the nasal septum when inserting.

To check for correct airway placement, first close the patient's mouth. Then place your finger over the tube's opening to detect air exchange. Also, depress the patient's tongue with a tongue blade and look for the airway tip behind the uvula.

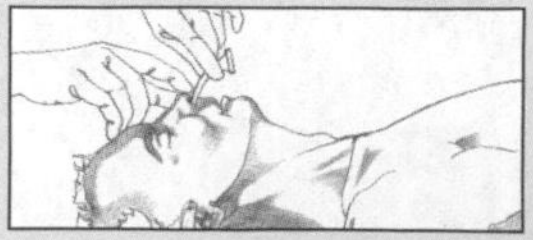

In... ting an oral airway (u... only in unconscious patien...

Un... this position is contraindicated, h... ext... the patient's head (as show... bef... using either the cross-f... bla... insertion method

T... nsert an oral a... fing... r method... tien... 's l... his ...

Performing Allen's test

Perform an Allen's test before puncturing a radial artery to ascertain adequate perfusion to the hand.

Rest the patient's arm on the mattress or bedside stand, and support his wrist with a rolled towel. Have him clench his fist. Then, using your index and middle fingers, press on the radial and ulnar arteries. Hold this position for a few seconds.

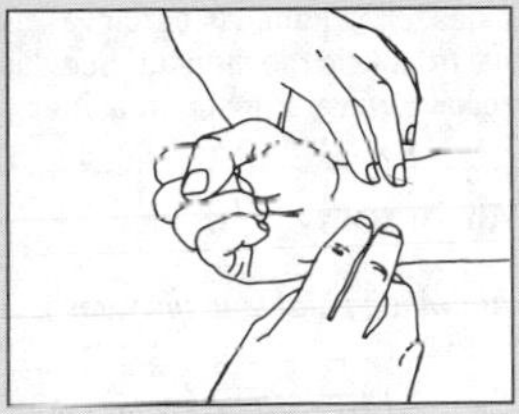

Without removing your fingers from the patient's arteries, ask him to unclench his fist and hold his hand in a relaxed position. The palm will be blanched because pressure from your fingers has impaired the normal blood flow.

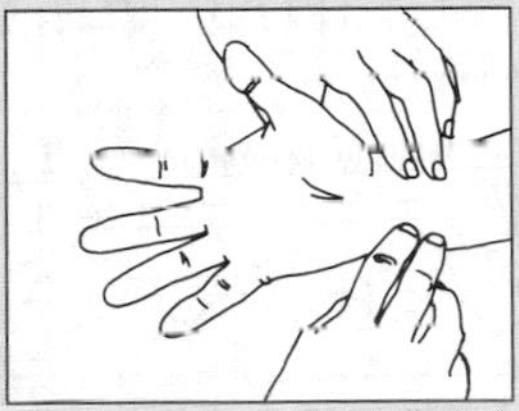

Release pressure on the patient's ulnar artery. If the hand becomes flushed, which indicates blood filling the vessels, you can safely proceed with the radial artery puncture. If the hand doesn't flush, perform the test on the other arm.

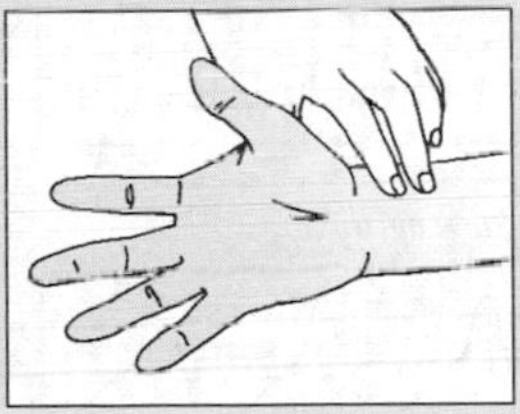

Recognizing an abnormal arterial waveform

Understanding a normal arterial waveform is relatively straightforward; however, an abnormal waveform is more difficult to decipher. Abnormal patterns and markings may provide important diagnostic clues to the patient's cardiovascular status, or they may simply signal trouble in the monitor. Use this table to help you recognize and resolve waveform abnormalities.

Abnormality	Possible causes
Alternating high and low waves in a regular pattern 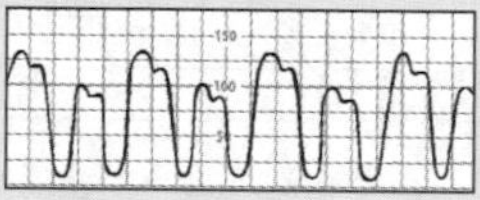	• Ventricular bigeminy
Flattened waveform 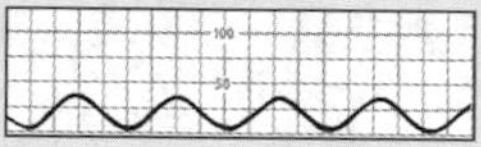	• Overdampened waveform or hypotensive patient
Slightly rounded waveform with consistent variations in systolic height 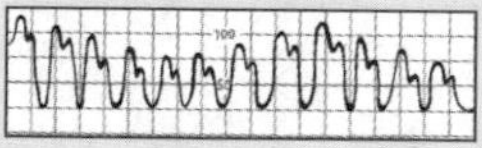	• Patient on ventilator with positive end-expiratory pressure
Slow upstroke 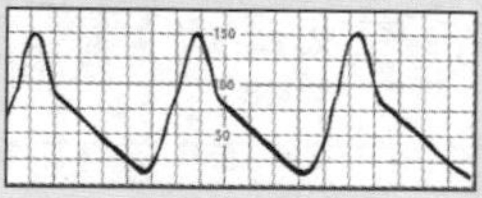	• Aortic stenosis
Diminished amplitude on inspiration 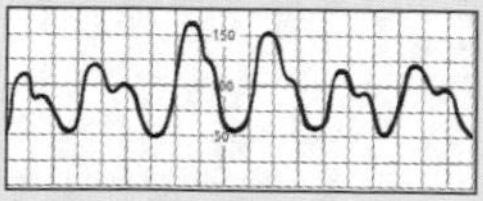	• Pulsus paradoxus, possibly from cardiac tamponade, constrictive pericarditis, or lung disease

Nursing interventions

• Check the patient's electrocardiogram to confirm ventricular bigeminy. The tracing should reflect premature ventricular contractions every second beat.

• Check the patient's blood pressure with a sphygmomanometer. If you obtain a reading, suspect overdampening. Correct the problem by trying to aspirate the arterial line. If you succeed, flush the line. If the reading is very low or absent, suspect hypotension.

• Check the patient's systolic blood pressure regularly. The difference between the highest and lowest systolic pressure reading should be less than 10 mm Hg. If the difference exceeds that amount, suspect pulsus paradoxus, possibly from cardiac tamponade.

• Check the patient's heart sounds for signs of aortic stenosis. Also, notify the practitioner, who will document suspected aortic stenosis in his notes.

• Note systolic pressure during inspiration and expiration. If inspiration pressure is at least 10 mm Hg less than expiratory pressure, call the practitioner.
• If you're also monitoring pulmonary artery pressure, observe for a diastolic plateau. This occurs when the mean central venous pressure (right arterial pressure), mean pulmonary artery pressure, and mean pulmonary artery wedge pressure are within 5 mm Hg of one another.

Skills

Arterial puncture technique

The angle of needle penetration in arterial blood gas sampling depends on which artery will be sampled. For the radial artery, which is used most commonly, the needle should enter bevel up at a 30- to 45-degree angle over the radial artery. After collecting the sample, apply pressure to the site for at least 5 minutes.

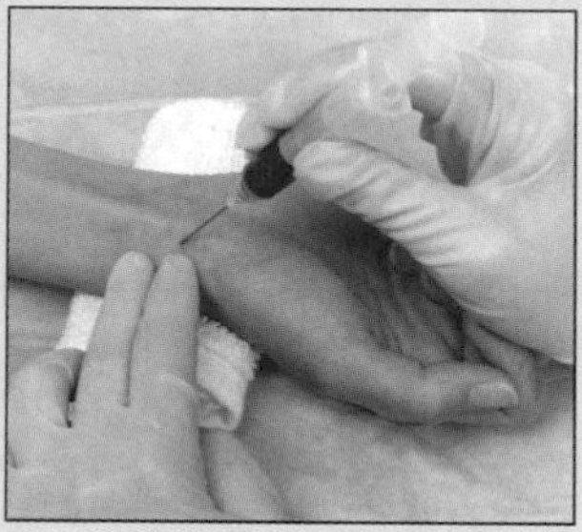

Using a bag-valve-mask device

Place the mask over the patient's face so that the apex of the triangle covers the bridge of the nose and the base lies between the lower lip and chin.

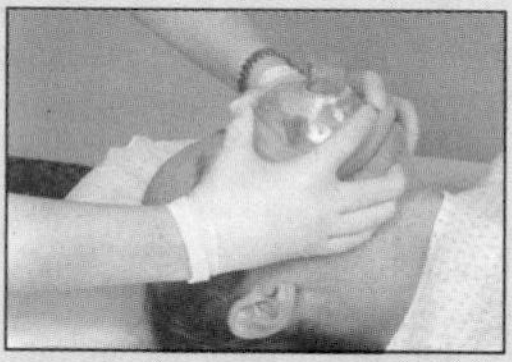

Make sure that the patient's mouth remains open underneath the mask. Attach the bag to the mask and to the tubing leading to the oxygen source.

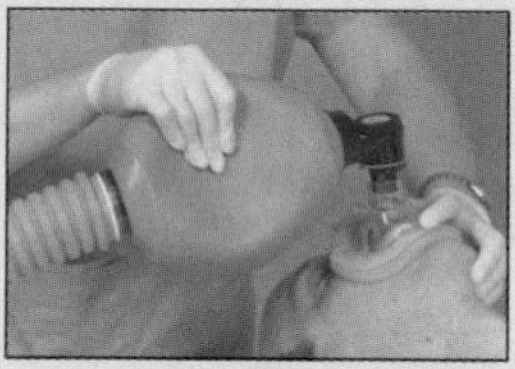

Or, if the patient has a tracheostomy or endotracheal tube in place, remove the mask from the bag and attach the device directly to the tube.

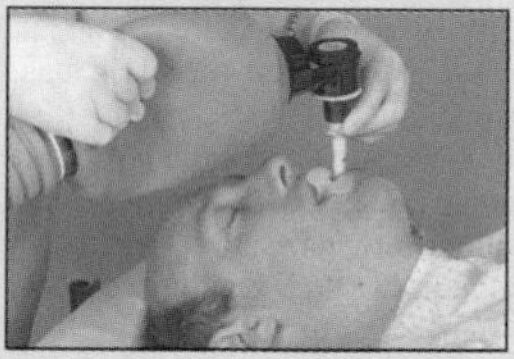

Transfusing blood

The most common cause of a severe transfusion reaction is receiving the wrong blood. You can protect your patients against this possibility by taking the following steps before administering blood or blood products.

Check

Check the practitioner's order for transfusion. Then check to make sure an informed consent form was signed. Then double-check the patient's name, medical record number, ABO blood group, Rh status (and other compatibility factors), and blood bank identification number against the label on the blood bag. Also check the expiration date on the bag. Then check and record the patient's vital signs.

Verify

Ask another nurse to verify all information, according to your facility's policy. (Most facilities require double identification.) Make sure that you and the nurse who checked the blood or blood product sign the blood confirmation slip. If even one discrepancy exists, don't administer the blood or blood product. Instead, immediately notify the blood bank.

Inspect

Inspect the blood or blood product to detect abnormalities. Then confirm the patient's identity by checking the name and medical record number on his wristband.

Transfusion don'ts

A blood transfusion requires extreme care. Here are some tips on what *not* to do when administering a transfusion:

- Don't add medications to the blood bag.
- Don't give blood products without checking the order against the blood bag label—the only way to tell whether the request form has been stamped with the wrong name. Most life-threatening reactions occur when this step is omitted.
- Don't transfuse the blood product if you discover a discrepancy in the blood number, blood slip type, or patient identification number.
- Don't piggyback blood into the port of an existing infusion set. Most solutions, including dextrose in water, are incompatible with blood. Administer blood only with normal saline solution.
- Don't hesitate to stop the transfusion if your patient shows changes in vital signs, is dyspneic or restless, or develops chills, hematuria, or pain in the flank, chest, or back. Your patient could go into shock, so don't remove the I.V. device that's in place. Keep it open with a slow infusion of normal saline solution; call the practitioner and the laboratory.
- Don't transfuse blood that has been out of the refrigerator for more than 4 hours. Once started, a transfusion must be infused within 4 hours.

Monitoring a blood transfusion

To help avoid transfusion reactions and safeguard your patient, follow these guidelines:

- Record vital signs before the transfusion, 15 minutes after the start of the transfusion, just after the transfusion is complete, and more frequently if warranted by the patient's condition, transfusion history, or your facility's policy. Most acute hemolytic reactions occur during the first 30 minutes of the transfusion, so monitor your patient carefully during that time.
- Always have sterile normal saline solution—an isotonic solution—set up as a primary line along with the transfusion.
- Act promptly if your patient develops wheezing and bronchospasm. These signs may indicate an allergic reaction or anaphylaxis. If the patient becomes dyspneic and shows generalized flushing and chest pain (with or without vomiting and diarrhea), he could be having an anaphylactic reaction. Stop the blood transfusion immediately, start the normal saline solution, check and document vital signs, call the practitioner, and follow your facility's policy for a transfusion reaction. Provide supportive care as indicated.
- If the patient develops a transfusion reaction, return the remaining blood together with a posttransfusion blood sample and any other required specimens to the blood bank.

Transfusing blood products: Plasma or plasma fractions

- Obtain baseline vital signs.
- Flush the patient's venous access device with normal saline solution.
- Attach the plasma, fresh frozen plasma, albumin, factor VIII concentrate, prothrombin complex, platelets, or cryoprecipitate to the patient's venous access device, after proper verification of patient and product, per your facility's policy.
- Begin the transfusion, and adjust the flow rate as ordered.
- Take the patient's vital signs, and assess him frequently for signs or symptoms of a transfusion reaction, such as fever, chills, or nausea.
- After the infusion, flush the line with 20 to 30 ml of normal saline solution. Then disconnect the I.V. line. If therapy is to continue, resume the prescribed infusate and adjust the flow rate as ordered.
- Record the type and amount of plasma or plasma fraction administered, duration of the transfusion, baseline and posttransfusion vital signs, and any adverse reactions.

Positioning cardiac monitoring leads

This chart shows the correct electrode positions for some of the monitoring leads you'll use most often. For each lead, you'll see electrode placement for two hardwire systems (the five-and the three-leadwire systems) and a telemetry system.

In the two hardwire systems, the electrode positions for one lead may be identical to the electrode positions for another lead. In this case, you simply change the lead selector switch to the setting that corresponds to the lead you want. In some cases, you'll need to reposition the electrodes.

In the telemetry system, you can create the same lead with two electrodes that you do with three by eliminating the ground electrode.

The illustrations below use these abbreviations: RA, right arm; LA, left arm; RL, right leg; LL, left leg; C, chest; and G, ground.

Five-leadwire system	Three-leadwire system	Telemetry system

Lead I

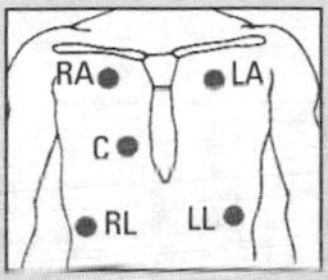

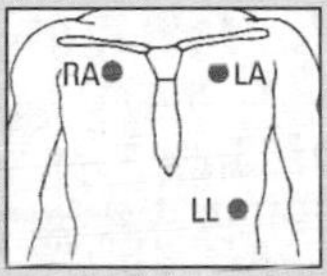

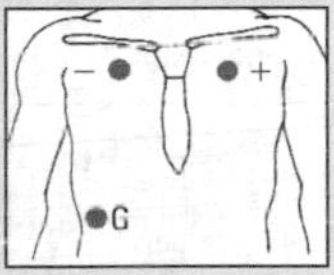

Lead II

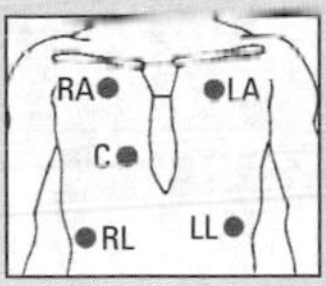

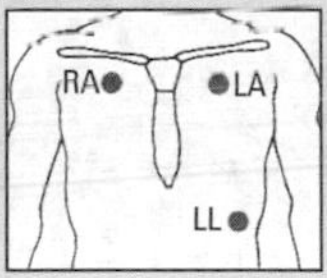

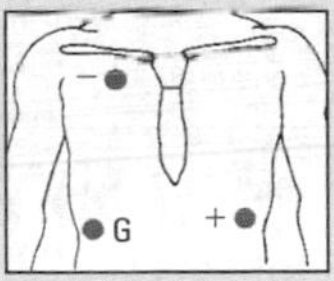

Lead III

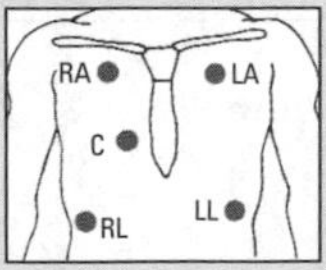

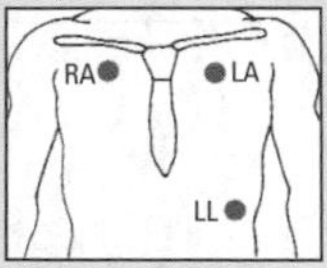

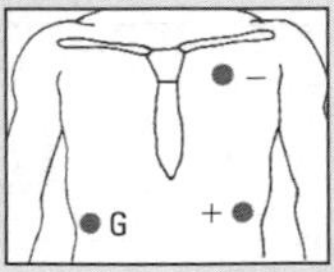

(continued)

Positioning cardiac monitoring leads *(continued)*

Five-leadwire system	Three-leadwire system	Telemetry system
Lead MCL_1		
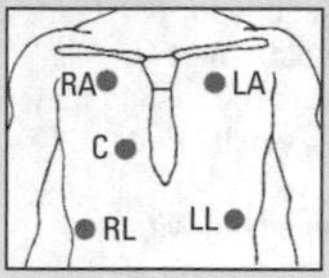	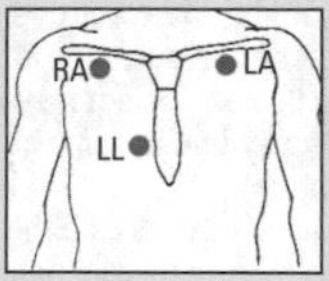	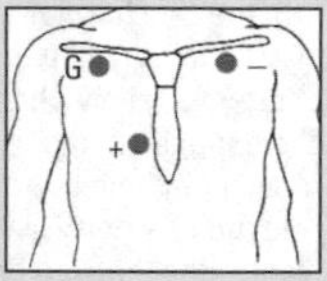
Lead MCL_6		
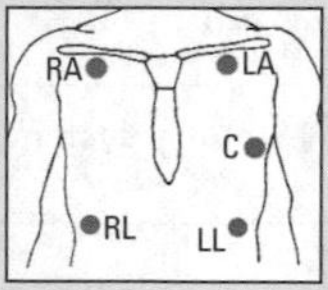	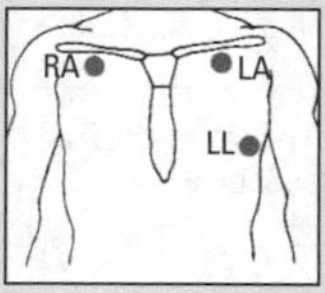	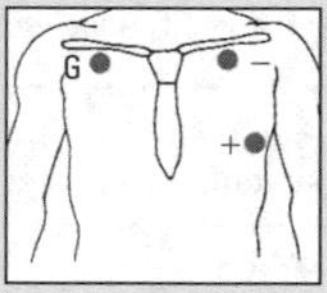
Sternal lead		
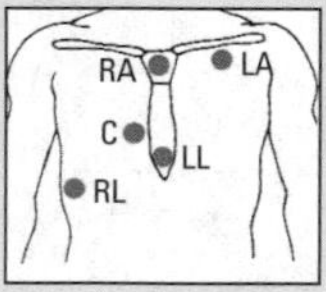	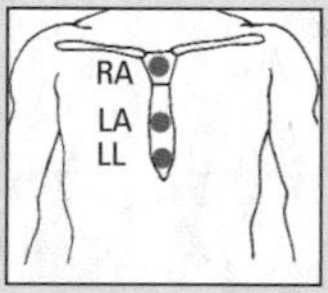	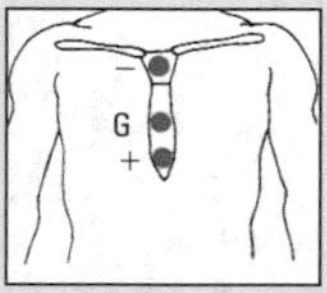
Lewis lead		
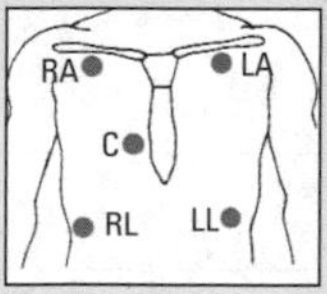	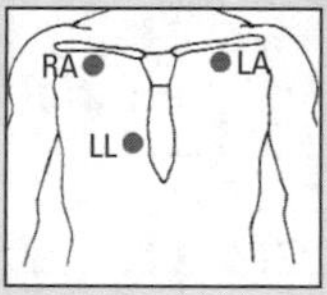	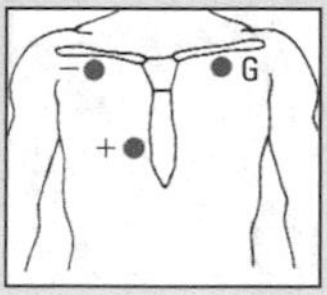

Identifying cardiac monitor problems

Problem	Possible causes	Nursing interventions
False-high-rate alarm	• Monitor interpreting large T waves as QRS complexes, which double the rate • Skeletal muscle activity	• Reposition electrodes to lead where QRS complexes are taller than T waves. • Place electrodes away from major muscle masses.
False-low-rate alarm	• Shift in electrical axis from patient movement, making QRS complexes too small to register • Low amplitude of QRS • Poor contact between electrode and skin	• Reapply electrodes. Set gain so height of complex is greater than 1 mV. • Increase gain. • Reapply electrodes.
Low amplitude	• Gain dial set too low • Poor contact between skin and electrodes; dried gel; broken or loose leadwires; poor connection between patient and monitor; malfunctioning monitor; physiologic loss of QRS amplitude	• Increase gain. • Check connections on all leadwires and monitoring cable. Replace electrodes as necessary. Reapply electrodes, if required.
Wandering baseline	• Poor position or contact between electrodes and skin • Thoracic movement with respirations	• Reposition or replace electrodes. • Reposition electrodes.
Artifact (waveform interference)	• Patient having seizures, chills, or anxiety • Patient movement • Electrodes applied improperly • Static electricity	• Notify practitioner and treat patient as ordered. Keep patient warm and reassure him. • Help patient relax. • Check electrodes and reapply, if necessary.

(continued)

Identifying cardiac monitor problems *(continued)*

Problem	Possible causes	Nursing interventions
Artifact (waveform interference) *(continued)*	• Electrical short circuit in leadwires or cable • Interference from decreased room humidity	• Make sure cables don't have exposed connectors. Change patient's static-causing gown or pajamas. • Replace broken equipment. Use stress loops when applying leadwires. • Regulate humidity to 40%.
Broken leadwires or cable	• Stress loops not used on leadwires • Cables and leadwires cleaned with alcohol or acetone, causing brittleness	• Replace leadwires and retape them, using stress loops. • Clean cable and leadwires with soapy water. Don't allow cable ends to become wet. Replace cable as necessary.
60-cycle interference (fuzzy baseline)	• Electrical interference from other equipment in room • Patient's bed improperly grounded	• Attach all electrical equipment to common ground. Check plugs to make sure prongs aren't loose. • Attach bed ground to the room's common ground.
Skin excoriation under electrode	• Patient allergic to electrode adhesive • Electrode on skin too long	• Remove electrodes and apply nonallergenic electrodes and nonallergenic tape. • Remove electrode, clean site, and reapply

Measuring cardiac output

ALERT Maintain consistency of technique and patient body positioning for serial cardiac output measurements.

- Verify the presence of a pulmonary artery (PA) waveform on the cardiac monitor.
- Unclamp the I.V. tubing and withdraw exactly 10 ml of solution.
- Reclamp the tubing.
- Turn the stopcock at the catheter injectant hub to open a fluid path between the injectant lumen of the PA catheter and the syringe.

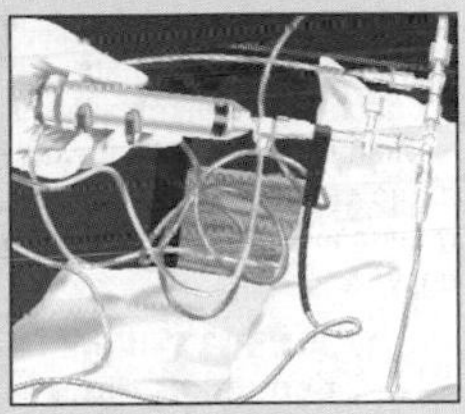

- Press the START button on the cardiac output computer or wait for the "Inject" message to flash.
- Inject solution smoothly within 4 seconds, making sure it doesn't leak at the connectors.
- If available, analyze the contour of the thermodilution washout curve on a strip chart recorder for a rapid upstroke and a gradual, smooth return to baseline.

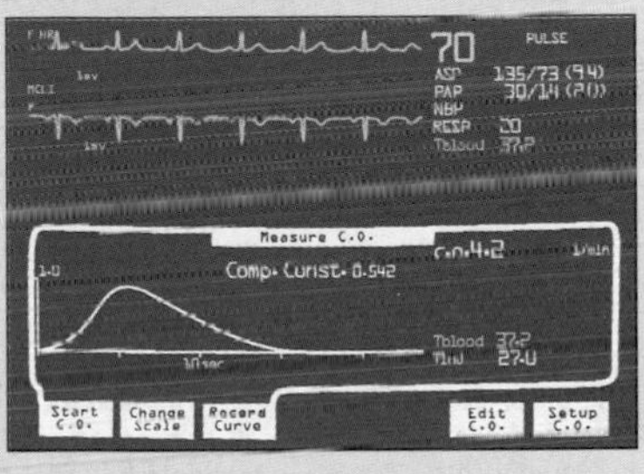

- Repeat steps until three values are within 10% to 15% of the median value.
- Compute the average of three values, and record the patient's cardiac output.
- Return the stopcock to the original position, and make sure the injectant delivery system tubing is clamped.
- Verify the presence of a PA waveform on the cardiac monitor.
- Discontinue cardiac output measurements when the patient is hemodynamically stable and weaned from vasoactive and inotropic drugs, as ordered.

Performing synchronized cardioversion

- Confirm the patient's identity using two patient identifiers according to your facility's policy.
- Explain the procedure to the patient, and make sure he has signed a consent form.
- Check his recent serum potassium and magnesium levels and arterial blood gas results.
- Check recent digoxin levels.
- Digitalized patients may undergo cardioversion, but tend to require lower energy levels to convert.

ALERT If the patient takes digoxin, withhold the dose on the day of the procedure.

- Withhold food and fluids for 6 to 12 hours before the procedure.
- Obtain a 12-lead electrocardiogram (ECG) to serve as a baseline.
- Check to see if the practitoner has ordered cardiac drugs before the procedure.
- Verify that the patient has a patent I.V. site in case drugs become necessary.
- Connect the patient to a pulse oximeter and automatic blood pressure cuff, if available.
- Consider giving oxygen for 5 to 10 minutes before cardioversion to promote myocardial oxygenation.
- If the patient wears dentures, evaluate whether they support his airway or may cause airway obstruction. If they may cause an obstruction, remove them.
- Place the patient in the supine position, and assess vital signs, level of consciousness (LOC), cardiac rhythm, and peripheral pulses.
- Remove the oxygen delivery device before cardioversion to prevent combustion.
- Have epinephrine (Adrenalin), lidocaine (Xylocaine), and atropine at the patient's bedside.
- Make sure the resuscitation bag is at the bedside.
- Give a sedative, as ordered. The sedation is considered moderate to deep with reflexes intact and with the patient still able to breathe adequately.
- Carefully monitor blood pressure and respiratory rate until he recovers.
- Press the POWER button to turn on the defibrillator.
- Push the SYNC button to synchronize the machine with the patient's QRS complexes.
- Make sure the SYNC button flashes with each of the patient's QRS complexes.
- You should see a bright green flag flash on the monitor.
- Turn the ENERGY SELECT dial to the ordered amount of energy.

ALERT Advanced cardiac life support protocols call for a monophasic energy dose of 50 to 100 joules for a patient with unstable supraventricular tachycardia, 100 to 200 joules for a patient with atrial fibrillation, 50 to 100 joules for a patient with atrial flutter, and 100 joules for a patient who has monomorphic ventricular tachycardia with

Skills

a pulse. If there's no response with the first shock, the health care provider should increase the joules in a step-wise manner.

- Remove the paddles from the machine, and prepare them as if you were defibrillating the patient.
- Place conductive gel pads or paddles in the same positions you would to defibrillate.
- Make sure everyone stands away from the bed; push the discharge buttons.
- Hold the paddles in place and wait for energy to be discharged—the machine has to synchronize the discharge with the QRS complex.
- Check the waveform on the monitor.
- If the arrhythmia fails to convert, repeat the procedure two or three more times at 3-minute intervals.
- Gradually increase the energy level with each additional countershock.
- After cardioversion, frequently assess the patient's LOC and respiratory status, including airway patency, respiratory rate and depth, and need for supplemental oxygen.

ALERT The patient may require airway support because he's heavily sedated.

- Record a postcardioversion 12-lead ECG, and monitor the patient's ECG rhythm for 2 hours or per your facility's sedation protocol.
- Check for electrical burns and treat as needed.

Performing carotid sinus massage

Before applying manual pressure to the patient's right carotid sinus, locate the bifurcation of the carotid artery on the right side of the neck. Turn his head slightly to the left and hyperextend the neck, bringing the carotid artery closer to the skin and moving the sternocleidomastoid muscle away from the carotid artery.

Using a circular motion, massage the right carotid sinus between your fingers and the transverse processes of the spine for 3 to 5 seconds. Don't massage for more than 5 seconds to avoid risking life-threatening complications.

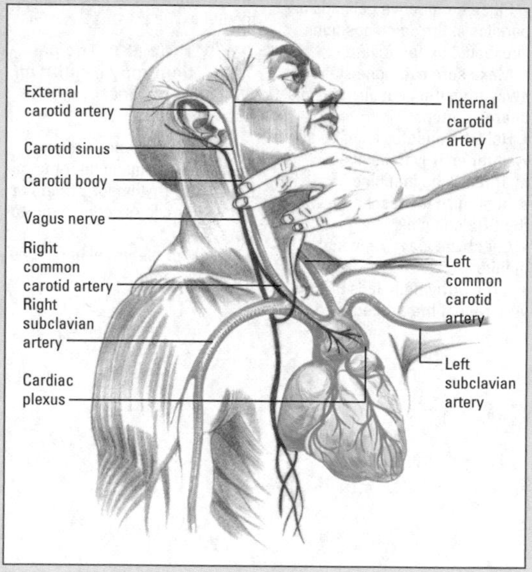

Skills

Inserting an arterial catheter

- The practitioner prepares and anesthetizes the insertion site and covers the surrounding area with sterile drapes.

ALERT Cannulation of the brachial artery isn't recommended because of the potential for thrombosis and ischemia of the lower arm and hand.

- The practitioner inserts the catheter into the artery and attaches it to the fluid-filled pressure tubing.
- While the practitioner holds the catheter in place, activate the fast-flush release (flushing 1 to 3 seconds) to flush blood from the catheter.
- After each fast flush, observe the drip chamber to verify a correct continuous flush rate.
- Observe the bedside monitor for a waveform.
- The practitioner may suture the catheter in place or secure it with hypoallergenic tape.
- Cover the insertion site with a sterile dressing.
- With a radial or brachial site, immobilize the insertion site according to your facility's policy.
- With a femoral site, assess the need for immobilization of the leg and maintain the patient on bed rest, with the head of the bed raised no more than 30 degrees, to prevent the catheter from kinking.
- Level the zeroing stopcock of the transducer with the phlebostatic axis, and then zero the transducer system to atmospheric pressure.
- Activate monitor alarms, as appropriate.

Removing an arterial catheter

- Determine if you're permitted to perform this procedure, according to your facility's policy.
- If you're permitted, record the patient's systolic, diastolic, and mean blood pressures.
- Obtain a manual blood pressure reading to establish a new baseline.
- Turn off the monitor alarms and the flow clamp to the flush solution.
- Carefully remove the dressing over the insertion site.
- Remove sutures using the suture removal kit.
- Withdraw the catheter using a gentle, steady motion, keeping the catheter parallel to the artery during withdrawal.
- Immediately apply pressure to the site with a sterile 4″ x 4″ gauze pad for at least 10 minutes (longer if bleeding or oozing persists) until hemostasis is obtained.
- If the patient has coagulopathy or is receiving anticoagulants, apply additional pressure to a femoral site.
- Cover the site with an appropriate dressing; secure the dressing with tape.
- Make a pressure dressing for a femoral site by folding four sterile 4″ x 4″ gauze pads in half. Place the dressing over the femoral site and cover with a tight adhesive bandage. Cover the bandage with a sandbag.
- Maintain the patient on bed rest for 6 hours with the sandbag in place.
- Observe the site for bleeding.
- Assess the extremity distal to the site by evaluating color, pulses, and sensation every 15 minutes for the first 4 hours, every 30 minutes for the next 2 hours, and hourly for the next 6 hours.

Catheter-tip culture

- If infection is suspected, obtain a culture of the catheter by cutting the tip so it falls into a sterile container. Label the specimen and send it to the laboratory.

Removing a central venous catheter

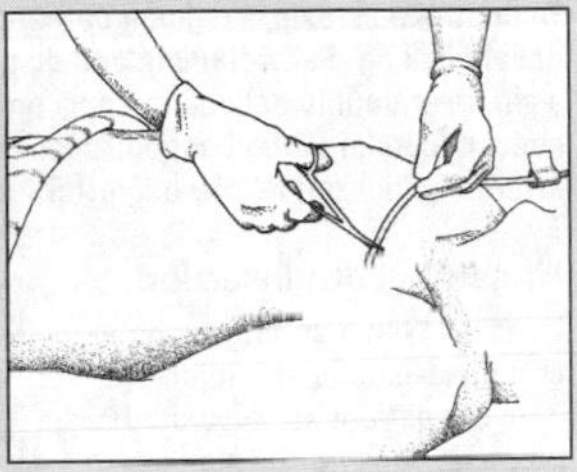

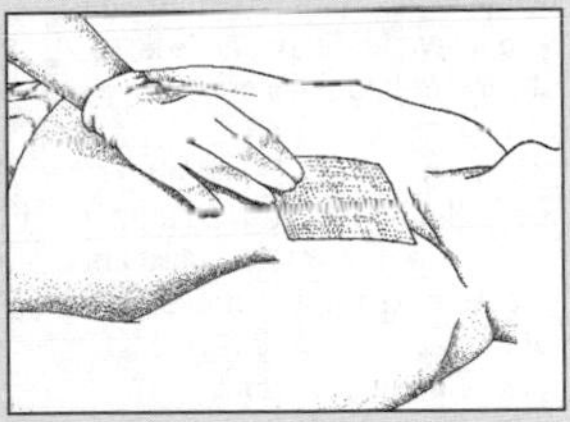

- Place the patient in a supine position to prevent an air embolism.
- Wash your hands, and put on clean gloves and a mask.
- Turn off all infusions.
- Remove and discard the old dressing, and change to sterile gloves.
- Inspect the site for signs of drainage and inflammation.
- Clip the sutures and, using forceps, remove the catheter in a slow and even motion. Have the patient perform Valsalva's maneuver as the catheter is withdrawn to prevent an air embolism.
- Apply pressure to the site until bleeding stops.
- Apply povidone-iodine ointment to the insertion site to seal it. Cover the site with a gauze pad, and apply a transparent semipermeable dressing over the gauze. Label the dressing with the date and time of the removal and your initials.
- Discard the catheter, soiled dressing, and gloves in the appropriate receptacle.

Using a nasal balloon catheter

To control epistaxis, a balloon catheter may be inserted instead of nasal packing. Self-retaining and disposable, the catheter may have a single or double balloon to apply pressure to bleeding nasal tissues. If bleeding is still uncontrolled, arterial ligation, cryotherapy, or arterial embolization may be performed.

Assisting with insertion

To assist with inserting a single- or double-balloon catheter, prepare the patient as you would for nasal packing. Be sure to discuss the procedure thoroughly to alleviate the patient's anxiety and promote his cooperation.

Explain that the catheter tip will be lubricated with an antibiotic or a water-soluble lubricant to ease passage and prevent infection.

Answer all questions.

Providing routine care

The tip of the single-balloon catheter will be inserted in the nostrils until it reaches the posterior pharynx. Then the balloon will be inflated with normal saline solution, pulled gently into the posterior nasopharynx, and secured at the nostrils with the collapsible bulb. With a double-balloon catheter, the posterior balloon is inflated with normal saline solution; then the anterior balloon is inflated.

To check catheter placement, mark the catheter at the nasal vestibule; then inspect for that mark and observe the oropharynx for the posteriorly placed balloon. Assess the nostrils for irritation or erosion. Remove secretions by gently suctioning the airway of a double-balloon catheter or by dabbing away crusted external secretions if the patient has a catheter with no airway.

To prevent damage to nasal tissue, the balloon may be deflated for 10 minutes every 24 hours. If bleeding recurs or remains uncontrolled, packing may be added.

Single-balloon catheter

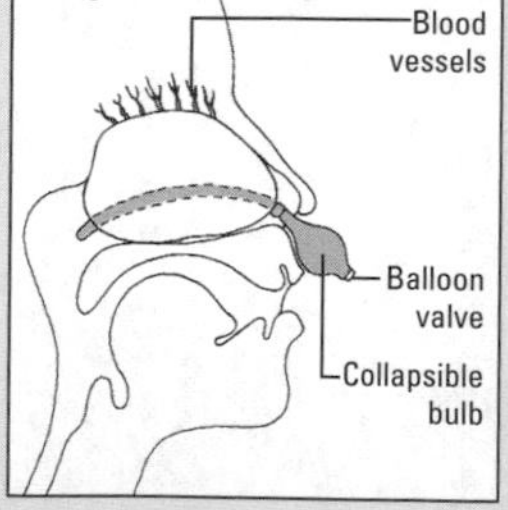

Double-balloon catheter

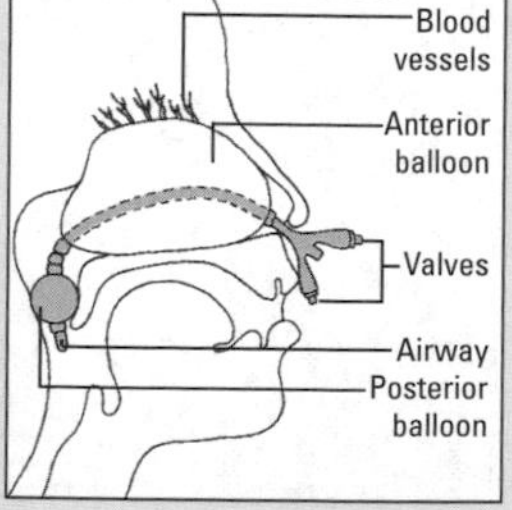

Skills

Measuring CVP with a manometer

To ensure accurate central venous pressure (CVP) readings, make sure the manometer base is aligned with the patient's right atrium (the zero reference point). The manometer set usually contains a leveling rod to allow you to determine this quickly.

After adjusting the manometer's position, examine the typical three-way stopcock. By turning it to any position shown here, you can control the direction of fluid flow. Four-way stopcocks also are available.

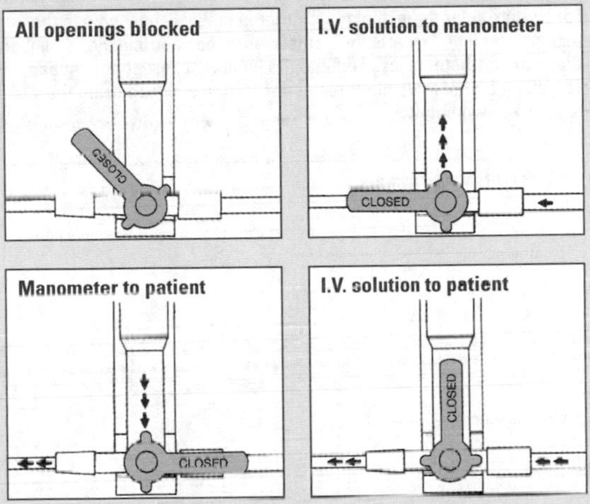

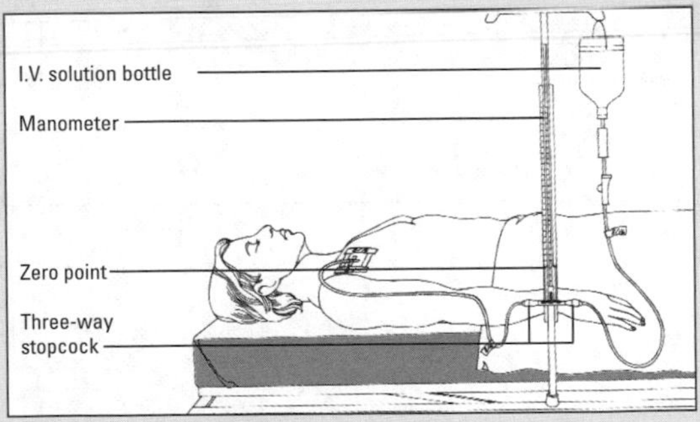

Using a cerebrospinal fluid drainage system

Cerebrospinal fluid (CSF) drainage aims to control intracranial pressure (ICP) during treatment for traumatic injury or other conditions that cause a rise in ICP. CSF can be withdrawn from the lateral ventricle (ventriculostomy) or lumbar subarachnoid space, depending on indication and desired outcome. Ventricular drainage is used to reduce increased ICP, whereas lumbar drainage is used to aid healing of the dura mater.

Drainage system setup

For a ventricular drain, the neurosurgeon makes a burr hole in the patient's skull and inserts the catheter into the ventricle. For a lumbar drain, the catheter is inserted into the lumbar subarachnoid space. The distal end of the catheter is connected to a closed drainage system, as shown below.

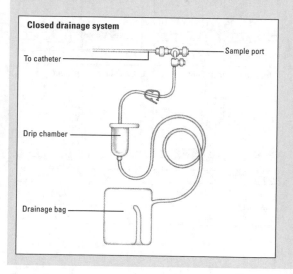

Closed drainage system

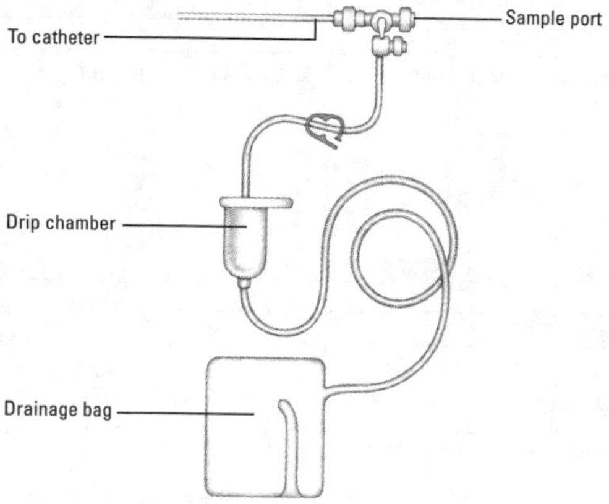

Skills

Monitoring CSF drainage

- Maintain a continuous hourly output of CSF by raising or lowering the drainage system drip chamber.
- To maintain CSF outflow, the drip chamber should be slightly lower than or at the level of the lumbar drain insertion site.
- You may need to carefully raise or lower the drip chamber to increase or decrease CSF flow.
- For a ventricular drain, ensure that the flow chamber of the ICP monitoring setup remains positioned as ordered.
- Correlate changes in ICP readings to the drainage.
- To drain CSF as ordered, put on gloves, and turn the main stopcock on to drainage to allow CSF to collect in the graduated flow chamber.
- Document the time and the amount of CSF obtained, and turn the stopcock off to drainage.
- To drain the CSF from this chamber into the drainage bag, release the clamp below the flow chamber.
- Check the dressing frequently for drainage, which could indicate CSF leakage.
- Check the tubing for patency by watching the CSF drops in the drip chamber.
- Observe CSF for color, clarity, amount, blood, and sediment.
- Obtain any CSF specimens for laboratory analysis from the collection port attached to the tubing, not from the collection bag.
- Change the collection bag when it's full or every 24 hours, according to your facility's policy.

ALERT Never empty the drainage bag. Instead, replace it when full, using sterile technique.

Assessing chest drainage system leaks

When attempting to locate a leak in a chest drainage system, try:

- clamping the chest tube momentarily at various points along its length, beginning at the patient's chest and working down toward the drainage system
- checking the seal around the connections
- pushing any loose connections back together and taping them securely.

The bubbling will stop when a clamp is placed between the air leak and the water seal. If you clamp along the tube's entire length and the bubbling doesn't stop, you may need to replace the drainage unit because it may be cracked.

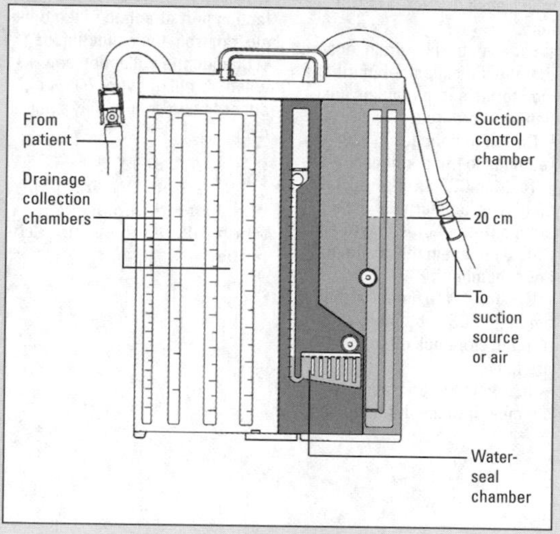

Troubleshooting chest drains

Problem	Interventions
Patient rolling over on drainage tubing, causing obstruction	• Reposition the patient, and remove kinks in the tubing. • Auscultate for decreased breath sounds, and percuss for dullness, which indicates a fluid accumulation, or for hyperresonance, which indicates air accumulation.
Dependent loops in tubing trapping fluids and preventing effective drainage	• Make sure the chest drainage unit is positioned below the patient's chest level. If necessary, raise the bed slightly to increase the gravity flow. Remove kinks in the tubing. • Monitor the patient for decreased breath sounds, and percuss for dullness.
No drainage appearing in collection chamber	• If draining blood or other fluid, suspect a clot or obstruction in the tubing. Gently milk the tubing to expel the obstruction, if your facility's policy permits. Do not completely occlude the tubing. • Monitor the patient for lung-tissue compression caused by accumulated pleural fluid.
Substantial increase in bloody drainage, indicating possible active bleeding or drainage of old blood	• Monitor the patient's vital signs. Look for an increased pulse rate, decreased blood pressure, and orthostatic changes that may indicate acute blood loss. • Measure drainage every 15 to 30 minutes to determine whether it's occurring continuously or if drainage increase occurred as a result of position change. Report drainage greater than 200 ml in 1 hour.
No bubbling in suction control chamber	• Check for obstructions in the tubing. Make sure all connections are tight. • Check that the suction apparatus is turned on. Increase the suction slowly until you see gentle bubbling.
Loud, vigorous bubbling in suction-control chamber	• Turn down the suction source until bubbling is just visible.

(continued)

Skills

Troubleshooting chest drains *(continued)*

Problem	Interventions
Constant bubbling in water-seal chamber	• Assess the chest drainage unit and tubing for an air leak. • If an air leak isn't noted in the external system, notify the practitioner immediately. Leaking and trapping of air in the pleural space can result in a tension pneumothorax.
Evaporation causing water level in suction-control chamber to drop below desired –20 cm H_2O	• Using a syringe and needle, add water or normal saline solution through a resealable diaphragm on the back of the suction-control chamber.
Trouble breathing immediately after special procedure due to obstructed drainage resulting from improper chest drainage unit positioning	• Raise the head of the bed, and reposition the unit so that gravity promotes drainage. • Perform a quick respiratory assessment, and take the patient's vital signs. Make sure enough water is in the water-seal and suction-control chambers.
Disconnected, contaminated chest drainage unit Patient transport to another department	• Clamp the chest tube proximal to the latex connecting tubing. • Insert the distal end of the chest tube into a container of sterile water or saline until the end is 1″ to 1½″ (2 to 4 cm) below the top of the water. Unclamp the chest tube. • Obtain a new closed chest drainage system and set it up. • Attach the chest tube to the new unit. • To prevent a tension pneumothorax (which may occur when clamping stops air and fluid from escaping), never leave the chest tube clamped for more than 1 minute. • Discontinue suction. Don't clamp the tube. The water seal in the drainage collection system will maintain the necessary negative pressure.

Removing a chest tube

After the patient's lung has reexpanded, you may assist the practitioner in removing the chest tube. First, obtain the patient's vital signs and perform a respiratory assessment. After explaining the procedure to the patient and answering all questions, administer an analgesic, as ordered, 30 minutes before tube removal. Then follow these steps.

- Place the patient in semi-Fowler's position or on his unaffected side.
- Place a linen-saver pad under the affected side to protect the bed linens from drainage and provide a place to put the chest tube after removal.
- Put on clean gloves and remove the chest tube dressings, taking care not to dislodge the chest tube. Discard soiled dressings.
- The practitioner puts on sterile gloves, holds the chest tube in place with sterile forceps, and cuts the suture anchoring the tube.
- The chest tube is securely clamped, and the patient is instructed to perform Valsalva's maneuver by exhaling fully and bearing down. Valsalva's maneuver effectively increases intrathoracic pressure.
- The practitioner holds an airtight dressing, usually petroleum gauze, so that he can cover the insertion site with it immediately after removing the tube. After he removes the tube and covers the insertion site, secure the dressing with tape. Be sure to cover the dressing completely with tape to make it as airtight as possible.
- Dispose of the chest tube, soiled gloves, and equipment according to your facility's policy.
- Take the patient's vital signs, and assess the depth and quality of his respirations. Assess him carefully for signs and symptoms of pneumothorax, subcutaneous emphysema, or infection.
- Assist with post-removal chest X-ray and report results to the practitioner.

Performing automated external defibrillation

- Firmly press the automated external defibrillator's (AED) ON button and wait while the machine performs a brief self-test.

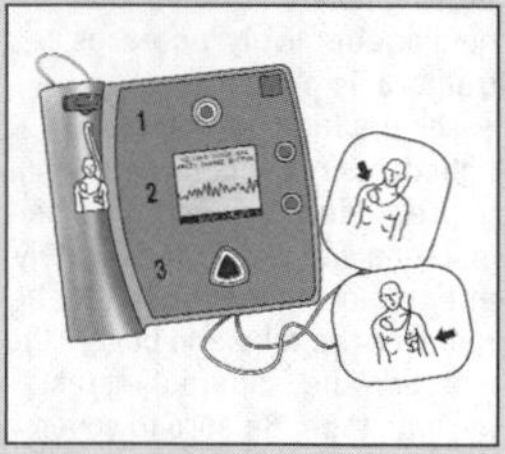

- Most AEDs signal readiness by a computerized voice that says, "Stand clear" or by emitting a series of loud beeps.
- If the AED is malfunctioning, it will convey the message "Don't use the AED. Remove and continue cardiopulmonary resuscitation (CPR)." Report AED malfunctions in accordance with your facility's procedure.
- Open the foil packets containing two electrode pads. Attach the electrode cable to the AED.
- Expose the patient's chest. Remove the plastic backing from the electrode pads and place the electrode pad on the right upper portion of the patient's chest, just beneath his clavicle. Place the second pad to the level of the heart's apex.
- Ask everyone to stand clear.
- Press the ANALYZE button when the machine prompts you to.

ALERT Be careful not to touch or move the patient while the AED is in analysis mode. (If you get the message "Check electrodes," make sure that the electrodes are correctly placed and the patient cable is securely attached; then press the ANALYZE button again.)

- In 15 to 30 seconds, the AED will analyze the patient's rhythm.
- If the patient needs a shock, the AED will display a "Stand clear" message and emit a beep that changes into a steady tone as it's charging.

• When the AED is fully charged and ready to deliver a shock, it will prompt you to press the SHOCK button. (Some fully automatic AED models automatically deliver a shock within 15 seconds after analyzing the patient's rhythm.)
• If a shock isn't needed, the AED will display "No shock indicated," and you should then continue CPR.
• Make sure that no one is touching the patient or his bed, and call out, "Stand clear."
• Press the SHOCK button on the AED.
• After the first shock at 360 joules (monophasic), the AED will automatically reanalyze the patient's rhythm.
• If no additional shock is needed, the machine will prompt you to check the patient. However, if he's still in ventricular fibrillation, perform CPR for 2 minutes and then press the ANALYZE button on the AED to identify the heart rhythm.
• If the patient is still in ventricular fibrillation, the AED will prompt you to press the SHOCK button. A second shock at 360 joules (monophasic) will be delivered.
• After five cycles of CPR (about 2 minutes), the AED should then analyze the cardiac rhythm and deliver another shock, if indicated.
• Repeat the steps performed earlier before delivering a shock to the patient.

ALERT If the patient is still in ventricular fibrillation after three shocks, resume CPR.

• Continue this sequence until the code team arrives.
• After the code, remove and transcribe the AED's computer memory module or tape, or prompt the AED to print a rhythm strip with code data.
• Follow your facility's policy for analyzing and storing code data.

ALERT Don't remove the pads until directed by the receiving practitioner or facility.

Performing defibrillation

• Defibrillation is performed on patients in ventricular tachycardia or ventricular fibrillation.

• Connect the monitoring leads of the defibrillator to the patient, and assess his cardiac rhythm.

• Expose the patient's chest and apply conductive pads or "hands off" pads at the appropriate positions: one to the right of the upper sternum, just below the right clavicle, and the other over the fifth or sixth intercostal space at the left anterior axillary line.

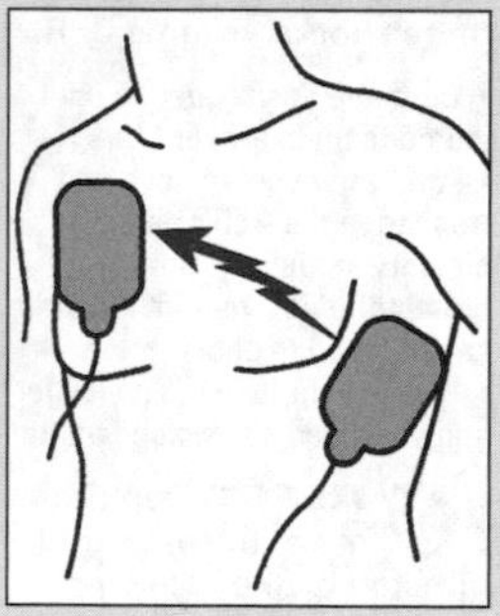

• Turn on the defibrillator and, if performing external defibrillation, set the energy level for the appropriate energy levels for the specific type of defibrillator or per the practitioner's order.

• Charge the paddles by pressing the charge buttons, located either on the machine or on the paddles.

• If using the paddles, place over the conductive pads and press firmly against the patient's chest, using 25 lb of pressure.

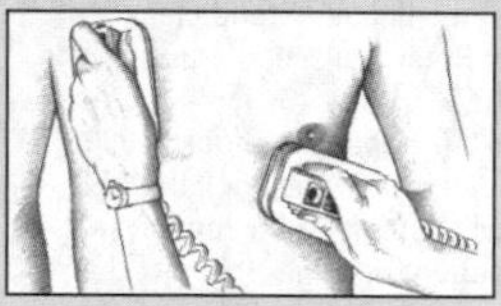

• Reassess the patient's cardiac rhythm on the defibrillator monitor.

• If the patient remains in ventricular fibrillation or pulseless ventricular tachycardia, tell all personnel to stand clear of the patient and the bed.

- Discharge the current by pressing both paddle charge buttons simultaneously or the "shock" button on the defibrillator.
- Perform five cycles (2 minutes) of CPR, and then check the patient's rhythm.
- Tell someone to reset the energy level on the defibrillator (or on the paddles) to 360 joules, or the biphasic energy equivalent, if necessary.
- Announce that you're preparing to defibrillate, and repeat the procedure.
- Perform five cycles (2 minutes) of CPR, and then check the patient's rhythm.
- If defibrillation is again necessary, tell someone to reset the energy level to 360 joules, or the biphasic energy equivalent.
- Follow the same procedure.
- When possible, secure an airway and confirm placement. Always minimize the amount of time chest compressions must be stopped.
- Give epinephrine or vasopressin as ordered.
- Consider possible causes for failure of the patient's rhythm to convert, such as acidosis or hypoxia.
- If defibrillation restores a normal rhythm, check the patient's central and peripheral pulses. If a pulse is present, obtain a blood pressure. If no pulse, follow the advanced cardiac life support algorithm for pulseless electrical activity.
- Assess the patient's level of consciousness, cardiac rhythm, breath sounds, skin color, and urine output.
- Obtain baseline arterial blood gas levels and a 12-lead electrocardiogram.
- Provide supplemental oxygen, ventilation, and drugs as needed.
- Check the patient's chest for electrical burns, and treat them, as ordered, with corticosteroid or lanolin-based creams.
- Prepare the defibrillator for immediate reuse.

Using a Doppler device

More sensitive than palpation for determining pulse rate, the Doppler ultrasound blood flow detector is especially useful when a pulse is faint or weak. Unlike palpation, which detects arterial wall expansion and retraction, this instrument detects the motion of red blood cells (RBCs) through a blood vessel.

- Apply a small amount of coupling gel or transmission gel (not water-soluble lubricant) to the ultrasound probe.
- Position the probe on the skin directly over the selected artery. In the illustration below left, the probe is over the posterior tibial artery.
- When using a Doppler model like the one in the illustration below left, turn the instrument on and, moving counterclockwise, set the volume control to the lowest setting. If your model doesn't have a speaker, plug in the earphones and slowly raise the volume. The Doppler ultrasound stethoscope shown in the illustration below right is basically a stethoscope fitted with an audio unit, volume control, and transducer, which amplifies the movement of RBCs.
- To obtain the best signals with either device, tilt the probe 45 degrees from the artery, being sure to put gel between the skin and the probe. Slowly move the probe in a circular motion to locate the center of the artery and the Doppler signal—a hissing noise at the heartbeat. Avoid moving the probe rapidly because this distorts the signal.
- Count the signals for 60 seconds to determine the pulse rate.
- After you've measured the pulse rate, clean the probe with a soft cloth soaked in antiseptic solution or soapy water. Don't immerse the probe or bump it against a hard surface.
- Wipe the area of skin covered with gel.
- Mark the site where the pulse was located if the site is to be rechecked.

Doppler probe with amplifier

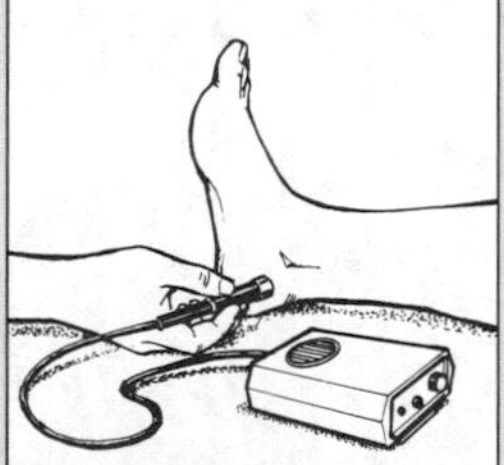

Doppler ultrasound stethoscope

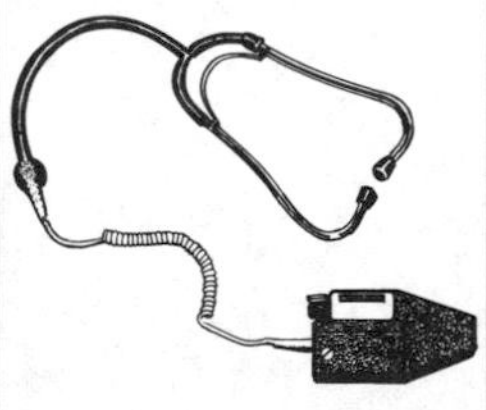

Skills

Changing a central venous dressing

Expect to change your patient's central venous dressing every 48 hours if it's gauze and at least every 7 days if it's transparent. Many facilities specify dressing changes whenever the dressing becomes soiled, moist, or loose. These illustrations show the key steps you'll perform.

First, put on clean gloves and a mask. Have the patient turn his head away from the insertion site, or ask him to also wear a mask. Remove the old dressing by pulling it toward the exit site of a long-term catheter or toward the insertion site of a short-term catheter. This technique helps you avoid pulling out the line. Remove and discard your gloves.

Next, put on sterile gloves and clean the skin around the site using an alcohol pad. Start at the center and move outward, using a circular motion.

Allow the skin to dry, and clean the site with chlorhexidine swabs using a vigorous side-to-side motion.

After the solution has dried, cover the site with a dressing, such as the transparent semi-permeable dressing shown here. Write the time and date on the dressing. Discard soiled materials appropriately.

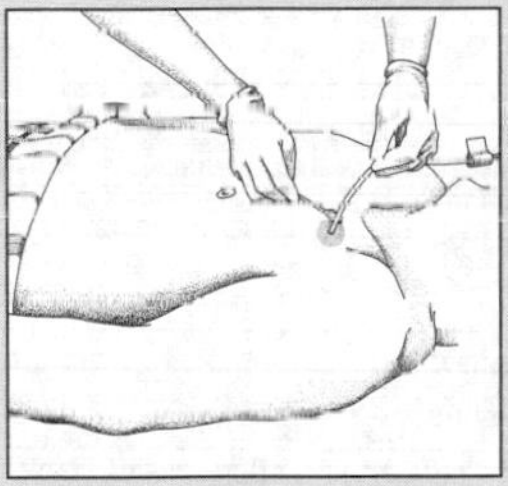

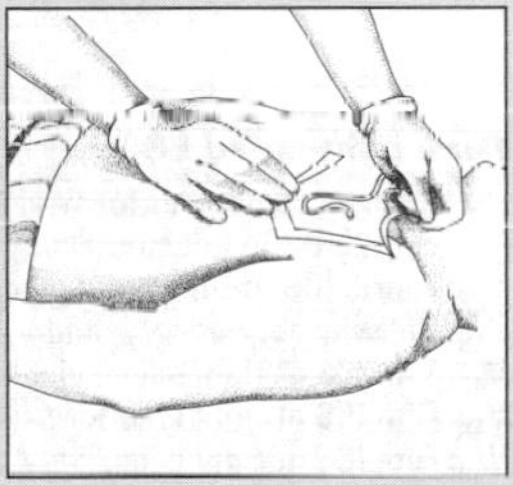

Skills

Positioning electrocardiography electrodes

For a standard electrocardiogram (ECG), position chest electrodes as follows:

V_1: Fourth intercostal space (ICS) at right sternal border
V_2: Fourth ICS at left sternal border
V_3: Halfway between V_2 and V_4
V_4: Fifth ICS at midclavicular line
V_5: Fifth ICS at anterior axillary line (halfway between V_4 and V_6)
V_6: Fifth ICS at midaxillary line, level with V_4

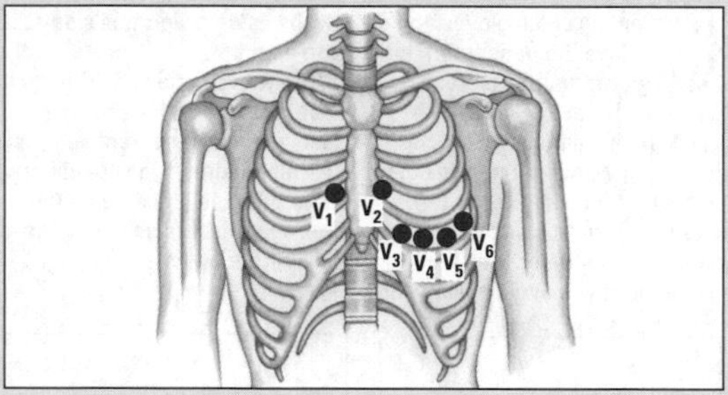

For a right-sided ECG

Place the electrodes as follows:

V_{1R}: Fourth ICS at left sternal border
V_{2R}: Fourth ICS at right sternal border
V_{3R}: Halfway between V_{2R} and V_{4R}
V_{4R}: Fifth ICS at right midclavicular line
V_{5R}: Fifth ICS at right anterior axillary line
V_{6R}: Fifth ICS at right midaxillary line

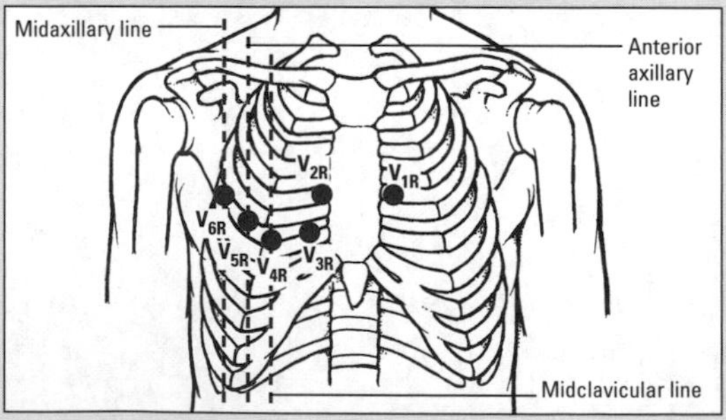

If asked to use posterior leads, make sure the posterior electrodes V_7, V_8, and V_9 are placed at the same level horizontally as the V_6 lead at the fifth ICS. Place lead V_7 at the posterior axillary line, lead V_9 at the paraspinal line, and lead V_8 halfway between leads V_7 and V_9.

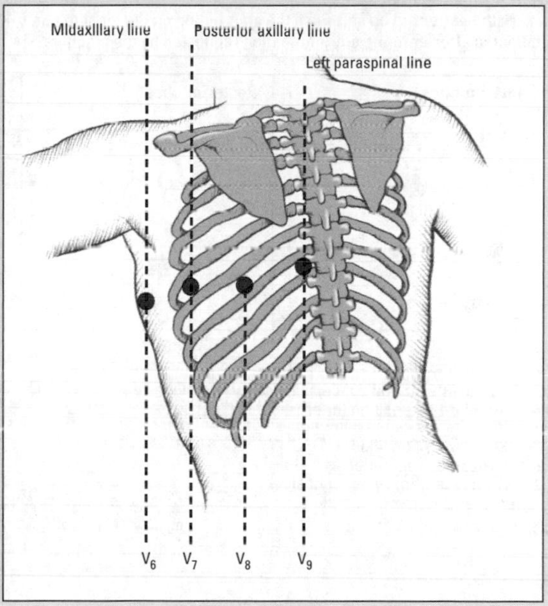

Skills

Performing signal-averaged electrocardiography

To prepare for signal-averaged electrocardiography, place the electrodes in the X, Y, and Z orthogonal positions shown here. These positions bisect one another to provide a three-dimensional, composite view of ventricular activation.

Ask the patient to be still. Push the start button on the machine as indicated after entering any information requested by the machine.

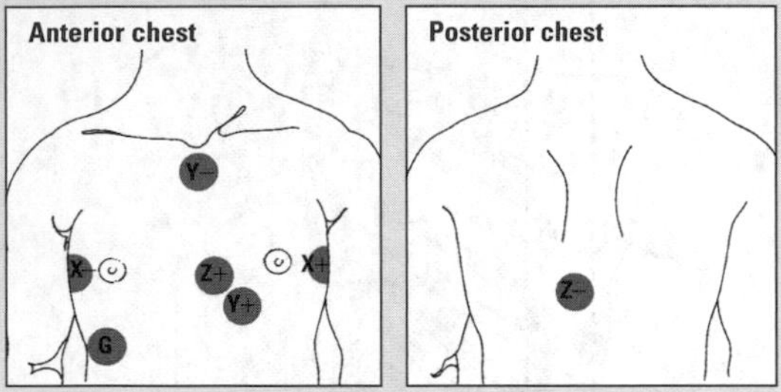

KEY

- **X+** Fourth intercostal space, midaxillary line, left side
- **X–** Fourth intercostal space, midaxillary line, right side
- **Y+** Standard V_3 position (or proximal left leg)
- **Y–** Superior aspect of manubrium
- **Z+** Standard V_2 position
- **Z–** V_2 position, posterior
- **G** Ground; eighth rib on right side

Repositioning an ET tube

- Get help from another nurse to prevent accidental extubation during the procedure if the patient coughs.

ALERT To prevent traumatic manipulation of the tube, instruct the assisting nurse to hold it as you carefully untape the tube or unfasten the Velcro tube holder.

- Hyperoxygenate the patient and then suction the trachea through the endotracheal (ET) tube to remove secretions, which can cause the patient to cough during the procedure.
- To prevent aspiration during cuff deflation, suction the patient's pharynx to remove secretions that may have accumulated above the tube cuff.
- When freeing the tube, note the centimeter mark on the tube at the lip.
- Deflate the cuff by attaching a 10-ml syringe to the pilot balloon port and aspirating air until you meet resistance and the pilot balloon deflates.

ALERT Deflate the cuff before moving the ET tube because the cuff forms a seal within the trachea; moving an inflated cuff can damage the tracheal wall and vocal cords.

- Reposition the tube as needed, checking that the tube is at the centimeter marking previously noted.
- To reinflate the cuff, have the patient inhale, and slowly inflate the cuff using a 10-ml syringe attached to the pilot balloon port.
- As you do this, use your stethoscope to auscultate the patient's neck to determine presence of an air leak.
- When air leakage ceases, stop cuff inflation; while still auscultating the neck, aspirate a small amount of air until you detect a minimal air leak, indicating the cuff is inflated at the lowest possible pressure for an adequate seal.
- If the patient is mechanically ventilated, aspirate to create a minimal air leak during the inspiratory phase because the positive pressure of the ventilator during inspiration will create a larger leak around the cuff.
- Note the amount of air required to achieve a minimal air leak.
- Measure cuff pressure; compare the reading with previous ones to prevent overinflation.
- Verify placement of the ET tube by auscultating both lung fields to verify breath sounds; listen over the epigastric area to confirm that the ET tube wasn't positioned in the stomach. Carbon dioxide levels may also be monitored to verify placement, and a chest X-ray may be required.
- Use tape to secure the tube, or refasten the Velcro tube holder.
- Make sure the patient is comfortable and the airway patent.
- Measure cuff pressure at least every 8 hours to avoid overinflation.

Removing an ET tube

- Check the practitioner's order before removing the endotracheal (ET) tube.
- To prevent traumatic manipulation of the tube, have another nurse help.
- Suction the patient's oropharynx and nasopharynx to remove accumulated secretions and help prevent aspiration when the cuff is deflated.
- Using a bag-valve-mask device or the mechanical ventilator, give the patient several deep breaths through the ET tube to hyperinflate his lungs and increase his oxygen reserve.
- Attach a 10-ml syringe to the pilot balloon port, and aspirate air until you meet resistance and the pilot balloon deflates.

ALERT If you don't detect an air leak around the deflated cuff, notify the practitioner immediately; don't proceed with extubation. Absence of an air leak can indicate marked tracheal edema, which can cause total airway obstruction if the ET tube is removed.

- If you detect the proper air leak, untape or unfasten the ET tube while the assisting nurse stabilizes it.
- Insert a sterile suction catheter through the ET tube.
- Apply suction. To reduce the risk of laryngeal trauma, ask the patient to take a deep breath, open his mouth fully, and pretend to cry out.
- Simultaneously remove the ET tube and suction catheter in one smooth, outward and downward motion, following the natural curve of the patient's mouth.

ALERT Suctioning during extubation removes secretions retained at the end of the tube and prevents aspiration.

- Give the patient supplemental oxygen. For humidity, use a cool-mist, large-volume nebulizer to decrease airway irritation and laryngeal edema.
- Encourage him to cough and deep-breathe.
- Make sure he's comfortable and his airway is patent.
- After extubation, auscultate his lungs frequently and be alert for stridor or other evidence of upper airway obstruction.
- If ordered, draw an arterial sample for blood gas analysis.

Securing an ET tube

Before taping an endotracheal (ET) tube in place, make sure the patient's face is clean, dry, and free from beard stubble. If possible, suction his mouth and dry the tube just before taping. Also, check the reference mark on the tube to ensure correct placement. After taping, always check for bilateral breath sounds to ensure that the tube hasn't been displaced by manipulation.

To tape the ET tube securely, use one of these three methods.

Method 1

Cut two 2" (5-cm) strips and two 15" (38-cm) strips of 1" cloth adhesive tape. Then cut a 13" (33-cm) slit in one end of each 15" strip (as shown).

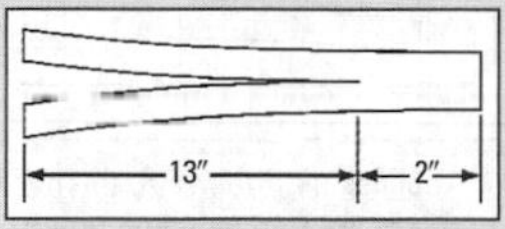

Apply skin adhesive to the patient's cheeks. Place the 2" strips on his cheeks, creating a new surface on which to anchor the tape securing the tube. When frequent retaping is necessary, this helps preserve the patient's skin integrity. If the patient's skin is excoriated or at risk, you can use a transparent semipermeable dressing to protect the skin.

Apply the adhesive to the tape on the patient's face and to the part of the tube where you'll be applying the tape. On the side of the mouth where the tube will be anchored, place the unslit end of the long tape on top of the tape on the patient's cheek.

Wrap the top half of the tape around the tube twice, pulling the tape tightly around the tube. Then, directing the tape over the patient's upper lip, place the end of the tape on his other cheek. Cut off excess tape. Use the lower half of the tape to secure an oral airway, if necessary (as shown below).

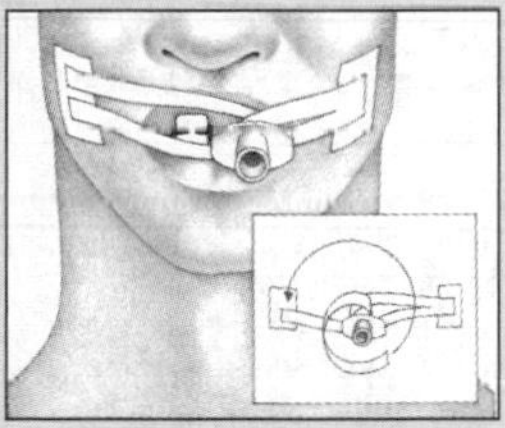

Or, twist the lower half of the tape around the tube twice and attach it to the original cheek (as shown above). Taping in opposite directions places equal traction on the tube.

If you've taped in an oral airway or are concerned about the tube's stability, apply the other 1" strip of tape in the same manner, starting on the other side of the patient's face. If the tape around the tube is too bulky, use only the upper part of the tape and cut off the lower part. If the patient has copious oral secretions, seal the tape by cutting a 1" piece of paper tape, coating it with benzoin tincture, and placing the paper tape over the adhesive tape.

(continued)

Skills

Securing an ET tube *(continued)*

Method 2

Cut one piece of 1″ cloth adhesive tape long enough to wrap around the patient's head and overlap in front. Then cut an 8″ (20.3-cm) piece of tape, and center it on the longer piece, sticky sides together. Next, cut a 5″ (12.7-cm) slit in each end of the longer tape (as shown below).

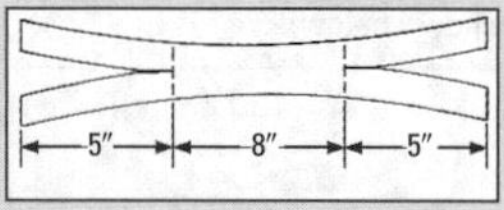

Apply skin adhesive to the patient's cheeks, under his nose, and under his lower lip.

Place the top half of one end of the tape under the patient's nose, and wrap the lower half around the ET tube. Place the lower half of the other end of the tape along his lower lip, and wrap the top half around the tube (as shown below).

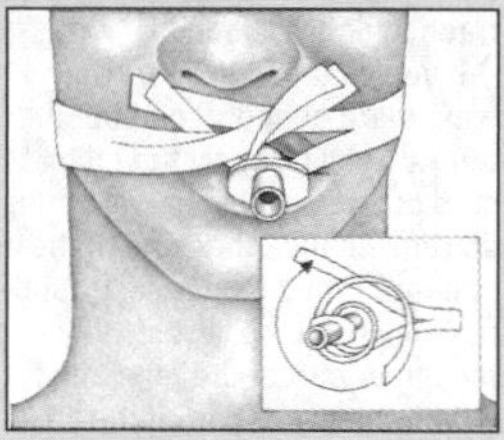

Method 3

Cut a tracheostomy tie in two pieces, one a few inches longer than the other, and cut two 6″ (15.2-cm) pieces of 1″ cloth adhesive tape. Then cut a 2″ (5.1-cm) slit in one end of both pieces of tape. Fold back the other end of the tape ½″ (1.3 cm) so that the sticky sides are together, and cut a small hole in it (as shown below).

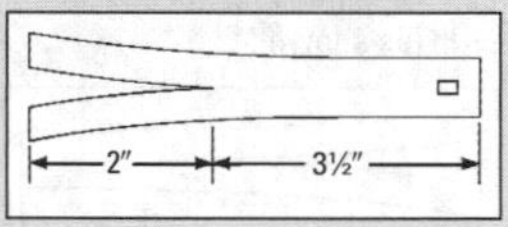

Apply skin adhesive to the part of the ET tube that will be taped. Wrap the split ends of each piece of tape around the tube, one piece on each side. Overlap the tape to secure it.

Apply the free ends of the tape to both sides of the patient's face. Then insert tracheostomy ties through the holes in the tape and knot the ties (as shown below).

Bring the longer tie behind the patient's neck. Knotting the ties on the side prevents him from lying on the knot and developing a pressure ulcer.

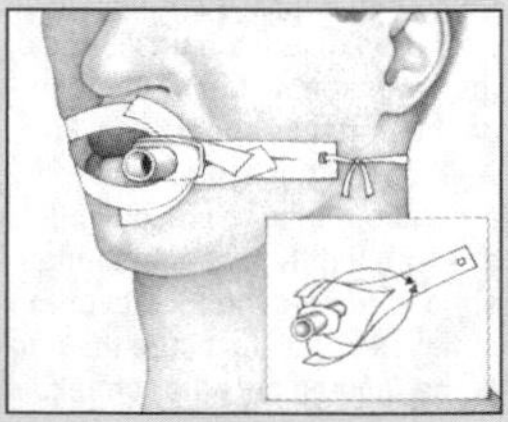

Using a femoral compression device

- Put on nonsterile gloves and protective eyewear; place the device strap under the patient's hips before sheath removal (if a sheath is necessary).
- After achieving hemostasis, put on sterile gloves and apply a sterile transparent dressing over the puncture site, using sterile technique.
- With the assistance of another nurse, position the compression arch over the puncture site.
- Apply manual pressure over the dome area while the straps are secured to the arch.
- When the dome is properly positioned over the puncture site, connect the pressure inflation device to the stopcock.
- Turn the stopcock to the open position and inflate the dome with the pressure inflation device to the ordered pressure.
- Turn the stopcock off and remove the pressure-inflation device.
- Assess the puncture site for proper placement of the device and for signs of bleeding or hematoma.
- Assess distal pulses and neurovascular condition according to your facility's policy.
- Confirm distal pulses after adjustments of the device.
- Deflate the device hourly and assess the puncture site for bleeding or hematoma. Assess for proper placement of the dome over the puncture site.
- Deflate and reposition the compression arch and dome as necessary; wear gloves and protective eyewear.

  Reinflate the device to the ordered pressure.
- When removing the device, put on nonsterile gloves and protective eyewear, remove the air from the dome, loosen the straps, and remove the device.
- Assess the puncture site for bleeding or hematoma.
- Change the sterile transparent dressing according to your facility's policy.
- Check the puncture site and distal pulses, and perform neurovascular assessments every 15 minutes for the first half hour and every 30 minutes for the next 2 hours according to your facility's policy.
- Watch for signs of bleeding, hematoma, or infection.
- Dispose of the device and equipment according to your facility's policy.

Skills

Setting up an ICP monitoring system

- Begin by opening a sterile towel. On the sterile field, place a 20-ml luer-lock syringe, an 18G needle, a 250-ml bag filled with normal saline solution (with the outer wrapper removed), and a disposable transducer.
- Put on sterile gloves and gown according to your facility's policy, and fill the 20-ml syringe with normal saline solution from the I.V. bag.
- Remove the injection cap from the patient line, and attach the syringe. Turn the system stopcock off to the short end of the patient line, and flush through to the drip chamber (as shown below left). Allow a few drops to flow through the flow chamber (the manometer), the tubing, and the one-way valve into the drainage bag. (Fill the tubing and the manometer slowly to minimize air bubbles. If any air bubbles surface, be sure to force them from the system.) In some systems, the drainage system will prime itself with the patient's cerebrospinal fluid (CSF).

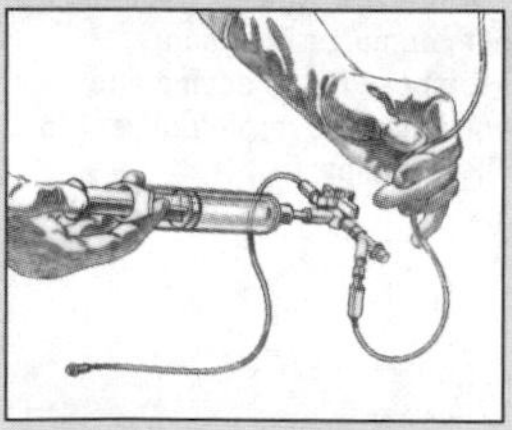

- Attach the manometer to the I.V. pole at the head of the bed.
- Slide the drip chamber onto the manometer, and align the chamber to the zero point, which should be at the inner canthus of the patient's eye.
- Next, connect the transducer to the monitor.
- Put on a clean pair of sterile gloves.
- Keeping one hand sterile, turn the patient stopcock off to the short end of the patient line.
- Align the zero point with the center line of the patient's head, level with the middle of the ear.
- Lower the flow chamber to zero, and turn the stopcock off to the dead-end cap. With a clean hand, balance the system according to monitor guidelines.
- Turn the system stopcock off to drainage, and raise the flow chamber to the ordered height (as shown below right).
- Return the stopcock to the ordered position, and observe the monitor for the return of intracranial pressure (ICP) patterns.
- The holder is raised and lowered to keep the patient's ICP at exact readings specified by the neurologist. If the neurologist orders CSF to drain if ICP reaches 10, then the chamber is raised to 10.

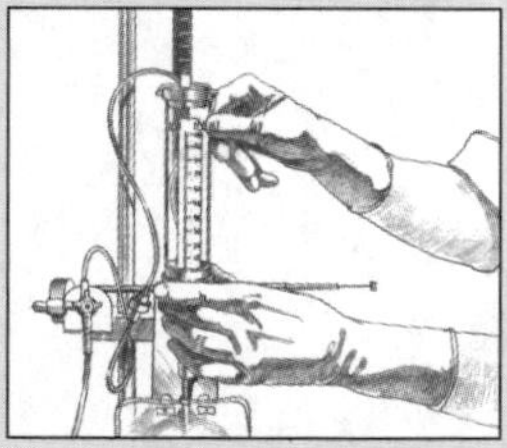

Skills

Inserting a nasogastric tube

- Help the patient into high Fowler's position unless contraindicated.
- Measure the tube by holding the end of the tube at the tip of the patient's nose, extending the tube to the patient's earlobe and then down to the xiphoid process.

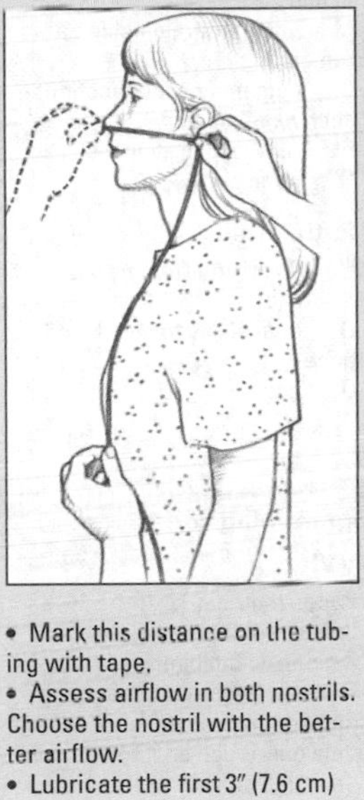

- Mark this distance on the tubing with tape.
- Assess airflow in both nostrils. Choose the nostril with the better airflow.
- Lubricate the first 3" (7.6 cm) of the tube with a water-soluble gel.
- Instruct the patient to hold her head straight and upright.
- Grasp the tube with the end pointing downward, and carefully insert it into the more patent nostril.
- Aim the tube downward and toward the ear closer to the chosen nostril, and advance it slowly.
- When the tube reaches the nasopharynx, you'll feel resistance. Instruct the patient to lower her head slightly; rotate the tube 180 degrees toward the opposite nostril.
- Unless contraindicated, direct the patient to sip water through a straw and swallow as you slowly advance the tube.
- Watch for respiratory distress as you advance the tube.
- Stop advancing the tube when the tape mark reaches the patient's nostril.
- Attach a catheter-tip or bulb syringe to the tube and inject air while listening over the stomach (you should hear a "sloosh").
- Then aspirate stomach contents.
- Place a small amount of aspirate on the pH test strip. Probability of gastric placement is increased if the aspirate has a typical gastric fluid appearance (grassy green, clear and colorless with mucus shreds, or brown) and a pH lower than 5.0.
- If you don't obtain stomach contents, position the patient on her left side to move the contents into the stomach's greater curvature, and aspirate again.
- If you still can't aspirate stomach contents, advance the tube 1" to 2" (2.5 to 5 cm).
- After placement is confirmed, secure the tube to the patient's nose with hypoallergenic tape.

Interpreting pacemaker codes

A permanent pacemaker uses a three- or five-letter programming code. The first letter represents the chamber that's paced. The second represents the chamber that's sensed. The third represents how the pulse generator responds. The fourth denotes the pacemaker's programmability. The fifth denotes the pacemaker's response to a tachyarrhythmia.

First letter

A = atrium
V = ventricle
D = dual (both chambers)
0 = not applicable

Second letter

A = atrium
V = ventricle
D = dual (both chambers)
0 = not applicable

Third letter

I = inhibited
T = triggered
D = dual (inhibited and triggered)
0 = not applicable

Fourth letter

P = basic functions programmable
M = multiprogrammable parameters
C = communicating functions such as telemetry
R = rate responsiveness
0 = none

Fifth letter

P = pacing ability
S = shock
D = dual ability to shock and pace
0 = none

Examples of two common programming codes

DDD

Pace: Atrium and ventricle
Sense: Atrium and ventricle
Response: Inhibited and triggered
This is the most common dual-chamber pacemaker setting, allowing the heart's intrinsic pacemaker cells to function whenever possible.

VVI

Pace: Ventricle
Sense: Ventricle
Response: Inhibited
This is a single-chamber pacemaker that will pace the ventricle only when an intrinsic contraction doesn't occur.

Skills

Applying a pneumatic antishock garment

After taking the patient's baseline vital signs and explaining the treatment, prepare to apply the antishock garment. On a smooth surface, open the garment with Velcro fasteners down.

Open all stopcock valves; then attach the foot pump tubing to the valve on the pressure control unit. Can the patient be turned from side to side? If not, slide the garment under him. If he can be turned, place the garment next to him and, with assistance, move him onto it.

Before closing the garment, remove any sharp objects, such as pieces of glass, stones, keys, or a buckle that could injure the patient or tear the garment. As appropriate, pad pressure points and apply lanolin to protect the patient's skin from irritation.

Place the upper edge of the garment just below the patient's lowest rib. Wrap the right leg compartment around the patient's right leg. Secure the compartment by fastening all the Velcro straps from ankle to thigh.

Repeat this procedure for the left leg; then wrap the abdomen. Double-check that all valves are properly positioned.

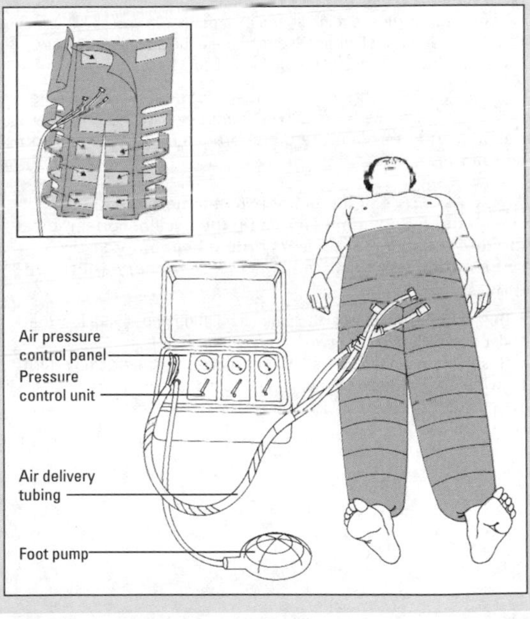

Skills

Obtaining a pulmonary artery wedge pressure reading

- Pulmonary artery wedge pressure (PAWP) is recorded by inflating the balloon and letting it float in a distal artery.
- Some facilities allow only practitioners or specially trained nurses to take a PAWP reading because of the risk of pulmonary artery rupture—a rare but life-threatening complication.
- If you're allowed to perform this procedure, do so with extreme caution, and make sure you're thoroughly familiar with intracardiac waveform interpretation.
- Verify that the transducer is properly leveled and zeroed.
- Detach the syringe from the balloon inflation hub.
- Draw 1.5 cc of air into the syringe; then reattach the syringe to the hub.
- Watching the monitor, inject the air through the hub slowly and smoothly.
- When you see a wedge tracing on the monitor, immediately stop inflating the balloon. Never inflate beyond the volume needed to obtain a wedge tracing.
- Take the pressure reading at end expiration.
- Note the amount of air needed to change the pulmonary artery tracing to a wedge tracing (normally, 1.25 to 1.5 cc).

ALERT If a wedge tracing appears with an injection of less than 1.25 cc, suspect that the catheter has migrated into a more distal branch and requires repositioning.

ALERT If the balloon is in a more distal branch, the tracings may move up the oscilloscope, indicating that the catheter tip is recording balloon pressure rather than PAWP. This may lead to pulmonary artery rupture.

- Detach the syringe from the balloon inflation port, and allow the balloon to deflate on its own.
- Observe the waveform tracing, and make sure the tracing returns from the wedge tracing to the normal pulmonary artery tracing.

Using pulse oximetry

- Select a finger for the test.
- Make sure the patient isn't wearing false fingernails or nail polish.
- Place the transducer (photodetector) probe over the patient's finger so that the light beams and sensors oppose each other.
- If the patient has long fingernails, position the probe perpendicular to the finger, if possible, or clip the fingernail.
- Always position the patient's hand at heart level to eliminate venous pulsations and to promote an accurate reading.
- Turn the power switch on; if the device is working properly, a beep will sound, a display will light momentarily, and the pulse searchlight will flash.
- After four to six heartbeats, the arterial oxygen saturation and pulse rate displays will supply information with each beat, and the pulse amplitude indicator will begin tracking the patient's pulse.

Using an ear probe

- Using an alcohol pad, massage the patient's earlobe for 10 to 20 seconds. Mild erythema indicates adequate vascularization.
- Following the manufacturer's instructions, attach the ear probe to the patient's earlobe or pinna.
- Be sure to establish good contact with the ear; an unstable probe may set off the low perfusion alarm.
- A saturation reading and pulse waveform will appear after a few seconds.
- Leave the ear probe in place for 3 or more minutes until readings stabilize at the highest point. An alternate method is to take three separate readings and average them.
- Make sure you revascularize the patient's earlobe each time.

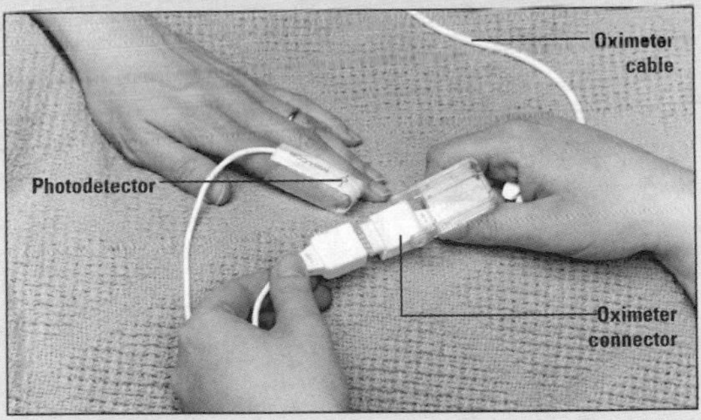

Skills

Troubleshooting pulse oximeter problems

To maintain a continuous display of arterial oxygen saturation (Spo_2) levels, you need to keep the monitoring site clean and dry. Make sure the skin doesn't become irritated from adhesives used to keep disposable probes in place. You may need to change the site if this happens. Disposable probes that irritate the skin can be replaced by nondisposable models that don't need tape.

A common problem with pulse oximeters is failure of the device to obtain a signal. If this happens, first check the patient's vital signs. If they're sufficient to produce a signal, check for the following problems.

Poor connection

Check that the sensors are properly aligned. Make sure that wires are intact and securely fastened and that the pulse oximeter is plugged into a power source.

Inadequate or intermittent blood flow to the site

Check the patient's pulse rate and capillary refill time, and take corrective action if blood flow to the site is decreased. This may require you to remove tight-fitting clothes, move a blood pressure cuff, check arterial and I.V. lines, or warm the site if it's cold. If none of these interventions works, you may need to find an alternate site. Finding a site with proper circulation may be a challenge when the patient is receiving vasoconstrictive drugs.

Equipment malfunction

Remove the pulse oximeter from the patient, and attempt to obtain an Spo_2 level on yourself or another healthy person. If you can obtain a normal value, the equipment is functioning properly. If you are unable to receive a signal, replace the machine.

Obtaining a nasopharyngeal specimen

Pass the swab into the nasopharynx about 3″ to 4″ (7.5 to 10 cm). Quickly but gently rotate the swab to collect the specimen. Then remove the swab, taking care not to injure the nasal mucous membrane. Insert the swab into the culture tube, label it, and send it to the laboratory.

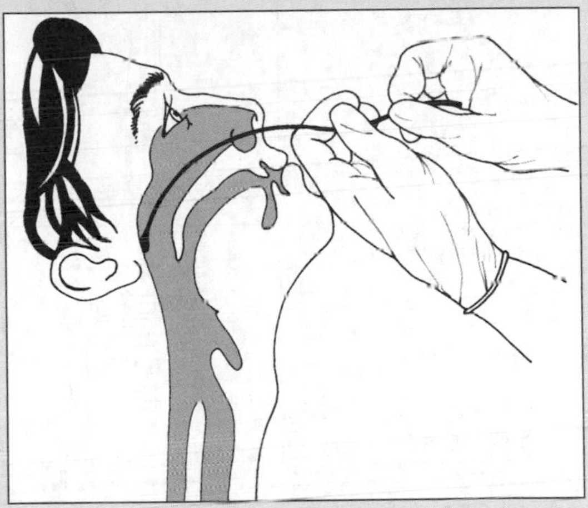

Obtaining a sputum specimen: Attaching specimen trap to suction catheter

Wearing gloves, push the suction tubing onto the male adapter of the in-line trap.

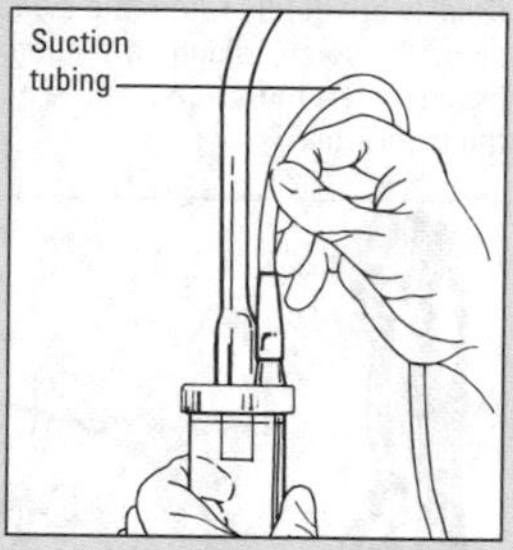

Insert the suction catheter into the rubber tubing of the trap.

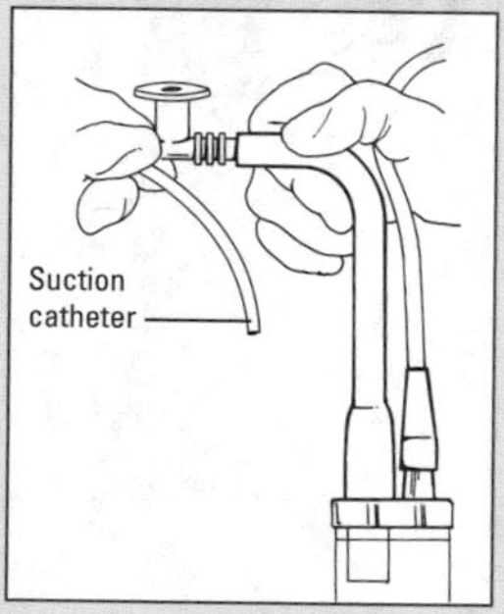

After suctioning, disconnect the in-line trap from the suction tubing and catheter. To seal the container, connect the rubber tubing to the male adapter of the trap.

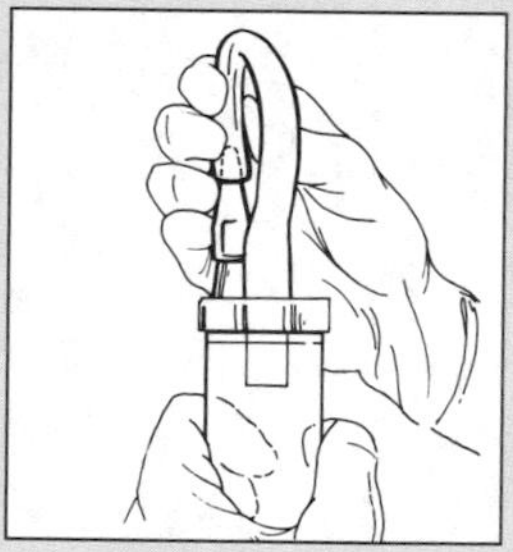

Skills

Measuring tracheal cuff pressure

- Attach the cuff pressure manometer to the pilot balloon port.
- Place the diaphragm of the stethoscope over the trachea, and listen for an air leak (a loud, gargling sound).

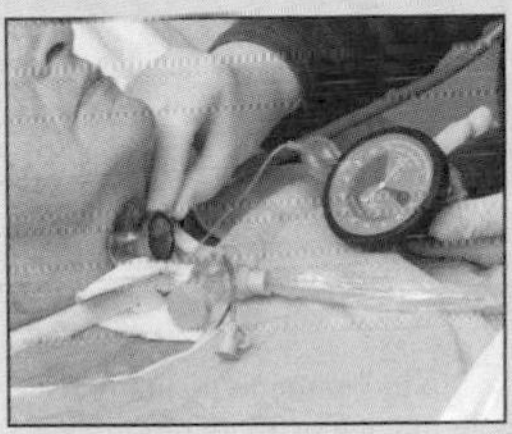

- If you don't hear an air leak, press the red button under the dial of the cuff pressure manometer to slowly release air from the balloon on the tracheal tube (as shown below). Auscultate for an air leak.

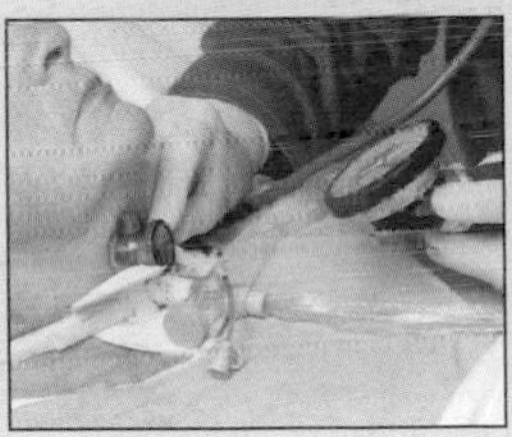

- As soon as you hear an air leak, release the red button and gently squeeze the handle of the cuff pressure manometer to inflate the cuff (as shown below). Continue to add air to the cuff until you no longer hear an air leak.

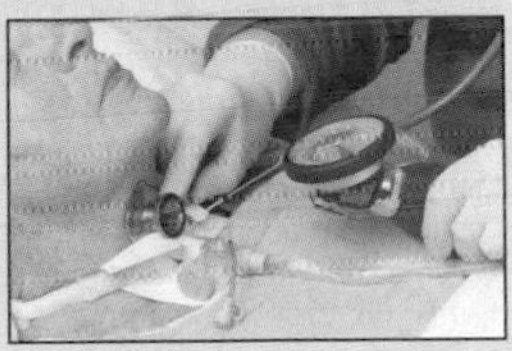

- When the air leak ceases, read the dial on the cuff pressure manometer (as shown below). This is the minimal pressure required to effectively occlude the trachea around the tracheal tube. In many cases, this pressure will fall within the green area (16 to 24 cm H_2O) on the manometer dial.

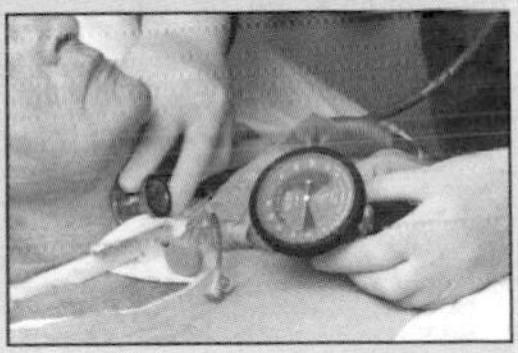

Performing open tracheal suctioning

- Remove the top from the normal saline solution or water bottle.
- Open the package containing the sterile solution container.
- Using strict sterile technique, open the suction catheter kit and put on the gloves. If using individual supplies, open the suction catheter and the gloves, placing the nonsterile glove on your nondominant hand and then the sterile glove on your dominant hand.
- Using your nondominant (nonsterile) hand, pour the normal saline solution or sterile water into the solution container.
- Place a small amount of water-soluble lubricant on the sterile area. Lubricant may be used to facilitate passage of the catheter during nasotracheal suctioning.
- Using your dominant (sterile) hand, remove the catheter from its wrapper. Keep it coiled so it can't touch a nonsterile object. Using your other hand to manipulate the connecting tubing, attach the catheter to the tubing.

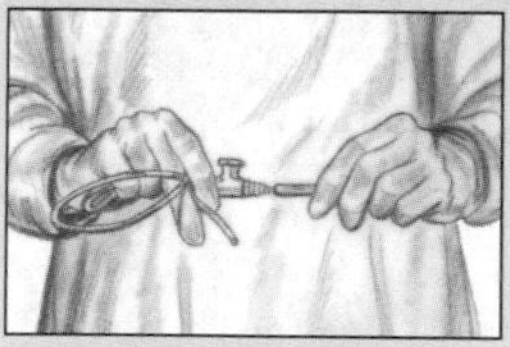

- Using your nondominant hand, set the suction pressure according to your facility's policy. Typically, pressure may be set between 80 and 120 mm Hg. Higher pressures don't enhance secretion removal and may cause traumatic injury. Occlude the suction port to assess suction pressure (as shown here).

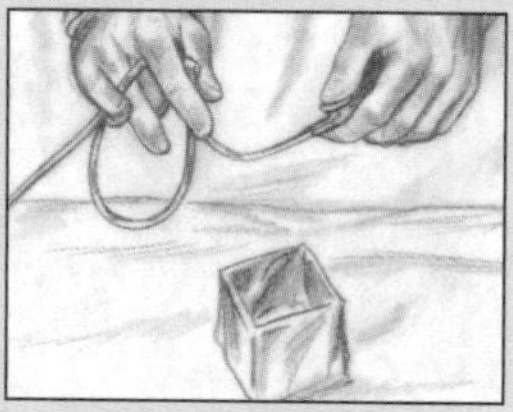

- Dip the catheter tip in the saline solution to lubricate the outside of the catheter and reduce tissue trauma during insertion.
- With the catheter tip in the sterile solution, occlude the control valve with the thumb of your nondominant hand. Then suction a small amount of solution through the catheter to lubricate the inside of the catheter, thus facilitating passage of secretions through it.

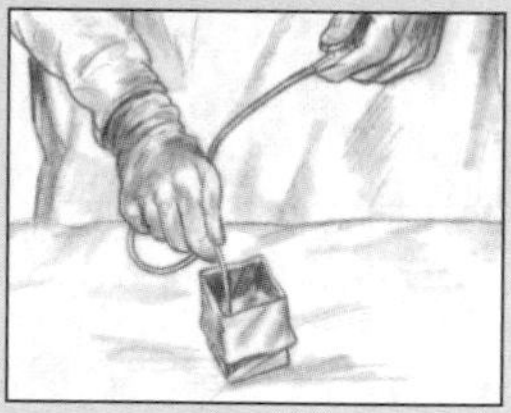

- For nasal insertion of the catheter, lubricate the tip of the catheter with the sterile, water-

Skills

soluble lubricant to reduce tissue trauma during insertion.

- Insert the catheter into the patient's nostril while gently rolling it between your fingers to help it advance through the turbinates.
- As the patient inhales, quickly advance the catheter as far as possible. To avoid oxygen loss and tissue trauma, don't apply suction during insertion.
- If the patient coughs as the catheter passes through the larynx, briefly hold the catheter still and then resume advancement when the patient inhales.
- If the patient isn't intubated or is intubated but isn't receiving supplemental oxygen or aerosol, instruct him to take three to six deep breaths to help minimize or prevent hypoxia during suctioning.
- If the patient is being mechanically ventilated, preoxygenate him using either a handheld resuscitation bag or the sigh mode on the ventilator.

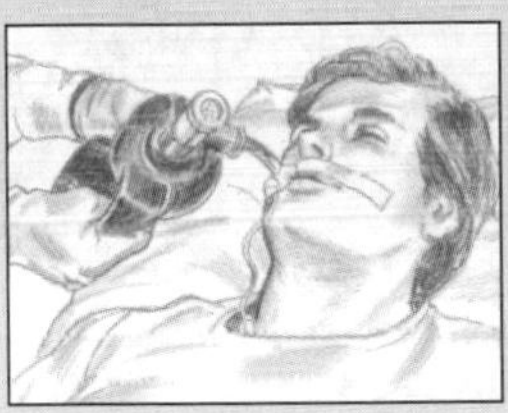

- Using your sterile hand, gently insert the suction catheter into the artificial airway (as shown below). Advance the catheter, without applying suction, until you meet resistance. If the patient coughs, pause briefly, and then resume advancement.

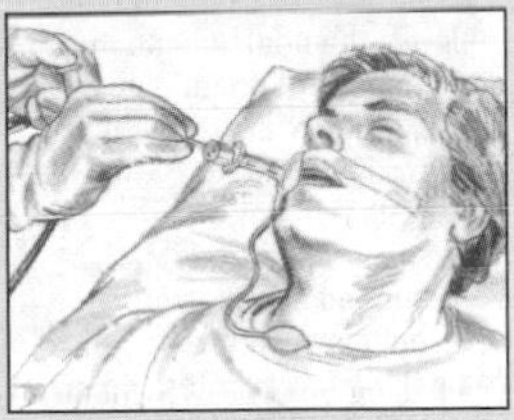

- Using your nonsterile hand, disconnect the patient from the ventilator.
- After inserting the catheter, apply suction intermittently by removing and replacing the thumb of your nondominant hand over the control valve. Simultaneously use your dominant hand to withdraw the catheter as you roll it between your thumb and forefinger. This rotating motion prevents the catheter from pulling tissue into the tube as it exits, thus avoiding tissue trauma. Never suction for more than 10 seconds at a time, to prevent hypoxia.

Performing closed tracheal suctioning

The closed tracheal suction system can ease removal of secretions and reduce patient complications. The system consists of a sterile suction catheter in a clear plastic sleeve, and permits the patient to remain connected to the ventilator during suctioning.

As a result, the patient can maintain the tidal volume, oxygen concentration, and positive end-expiratory pressure delivered by the ventilator, while being suctioned. This, in turn, reduces the occurrence of suction-induced hypoxemia.

Using this system also helps reduce the risk of infection, even when the same catheter is used many times. The caregiver doesn't need to touch the catheter, and the ventilator circuit remains closed.

Implementation

To perform the procedure, gather a closed suction control valve, a T-piece to connect the artificial airway to the ventilator breathing circuit, and a catheter sleeve that encloses the catheter and has connections at each end for the control valve and the T-piece. Then follow these steps:

- Remove the closed suction system from its wrapping. Attach the control valve to the connecting tubing.
- Depress the thumb suction control valve, and keep it de-

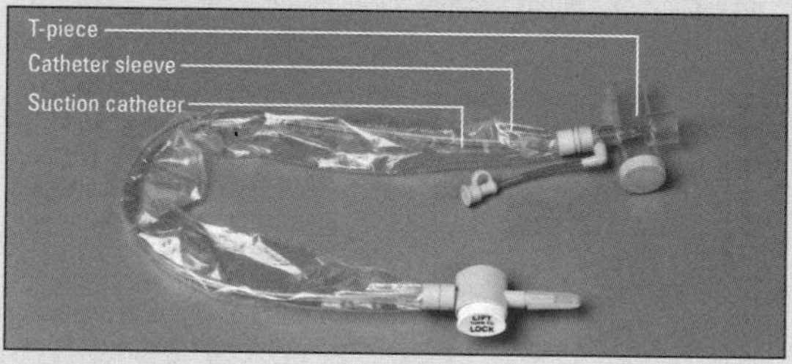

Skills

pressed while setting the suction pressure to the desired level.

• Connect the T-piece to the ventilator breathing circuit, making sure that the irrigation port is closed; then connect the T-piece to the patient's endotracheal or tracheostomy tube (as shown below).

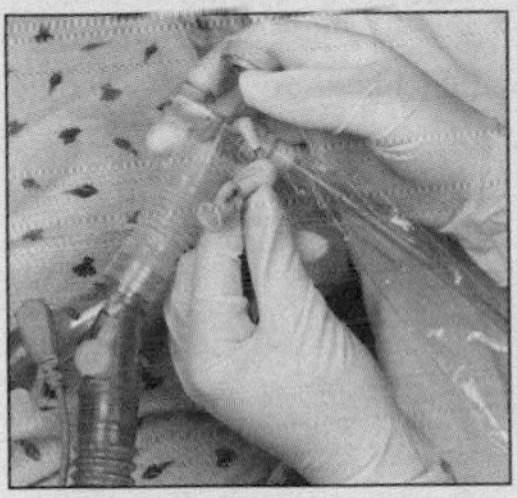

• Use one hand to keep the T-piece parallel to the patient's chin, and the thumb and index finger of the other hand to advance the catheter through the tube and into the patient's tracheobronchial tree (as shown top right).

• It may be necessary to gently retract the catheter sleeve as you advance the catheter.

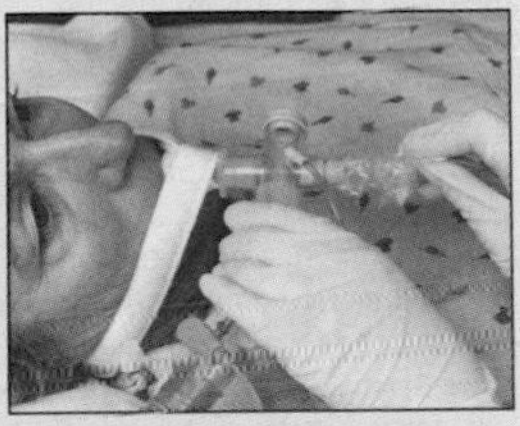

• As you continue to hold the T-piece and control valve, apply intermittent suction and withdraw the catheter until it reaches its fully extended length in the sleeve. Repeat the procedure as necessary.

• After you've finished suctioning, flush the catheter by maintaining suction while slowly introducing normal saline solution or sterile water into the irrigation port.

• Place the thumb control valve in the off position.

• Dispose of and replace the suction equipment and supplies according to your facility's policy.

• Change the closed suction system per the manufacturer's and your facility's policy.

Skills

Assisting with a bedside tracheotomy

To perform a tracheotomy, the surgeon will first clean the area from the chin to the nipples with povidone-iodine solution. Next, he'll place sterile drapes on the patient and locate the area for the incision—usually 1 to 2 cm below the cricoid cartilage. Then he'll inject a local anesthetic.

He'll make a horizontal or vertical incision in the skin. (A vertical incision helps avoid arteries, veins, and nerves on the lateral borders of the trachea.) Then he'll dissect subcutaneous fat and muscle and move the muscle aside with vein retractors to locate the tracheal rings. He'll make an incision between the second and third tracheal rings (as shown below) and use hemostats to control bleeding.

Incision site

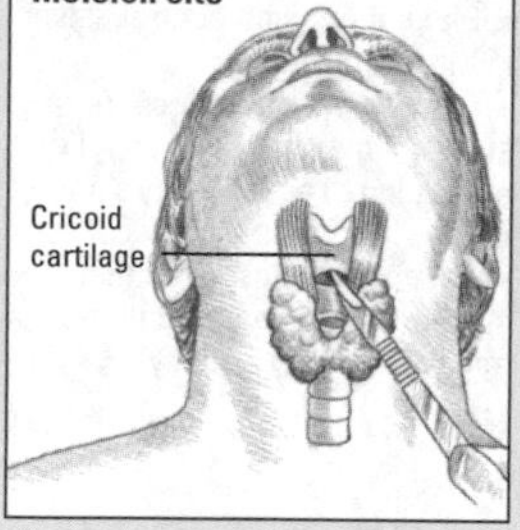

He'll inject a local anesthetic into the tracheal lumen to suppress the cough reflex, and then he'll create a stoma in the trachea. When this is done, carefully apply suction to remove blood and secretions that may obstruct the airway or be aspirated into the lungs. The surgeon then will insert the tracheostomy tube and obturator into the stoma (as shown below). After inserting the tube, he'll remove the obturator.

Tube insertion

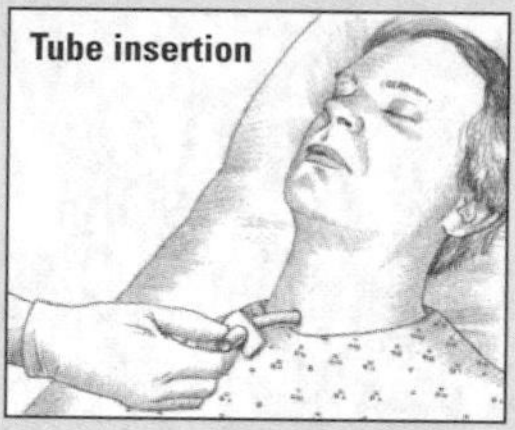

Apply a sterile tracheostomy dressing, and anchor the tube with tracheostomy ties (as shown below). Check for air movement through the tube, and auscultate the lungs to ensure proper placement.

Sterile dressing

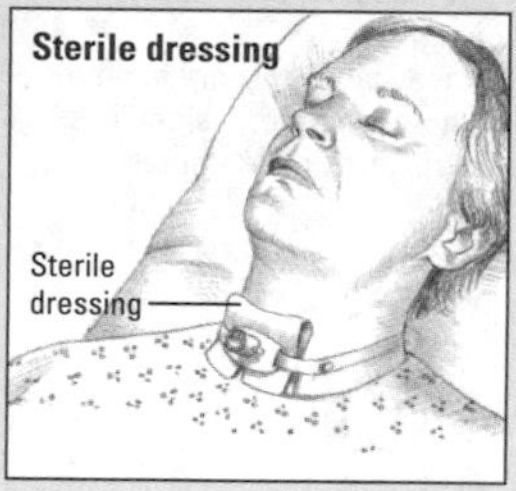

Skills

An alternative approach

In another approach, the surgeon inserts the tracheostomy tube percutaneously. Using either a series of dilators or a pair of forceps, he creates a stoma for tube insertion. Unlike the surgical technique, this method dilates rather than cuts the tissue structures.

After the skin is prepared and anesthetized, the surgeon makes a 1-cm midline incision. When the stoma reaches the desired size, the surgeon inserts the tracheostomy tube. When the tube is in place, inflate the cuff, secure the tube, and check the patient's breath sounds. Next, obtain a portable chest X-ray.

Deflating and inflating a tracheostomy cuff

As part of tracheostomy care, you may be required to deflate and inflate a tracheostomy cuff. If so, gather a 5-ml or 10-ml syringe, padded hemostat, and stethoscope, and follow these steps.

- Confirm the patient's identity using two different patient identifiers according to your facility's policy.
- Read the cuff manufacturer's instructions because cuff types and procedures vary.
- Assess the patient's condition, explain the procedure to him, and reassure him. Wash your hands thoroughly.
- Help the patient into semi-Fowler's position, if possible, or place him in a supine position so secretions above the cuff site will be pushed up into his mouth if he's receiving positive-pressure ventilation.
- Suction the oropharyngeal cavity to prevent pooled secretions from descending into the trachea after cuff deflation.
- Release the padded hemostat clamping the cuff inflation tubing if a hemostat is present.
- Insert a 5-ml or 10-ml syringe into the cuff pilot balloon, and very slowly withdraw all air from the cuff. Leave the syringe attached to the tubing for later reinflation of the cuff.
- Remove the ventilation device. Suction the lower airway through the existing tube to remove all secretions, and then reconnect the patient to the ventilation device.
- Maintain cuff deflation for the prescribed time. Observe the patient for adequate ventilation, and suction as necessary. If the patient has difficulty breathing, reinflate the cuff immediately by depressing the syringe plunger very slowly. Use a stethoscope to listen over the trachea for the air leak, and then inject the least amount of air needed to achieve an adequate tracheal seal.
- When inflating the cuff, you may use the minimal-leak technique or the minimal occlusive-volume technique to help gauge the proper inflation point.
- If you're inflating the cuff using cuff pressure measurement, be careful not to exceed 25 mm Hg.
- After you've inflated the cuff, if the tubing doesn't have a one-way valve at the end, clamp the inflation line with a padded hemostat (to protect the tubing) and remove the syringe.
- Check for a minimal-leak cuff seal. You shouldn't feel air coming from the patient's mouth, nose, or tracheostomy site, and a conscious patient shouldn't be able to speak. Be alert for air leaks from the cuff itself.
- Note the exact amount of air used to inflate the cuff to detect tracheal malacia if more air is consistently needed.
- Make sure the patient is comfortable and can easily reach the call button and communication aids.
- Properly clean or dispose of all equipment, supplies, and trash according to your facility's policy. Replenish used supplies, and make sure all necessary emergency supplies are at the bedside.

Setting up a transducer system

- Put the pressure module into the monitor, if necessary, connecting the transducer cable to the monitor.
- Remove the preassembled pressure tubing from the package.
- If necessary, connect the pressure tubing to the transducer and tighten all tubing connections.
- Position all stopcocks so the flush solution flows through the entire system.
- Roll the tubing's flow regulator to the OFF position.
- Spike the flush solution bag with the tubing, invert the bag, open the roller clamp, and squeeze all the air through the drip chamber.
- Compress the tubing's drip chamber, filling it no more than halfway with the flush solution.
- Hang the pressure infuser bag on the I.V. pole, and then position the flush solution bag inside the pressure infuser bag.
- Open the flow regulator, uncoil the tube if not already done, and remove the protective cap.
- Squeeze the continuous flush device slowly to prime the entire system, including the stopcock ports, with the flush solution.
- As the solution nears the disposable transducer, hold the transducer at a 45 degree angle (as shown top of next column) to force solution to flow upward to the transducer. This forces air out of the system.
- When the stopcock fills, close it to air, and turn it open to the remainder of the tubing. Do this for each stopcock.

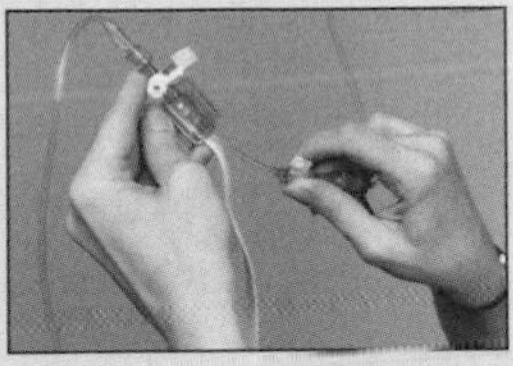

- When the solution nears a stopcock, open the stopcock to air, allowing the solution to flow into the stopcock (as shown below).

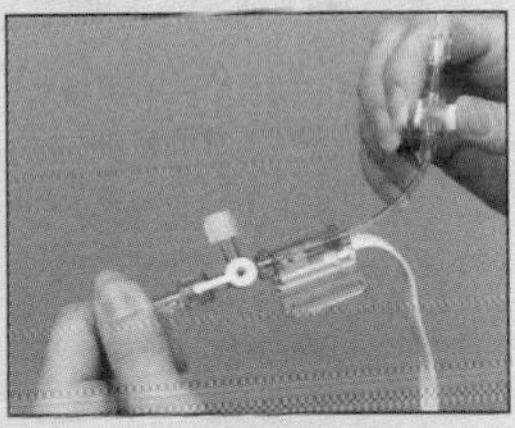

- After you've primed the system, replace the protective cap at the tubing end.
- Inflate the pressure infuser bag to 300 mm Hg. This bag keeps the pressure in the arterial line higher than the patient's systolic pressure, preventing blood backflow into the tubing and ensuring a continuous flow rate.

ALERT Never inflate the pressure infuser bag prior to priming the tubing because this could cause microbubbles.

- When inflating the pressure bag, don't let the drip chamber completely fill with fluid. After-

(continued)

Skills

ward, flush the system again to remove air bubbles.

- Replace the vented caps on the stopcocks with sterile non-vented caps. If you're going to mount the transducer on an I.V. pole, insert the device into its holder.

Zeroing the system

- To ensure accuracy, position the patient and the transducer on the same level each time you zero the transducer or record a pressure. Typically, the patient lies flat in bed, if possible.
- Use the carpenter's level to position the air-reference stopcock or the air-fluid interface of the transducer level with the phlebostatic axis (midway between the posterior chest and sternum at the fourth intercostal space, midaxillary line).
- You may level the air-reference stopcock or the air-fluid interface to the same position as the catheter tip; then turn the stopcock next to the transducer so that it's closed to the patient and open to air.
- Remove the cap to the stopcock port.
- Place the cap inside an opened sterile gauze package to prevent contamination.
- Now zero the transducer, following the manufacturer's directions for zeroing.
- Turn the stopcock on the transducer so that it's closed to air and open to the patient (monitoring position).
- Replace the cap on the stopcock.
- Attach the single-pressure transducer to the patient's catheter to finish assembling the system (as shown below).

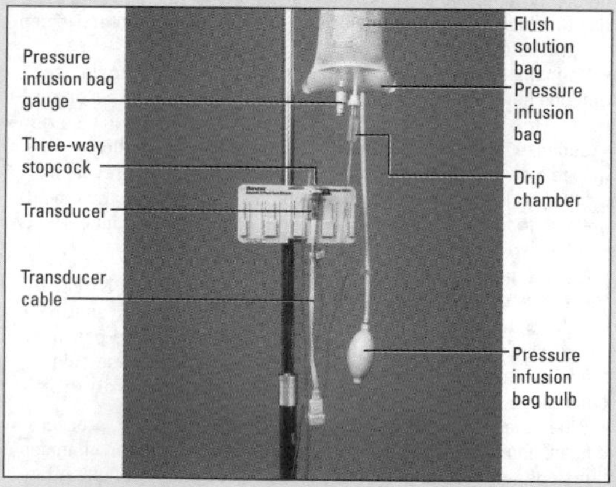

Skills

Responding to ventilator alarms

Signal	Possible causes	Nursing interventions
Low-pressure alarm	• Tube disconnected from ventilator	• Reconnect tube to ventilator.
	• Endotracheal (ET) tube displaced above vocal cords or tracheostomy tube extubated	• Check tube placement and reposition if needed. If extubation or displacement has occurred, ventilate the patient manually and call the practitioner immediately.
	• Leaking tidal volume from low cuff pressure (from an underinflated or ruptured cuff or a leak in the cuff or one-way valve)	• Listen for a whooshing sound around tube, indicating an air leak. If you hear one, check cuff pressure. If you can't maintain pressure, call the practitioner; he may need to insert a new tube.
	• Ventilator malfunction	• Disconnect the patient from the ventilator and ventilate him manually if necessary. Obtain another ventilator.
	• Leak in ventilator circuitry (from loose connection or hole in tubing, loss of temperature-sensitive device, or cracked humidification jar)	• Make sure all connections are intact. Check for holes or leaks in tubing and replace if necessary. Check the humidification jar and replace if cracked.
High-pressure alarm	• Increased airway pressure or decreased lung compliance caused by worsening disease	• Auscultate the lungs for evidence of increasing lung consolidation, barotrauma, or wheezing. Call the practitioner if indicated.
	• Patient biting on oral ET tube	• Insert a bite block if needed. • Consider an analgesic or sedation, if appropriate.

(continued)

Skills

Responding to ventilator alarms *(continued)*

Signal	Possible causes	Nursing interventions
High-pressure alarm *(continued)*	• Secretions in airway	• Look for secretions in the airway. To remove them, suction the patient or have him cough.
	• Condensate in large-bore tubing	• Check tubing for condensate and remove any fluid.
	• Intubation of right mainstem bronchus	• Auscultate the lungs for evidence of diminished or absent breath sounds in the left lung fields. • Check tube position. If it has slipped, call the practitioner; he may need to reposition it.
	• Patient coughing, gagging, or attempting to talk	• If the patient fights the ventilator, the practitioner may order a sedative or neuromuscular-blocking agent.
	• Chest wall resistance	• Reposition the patient to improve chest expansion. If repositioning doesn't help, administer the prescribed analgesic.
	• Failure of high-pressure relief valve	• Have faulty equipment replaced.
	• Bronchospasm	• Assess the patient for the cause. Report to the practitioner, and treat as ordered.

Using a warming system

Shivering, the compensatory response to falling body temperature, may use more oxygen than the body can supply—especially in a surgical patient. In the past, patients were covered with blankets to warm their bodies. Now, health care facilities may supply a warming system, such as the Bair Hugger patient-warming system (shown below).

This system helps to gradually increase body temperature by drawing air through a filter, warming the air to the desired temperature, and circulating it through a hose to a warming blanket placed over the patient.

When using the warming system, follow these guidelines:

- Place the warming blanket directly over the patient with the paper side facing down and the clear tubular side facing up.
- Use a bath blanket in a single layer over the warming blanket to minimize heat loss.
- Make sure the connection hose is at the foot of the bed.
- Take the patient's temperature during the first 15 to 30 minutes and at least every 30 minutes while the warming blanket is in use.

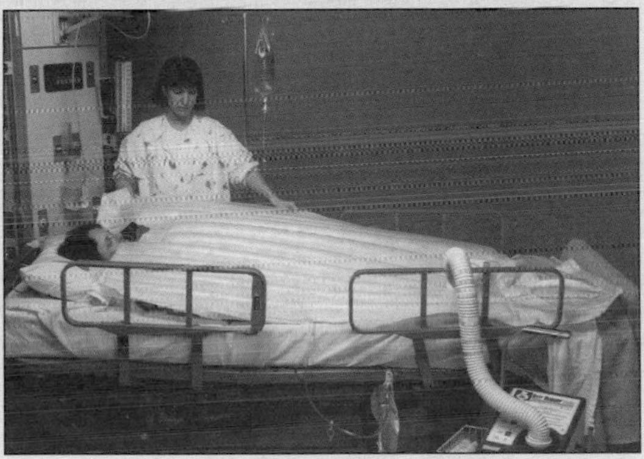

Monitoring blood glucose

- Before using a blood glucose meter, follow the manufacturer's instructions for calibration.
- Explain the procedure to the patient.
- Wash your hands and put on gloves.
- Select the puncture site—usually the lateral side of a fingertip.
- Avoid selecting cold, cyanotic, or swollen puncture sites to ensure an adequate blood sample. If you can't obtain a capillary sample, perform venipuncture and place a large drop of venous blood on the reagent strip.
- If necessary, dilate the capillaries by applying a warm, moist compress to the area for about 10 minutes.
- Wipe the puncture site with an alcohol pad, and dry it thoroughly with a gauze pad.
- To collect a sample from the fingertip with a disposable lancet, position the lancet on the side of the patient's fingertip perpendicular to the lines of the fingerprints. Pierce the skin sharply and quickly. Alternatively, you can use a mechanical blood-letting device, which uses a spring-loaded lancet.
- Don't squeeze the puncture site, to avoid diluting the sample with tissue fluid.
- Touch a drop of blood to the reagent patch on the strip; make sure you cover the entire patch.
- Briefly apply pressure to the puncture site. Ask the adult patient to hold a gauze pad firmly over the puncture site until bleeding stops.
- Insert the strip into the meter, and watch for the digital display of the resulting glucose level.
- Apply a small adhesive bandage to the puncture site, if needed.

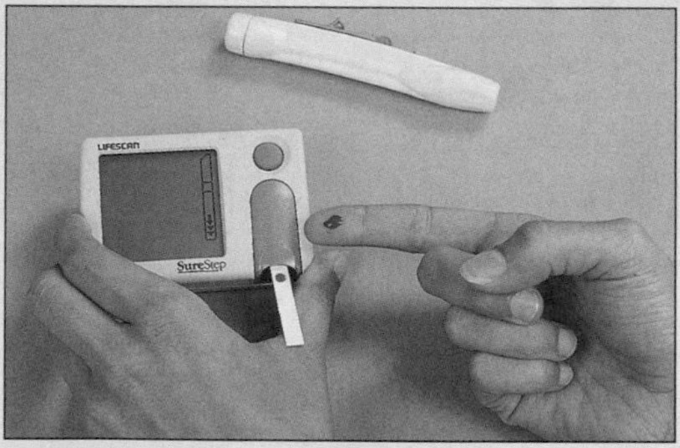

Medications & I.V.s

Medications & I.V.s

Drug administration guidelines

Precautions for drug administration

Whenever you administer medication, observe these precautions to ensure that you're giving the right drug in the right dose to the right patient at the right time by the right route.

Check the order
Check the order on the patient's medication record against the practitioner's order.

Check the label
Check the label on the medication three times before administering it to the patient to ensure that you're administering the prescribed medication in the prescribed dose by the prescribed route. Check it when you take the container from the shelf or drawer, right before pouring the medication into the medication cup or drawing it into the syringe, and before returning the container to the shelf or drawer. If you're administering a unit-dose medication, check the label for the third time immediately after pouring the medication and again before discarding the wrapper. Don't open a unit-dose medication until you're at the patient's bedside.

Confirm the patient's identity
Before giving the medication, confirm the patient's identity by checking two patient identifiers. Then make sure that you have the correct medication.

Explain the procedure to the patient and provide privacy.

Have a written order
Make sure that you have a written order for every medication that's to be given. If the order is verbal, make sure that the practitioner signs for it within the specified time according to your facility's policy.

Give labeled medication
Don't give medication from a poorly labeled, soiled, or unlabeled container. Furthermore, don't attempt to label drugs or reinforce drug labels yourself; a pharmacist must do that.

Monitor medication
Never give a medication that someone else has poured or prepared. Never allow your medication cart or tray out of your sight. Never return unwrapped or prepared medications to stock containers. Instead, dispose of them and notify the pharmacy.

Respond to the patient's questions
If the patient questions you about his medication or the dosage, check his medication record again. If the medication is correct, reassure him that it's correct. Be sure to tell him about changes in his medication or dosage. Instruct him, as appropriate, about possible adverse reactions, and encourage him to report any that he experiences.

Identifying the most dangerous drugs

Almost any drug can cause an adverse reaction in some patients, but the following drugs cause about 90% of all reported reactions.

Anticoagulants
- Heparin
- Warfarin

Antimicrobials
- Cephalosporins
- Penicillins
- Sulfonamides

Bronchodilators
- Sympathomimetics
- Theophylline

Cardiac drugs
- Antihypertensives
- Digoxin
- Diuretics
- Quinidine

Central nervous system drugs
- Analgesics
- Anticonvulsants
- Neuroleptics
- Sedative-hypnotics

Diagnostic agents
- X-ray contrast media

Hormones
- Corticosteroids
- Estrogens
- Insulin

Dangerous abbreviations

The Joint Commission has approved the following "minimum required list" of dangerous abbreviations, acronyms, and symbols that shouldn't be used by accredited organizations. They have also provided a list of other abbreviations that medical personnel should consider not using. Avoiding use of all of these abbreviations, acronyms, and symbols should help protect patients from the effects of miscommunication in clinical documentation.

Abbreviation	Potential problem	Preferred term
U (for unit)	Mistaken as zero, four, or cc	Write "unit."
IU (for international unit)	Mistaken as IV (intravenous) or 10	Write "international unit."
Q.D., Q.O.D. (Latin abbreviations for "once daily" and "every other day")	Mistaken for each other; the period after the "Q" can be mistaken for an "I"; the "O" can also be mistaken for an "I"	Write "daily" and "every other day."
Trailing zero (X.0 mg); lack of leading zero (.X mg)	Decimal point is missed	Never write a zero by itself after a decimal point (X mg); always use a zero before a decimal point (0.X mg).
MS, MSO_4, $MgSO_4$	Confused with each other	Write "morphine sulfate" or "magnesium sulfate."
µg (for microgram)	Mistaken for mg (milligram), resulting in overdose	Write "mcg."
H.S. (for half-strength or Latin abbreviation for "bedtime")	Mistaken for either "half-strength" or "hour of sleep"; "q H.S." mistaken for "every hour"	Write "half-strength" or "at bedtime."

Dangerous abbreviations (continued)

Abbreviation	Potential problem	Preferred term
T.I.W. (for three times a week)	Mistaken for "three times a day" or "twice weekly"	Write "3 times weekly" or "three times weekly."
S.C. or S.Q. (for subcutaneous)	Mistaken for "SL" (sublingual) or "5 every"	Write "sub-Q," "subQ," or "subcutaneously."
D/C (for discharge)	Mistaken for discontinue whatever drugs follow	Write "discharge."
c.c. (for cubic centimeter)	Mistaken for U (units) when written poorly	Write "ml" (milliliter).
A.S., A.D., A.U. (Latin abbreviations for "left ear," "right ear," and "both ears")	Mistaken for OS, OD, OU	Write "left ear," "right ear," or "both ears."

Body surface area nomogram

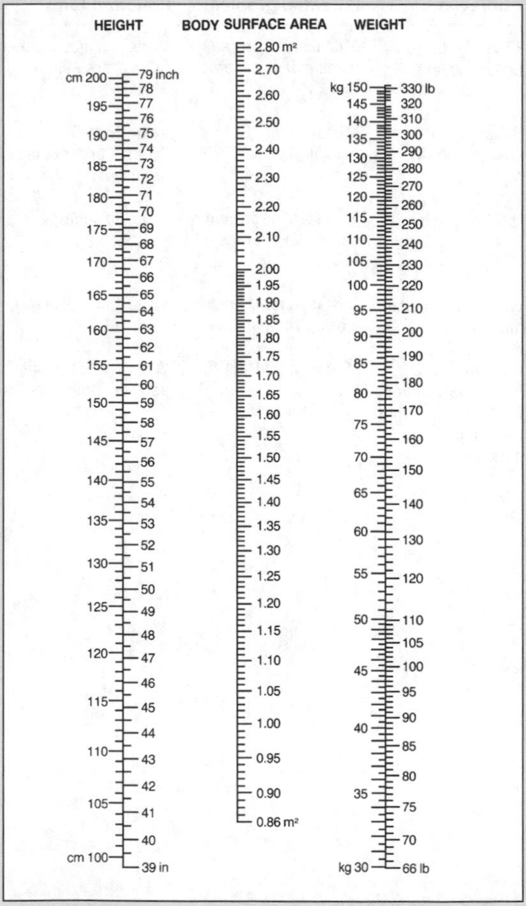

Reprinted with permission from *Geigy Scientific Tables,* 8th ed., vol. 5, p. 105.

Dosage calculation formulas and common conversions

Dosage calculation formulas

$$\text{Body surface area in m}^2 = \sqrt{\frac{\text{height in cm} \times \text{weight in kg}}{3{,}600}}$$

$$\text{mcg/ml} = \text{mg/ml} \times 1{,}000$$

$$\text{ml/minute} = \frac{\text{ml/hour}}{60}$$

$$\text{gtt/minute} = \frac{\text{volume to be infused in ml}}{\text{time in minutes}} \times \text{drip factor in gtt/ml}$$

$$\text{mg/minute} = \frac{\text{mg in bag} \times \text{flow rate} \div 60}{\text{ml in bag}}$$

$$\text{mcg/minute} = \frac{\text{mg in bag} \div 0.06 \times \text{flow rate}}{\text{ml in bag}}$$

$$\text{mcg/kg/minute} = \frac{\text{mcg/ml} \times \text{ml/minute}}{\text{weight in kg}}$$

Common conversions

1 kg	=	1,000 g
1 g	=	1,000 mg
1 mg	=	1,000 mcg
1"	=	2.54 cm
1 L	=	1,000 ml
1 ml	=	1,000 microliters
1 tsp	=	5 ml
1 tbs	=	15 ml
2 tbs	=	30 ml
8 oz	=	240 ml
1 oz	=	30 g
1 lb	=	454 g
2.2 lb	=	1 kg

Drip rate calculation

When calculating the flow rate of I.V. solutions, remember that the number of drops required to deliver 1 ml varies with the type of administration set. To calculate the drip rate, you must know the calibration of the drip rate for each manufacturer's product. As a quick guide, refer to the chart below. Use this formula to calculate specific drip rates:

$$\frac{\text{volume of infusion (in ml)}}{\text{time of infusion (in minutes)}} \times \text{drip factor (in drops/ml)} = \text{drops/minute}$$

	Ordered volume					
	500 ML/ 24 HR OR 21 ML/HR	1,000 ML/ 24 HR OR 42 ML/HR	1,000 ML/ 20 HR OR 50 ML/HR	1,000 ML/ 10 HR OR 100 ML/HR	1,000 ML/ 8 HR OR 125 ML/HR	1,000 ML/ 6 HR OR 167 ML/HR
Drops/ml	**Drops/minute to infuse**					
Macrodrip						
10	4	7	8	17	21	28
15	5	11	13	25	31	42
20	6	14	17	33	42	56
Microdrip						
60	21	42	50	100	125	167

Tips for high-risk drips

Patient-controlled analgesia (PCA), heparin, and insulin infusions can be especially dangerous if administered incorrectly. If possible, have another nurse independently check the practitioner's order, your calculations, and the pump settings for these drugs before starting them.

PCA

Be sure to note:

- strength of the drug solution in the syringe
- number of drug administrations during assessment period
- basal dose, if any
- amount of solution received (number of injections × volume of injections + basal doses)
- total amount of drug received (amount of solution × solution strength).

Heparin

Be sure to:

- determine the solution's concentration (Divide the units of drug added by the amount of the solution in milliliters.)
- state as a fraction: the desired dose over the unknown flow rate
- cross-multiply to find the flow rate.

Insulin

Be sure to:

- remember that regular insulin is the only type given by I.V. route
- always use an infusion pump
- use concentrations of 1 unit/ml.

Infusion flow rates

Epinephrine infusion rates

Mix 1 mg in 250 ml (4 mcg/ml).

Dose (MCG/MINUTE)	**Infusion rate** (ML/HOUR)
1	15
2	30
3	45
4	60
5	75
6	90
7	105
8	120
9	135
10	150
15	225
20	300
25	375
30	450
35	525
40	600

Isoproterenol infusion rates

Mix 1 mg in 250 ml (4 mcg/ml).

Dose (MCG/MINUTE)	**Infusion rate** (ML/HOUR)
1	15
2	30
3	45
4	60
5	75
6	90
7	105
8	120
9	135
10	150
15	225
20	300
25	375
30	450

Nitroglycerin infusion rates

Determine the infusion rate in ml/hour using the ordered dose and the concentration of the drug solution.

Dose (MCG/MINUTE)	**25 mg/ 250 ml** (100 MCG/ML)	**50 mg/ 250 ml** (200 MCG/ML)	**100 mg/ 250 ml** (400 MCG/ML)
5	3	2	1
10	6	3	2
20	12	6	3
30	18	9	5
40	24	12	6
50	30	15	8
60	36	18	9
70	42	21	10
80	48	24	12
90	54	27	14
100	60	30	15
150	90	45	23
200	120	60	30

Dobutamine infusion rates

Mix 250 mg in 250 ml of D_5W (1,000 mcg/ml). Determine the infusion rate in ml/hr using the ordered dose and the patient's weight in pounds or kilograms.

Dose (mcg/kg/min)	Patient's weight						
	LB KG	88 40	99 45	110 50	121 55	132 60	143 65
2.5		6	7	8	8	9	10
5		12	14	15	17	18	20
7.5		18	20	23	25	27	29
10		24	27	30	33	36	39
12.5		30	34	38	41	45	49
15		36	41	45	50	54	59
20		48	54	60	66	72	78
25		60	68	75	83	90	98
30		72	81	90	99	108	117
35		84	95	105	116	126	137
40		96	108	120	132	144	156

	154 70	165 75	176 80	187 85	198 90	209 95	220 100	231 105	242 110
	11	11	12	13	14	14	15	16	17
	21	23	24	26	27	29	30	32	33
	32	34	36	38	41	43	45	47	50
	42	45	48	51	54	57	60	63	66
	53	56	60	64	68	71	75	79	83
	63	68	72	77	81	86	90	95	99
	84	90	96	102	108	114	120	126	132
	105	113	120	128	135	143	150	158	165
	126	135	144	153	162	171	180	189	198
	147	158	168	179	189	200	210	221	231
	168	180	192	204	216	228	240	252	264

Dopamine infusion rates

Mix 400 mg in 250 ml of D_5W (1,600 mcg/ml). Determine the infusion rate in ml/hour using the ordered dose and the patient's weight in pounds or kilograms.

Dose (mcg/kg/min)	Patient's weight						
	LB	88	99	110	121	132	143
	KG	40	45	50	55	60	65
2.5		4	4	5	5	6	6
5		8	8	9	10	11	12
7.5		11	13	14	15	17	18
10		15	17	19	21	23	24
12.5		19	21	23	26	28	30
15		23	25	28	31	34	37
20		30	34	38	41	45	49
25		38	42	47	52	56	61
30		45	51	56	62	67	73
35		53	59	66	72	79	85
40		60	68	75	83	90	98
45		68	76	84	93	101	110
50		75	84	94	103	113	122

154 70	165 75	176 80	187 85	198 90	209 95	220 100	231 105
7	7	8	8	8	9	9	10
13	14	15	16	17	18	19	20
20	21	23	24	25	27	28	30
26	28	30	32	34	36	38	39
33	35	38	40	42	45	47	49
39	42	45	48	51	53	56	59
53	56	60	64	68	71	75	79
66	70	75	80	84	89	94	98
79	84	90	96	101	107	113	118
92	98	105	112	118	125	131	138
105	113	120	128	135	143	150	158
118	127	135	143	152	160	169	177
131	141	150	159	169	178	188	197

Nitroprusside infusion rates

Mix 50 mg in 250 ml of D_5W (200 mcg/ml). Determine the infusion rate in ml/hour using the ordered dose and the patient's weight in pounds or kilograms.

Dose (mcg/kg/min)	**Patient's weight**						
	LB KG	88 40	99 45	110 50	121 55	132 60	143 65
0.3		4	4	5	5	5	6
0.5		6	7	8	8	9	10
1		12	14	15	17	18	20
1.5		18	20	23	25	27	29
2		24	27	30	33	36	39
3		36	41	45	50	54	59
4		48	54	60	66	72	78
5		60	68	75	83	90	98
6		72	81	90	99	108	117
7		84	95	105	116	126	137
8		96	108	120	132	144	156
9		108	122	135	149	162	176
10		120	135	150	165	180	195

154 70	165 75	176 80	187 85	198 90	209 95	220 100	231 105	242 110
6	7	7	8	8	9	9	9	10
11	11	12	13	14	14	15	16	17
21	23	24	26	27	29	30	32	33
32	34	36	38	41	43	45	47	50
42	45	48	51	54	57	60	63	66
63	68	72	77	81	86	90	95	99
84	90	96	102	108	114	120	126	132
105	113	120	128	135	143	150	158	165
126	135	144	153	162	171	180	189	198
147	158	168	179	189	200	210	221	231
168	180	192	204	216	228	240	252	264
189	203	216	230	243	257	270	284	297
210	225	240	255	270	285	300	315	330

Insulin overview

Insulin type	Onset	Peak (hours)	Usual effective duration (hours)	Usual maximum duration (hours)
Animal				
Regular	0.5 to 2 hours	3 to 4	4 to 6	6 to 8
NPH	4 to 6 hours	8 to 14	16 to 20	20 to 24
Human				
Insulin aspart	5 to 10 minutes	1 to 3	3 to 5	4 to 6
Insulin lispro	< 15 minutes	0.5 to 1.5	2 to 4	4 to 6
Regular	0.5 to 1 hour	2 to 3	3 to 6	6 to 10
NPH	2 to 4 hours	4 to 10	10 to 16	14 to 18
Lente	3 to 4 hours	4 to 12	12 to 18	16 to 20
Ultralente	6 to 10 hours	—	18 to 20	20 to 24
Insulin glargine	1 hour	—	24	24

Insulin infusion pumps

A subcutaneous (subQ) insulin infusion pump provides continuous, long-term insulin therapy for patients with type 1 diabetes mellitus. Complications include site infection, catheter clogging, and insulin loss from loose reservoir-catheter connections. Insulin pumps work on either an open-loop or a closed-loop system.

Open-loop system

- Is the most common.
- Infuses insulin but can't respond to changes in the patient's serum glucose levels.
- Delivers insulin in small (basal) doses every few minutes; large (bolus) doses are set by the patient.
- Consists of reservoir containing insulin syringe, small pump, infusion-rate selector that allows insulin release adjustments, battery, and plastic catheter with attached needle leading from syringe to subQ injection site.
- Needle is held in place with waterproof tape.
- Pump is worn on a belt or in a pocket.
- Infusion line must have clear path to injection site.
- Infusion-rate selector releases about one-half the total daily insulin.
- The patient releases the remainder in bolus doses before meals and snacks.
- The patient must change the syringe daily.
- The patient must change needle, catheter, and injection site every other day.

Closed-loop system

- Self-contained; detects and responds to changing serum glucose levels.
- Includes glucose sensor, programmable computer, power supply, pump, and insulin reservoir.
- The computer triggers continuous insulin delivery in appropriate amounts.

Nonneedle catheter system

- Uses tiny plastic catheter inserted into the skin over a needle using a special insertion device.
- The needle is withdrawn, leaving the catheter in place (in the abdomen, thigh, or flank).
- Catheter is changed every 2 to 3 days.

50 common critical care drugs

This table provides information on drugs commonly used in critical care nursing, along with their indications.

Drug name	Indications
Abciximab (ReoPro)	• Adjunct to percutaneous transluminal coronary angioplasty or arterectomy • Unstable angina not responding to conventional medical therapy in patients scheduled for percutaneous coronary intervention within 24 hours
Adenosine (Adenocard)	• To convert paroxysmal supraventricular tachycardia to sinus rhythm
Alprazolam (Xanax)	• Anxiety
Alteplase (tissue plasminogen activator, recombinant) (Activase)	• Lysis of thrombi in acute myocardial infarction (MI), pulmonary emboli, or central venous access devices
Amiodarone (Cordarone)	• Cardiac arrest, pulseless ventricular tachycardia, ventricular fibrillation • Atrial fibrillation • Heart failure
Amlodipine (Norvasc)	• Chronic stable angina • Hypertension
Atenolol (Tenormin)	• Hypertension • Angina pectoris • Risk reduction of cardiovascular-related death and reinfarction postacute MI
Atropine sulfate (Sal-Tropine)	• Symptomatic bradycardia, bradyarrhythmia • Preoperatively to diminish secretions and block cardiac vagal reflexes
Bumetanide (Bumex)	• Heart failure

50 common critical care drugs *(continued)*

Drug name	Indications
Calcium chloride	• Hypocalcemic emergency • Hypocalcemic tetany • Hyperphosphatemia • Hyperkalemia with secondary cardiac toxicity
Clonidine (Catapres)	• Hypertension • Migraine prophylaxis • Opioid dependence • Alcohol dependence
Dexamethasone (Decadron)	• Cerebral edema • Inflammatory conditions, allergic reaction • Shock • Adrenocortical insufficiency
Diazepam (Valium)	• Anxiety • Acute alcohol withdrawal • Cardioversion • Status epilepticus, severe recurrent seizures
Digoxin (Lanoxin)	• Heart failure • Paroxysmal supraventricular tachycardia, atrial fibrillation and flutter
Diltiazem (Cardizem)	• Prinzmetal's or chronic stable angina pectoris • Hypertension • Atrial fibrillation or flutter, paroxysmal supraventricular tachycardia
Diphenhydramine (Benadryl)	• Sedation • Nighttime sleep aid • Allergy symptoms
Dobutamine (Dobutrex)	• Heart failure • Adjunctive therapy in cardiac surgery
Dopamine (Intropin)	• Shock • Hypotension • To increase organ perfusion

(continued)

50 common critical care drugs *(continued)*

Drug name	Indications
Drotrecogin alfa (Xigris)	• Sepsis
Enalaprilat (Vasotec)	• Hypertension • Heart failure • Asymptomatic left ventricular dysfunction
Enoxaparin (Lovenox)	• Pulmonary emboli (PE) and deep vein thrombosis (DVT) prophylaxis • Prevention of ischemic complications of unstable angina and non-Q-wave MI • DVT
Epinephrine (EpiPen)	• Bronchospasm, hypersensitivity reactions, anaphylaxis • Cardiac arrest • Acute asthma attack
Eptifibatide (Integrilin)	• Acute coronary syndrome
Furosemide (Lasix)	• Acute pulmonary edema • Edema • Hypertension
Heparin sodium (Heparin sodium injection)	• DVT • MI • PE • Atrial fibrillation with embolism
Lorazepam (Ativan)	• Anxiety • Status epilepticus
Magnesium sulfate	• Hypomagnesemia • Seizures
Mannitol (Osmitrol)	• Oliguria • Drug intoxication • Increased intraocular pressure • Increased intracranial pressure
Methylprednisolone (Solu-Medrol)	• Severe inflammation or immunosuppression • Shock

50 common critical care drugs *(continued)*

Drug name	Indications
Metoprolol (Lopressor)	• Hypertension • Early intervention in acute MI • Angina pectoris • Stable, symptomatic heart failure resulting from ischemia, hypertension, or cardiomyopathy
Midazolam (Versed)	• Preoperative sedation • Conscious sedation
Morphine sulfate (Duramorph)	• Pain
Naloxone (Narcan)	• Known or suspected opioid-induced respiratory depression
Nesiritide (Natrecor)	• Acute decompensated heart failure
Nitroglycerin (Nitrostat)	• Prophylaxis against chronic anginal attacks • Acute angina pectoris • Hypertension
Nitroprusside (Nipride)	• Hypertensive emergency • Cardiogenic shock
Norepinephrine (Levophed)	• Hypotension
Pancuronium	• Adjunct to anesthesia to relax skeletal muscle, facilitate intubation, assist with mechanical ventilation
Phenobarbital (Solfoton)	• Seizures, status epilepticus • Sedation
Phenylephrine (Neo-Synephrine)	• Hypotensive emergency • Shock
Phenytoin (Dilantin)	• Seizures, status epilepticus
Potassium chloride (K-Lor)	• Hypokalemia

(continued)

50 common critical care drugs *(continued)*

Drug name	Indications
Propranolol (Inderal)	• Angina pectoris • To decrease risk of death after MI • Supraventricular, ventricular, and atrial arrhythmias; tachyarrhythmias caused by excessive catecholamine action • Hypertension
Protamine sulfate	• Heparin overdose
Streptokinase (Streptase)	• Arteriovenous-cannula occlusion • Venous thrombosis, PE, arterial thrombosis and embolism • Lysis of coronary artery thrombi following acute MI
Vasopressin (Pitressin)	• Non-nephrogenic, non-psychogenic diabetes insipidus • GI bleeding
Vecuronium	• Adjunct to general anesthesia to facilitate endotracheal intubation and relax skeletal muscles during surgery or mechanical ventilation
Verapamil (Calan)	• Vasospastic angina, classic chronic stable angina • Chronic atrial fibrillation, supraventricular arrhythmias • Hypertension
Vitamin K analogue (AquaMEPHYTON)	• Hypoprothrombinemia
Warfarin (Coumadin)	• PE with DVT • MI • Rheumatic heart disease with heart valve damage, prosthetic heart valves • Chronic atrial fibrillation

Common antidotes

Drug or toxin	Antidote
Acetaminophen	Acetylcysteine (Mucomyst)
Anticholinergics	Physostigmine (Antilirium)
Benzodiazepines	Flumazenil (Romazicon)
Calcium channel blockers	Calcium chloride
Cyanide	Amyl nitrate, sodium nitrite, and sodium thiosulfate (Cyanide Antidote Kit); methylene blue
Digoxin, cardiac glycosides	Digoxin immune fab (Digibind)
Ethylene glycol	Ethanol
Heparin	Protamine sulfate
Insulin-induced hypoglycemia	Glucagon
Iron	Deferoxamine mesylate (Desferal)
Lead	Edetate calcium disodium (Calcium Disodium Versenate)
Opioids	Naloxone (Narcan), nalmefene (Revex), naltrexone (ReVia)
Organophosphates, anticholinesterases	Atropine, pralidoxime (Protopam)
Warfarin	Vitamin K

Antidotes for extravasation

Antidote	Extravasated drug
Ascorbic acid injection	• dactinomycin
Edetate calcium disodium (calcium EDTA)	• cadmium • copper • manganese • zinc
Hyaluronidase 15 units/ml	• aminophylline • calcium solutions • contrast media • dextrose solutions (concentrations of 10% or more) • nafcillin • potassium solutions • total parenteral nutrition solutions • vinblastine • vincristine • vindesine
Hydrocortisone sodium succinate 100 mg/ml Usually followed by topical application of hydrocortisone cream 1%	• doxorubicin • vincristine
Phentolamine	• dobutamine • dopamine • epinephrine • metaraminol bitartrate • norepinephrine
Sodium bicarbonate 8.4%	• carmustine • daunorubicin • doxorubicin • vinblastine • vincristine
Sodium thiosulfate 10%	• cisplatin • dactinomycin • mechlorethamine • mitomycin

Dangerous effects of drug combinations

If possible, avoid administering these drug combinations to prevent dangerous drug interactions.

Drug	Interacting drug	Possible effect
Aminoglycosides amikacin gentamicin kanamycin neomycin netilmicin streptomycin tobramycin	Parenteral cephalosporins • ceftazidime • ceftizoxime	Possible enhanced nephrotoxicity
	Loop diuretics • bumetanide • ethacrynic acid • furosemide	Possible enhanced ototoxicity
Amphetamines amphetamine benzphetamine dextroampheta-mine methampheta-mine	Urine alkalinizers • potassium citrate • sodium acetate • sodium bicarbon-ate • sodium citrate • sodium lactate • tromethamine	Decreased urinary ex-cretion of amphetamine
Angiotensin-converting enzyme (ACE) inhibitors benazepril captopril enalapril fosinopril lisinopril quinapril ramipril	Indomethacin Nonsteroidal anti-inflammatory drugs (NSAIDs)	Decreased or abolished effectiveness of antihy-pertensive action of ACE inhibitors
Barbiturate anesthetics methohexital thiopental	Opiate analgesics	Enhanced central nerv-ous system and respira-tory depression

(continued)

Dangerous effects of drug combinations *(continued)*

Drug	Interacting drug	Possible effect
Barbiturates amobarbital aprobarbital butabarbital mephobarbital pentobarbital phenobarbital primidone secobarbital	Valproic acid	Increased serum barbiturate levels
Beta-adrenergic blockers acebutolol atenolol betaxolol carteolol esmolol levobunolol metoprolol nadolol penbutolol pindolol propranolol timolol	Verapamil	Enhanced pharmacologic effects of both beta-adrenergic blockers and verapamil
Carbamazepine	Erythromycin	Increased risk of carbamazepine toxicity
Carmustine	Cimetidine	Enhanced risk of bone marrow toxicity
Ciprofloxacin	Antacids that contain magnesium or aluminum hydroxide, iron supplements, sucralfate, multivitamins that contain iron or zinc	Decreased plasma levels and effectiveness of ciprofloxacin
Clonidine	Beta-adrenergic blockers	Enhanced rebound hypertension following rapid clonidine withdrawal

Dangerous effects of drug combinations *(continued)*

Drug	Interacting drug	Possible effect
Cyclosporine	Carbamazepine, isoniazid, phenobarbital, phenytoin, rifabutin, rifampin	Reduced plasma levels of cyclosporine
Cardiac glycosides	Loop and thiazide diuretics	Increased risk of cardiac arrhythmias due to hypokalemia
	Thiazide-like diuretics	Increased therapeutic or toxic effects
Digoxin	Amiodarone	Decreased renal clearance of digoxin
	Quinidine	Enhanced clearance of digoxin
	Verapamil	Elevated serum digoxin levels
Dopamine	Phenytoin	Hypertension and bradycardia
Epinephrine	Beta-adrenergic blockers	Increased systolic and diastolic pressures; marked decrease in heart rate
Erythromycin	Carbamazepine	Decreased carbamazepine clearance
	Theophylline	Decreased hepatic clearance of theophylline
Ethanol	Disulfiram Furazolidone Metronidazole	Acute alcohol intolerance reaction

(continued)

Dangerous effects of drug combinations *(continued)*

Drug	Interacting drug	Possible effect
Furazolidone	Amine-containing foods Anorexiants	Inhibits monoamine oxidase (MAO), possibly leading to hypertensive crisis
Heparin	Salicylates NSAIDs	Enhanced risk of bleeding
Levodopa	Furazolidone	Enhanced toxic effects of levodopa
Lithium	Thiazide diuretics NSAIDs	Decreased lithium excretion
Meperidine	MAO inhibitors	Cardiovascular instability and increased toxic effects
Methotrexate	Probenecid	Decreased methotrexate elimination
	Salicylates	Increased risk of methotrexate toxicity
MAO inhibitors	Amine-containing foods Anorexiants Meperidine	Risk of hypertensive crisis
Nondepolarizing muscle relaxants	Aminoglycosides Inhaled anesthetics	Enhanced neuromuscular blockade
Potassium supplements	Potassium-sparing diuretics	Increased risk of hyperkalemia
Quinidine	Amiodarone	Increased risk of quinidine toxicity
Sympathomimetics	MAO inhibitors	Increased risk of hypertensive crisis

Dangerous effects of drug combinations *(continued)*

Drug	Interacting drug	Possible effect
Tetracyclines	Antacids containing magnesium, aluminum, or bismuth salts Iron supplements	Decreased plasma levels and effectiveness of tetracyclines
Theophylline	Carbamazepine	Reduced theophylline levels
	Cimetidine	Increased theophylline levels
	Ciprofloxacin	Increased theophylline levels
	Erythromycin	Increased theophylline levels
	Phenobarbital	Reduced theophylline levels
	Rifampin	Reduced theophylline levels
Warfarin	Testosterone	Possible enhanced bleeding caused by increased hypoprothrombinemia
	Barbiturates Carbamazepine	Reduced effectiveness of warfarin
	Amiodarone Cephalosporins (certain ones) Chloral hydrate Cholestyramine Cimetidine Clofibrate Co-trimoxazole Dextrothyroxine Disulfiram	Increased risk of bleeding

(continued)

Dangerous effects of drug combinations *(continued)*

Drug	Interacting drug	Possible effect
Warfarin (continued)	Erythromycin Glucagon Metronidazole Phenylbutazone Quinidine Quinine Salicylates Sulfinpyrazone Thyroid drugs Tricyclic antidepressants	Increased risk of bleeding
	Chlordiazepoxide Carbamazepine Vitamin K	Decreased pharmacologic effect
	Rifampin Trazodone	Decreased risk of bleeding
	Methimazole Propylthiouracil	Increased or decreased risk of bleeding

Herb-drug interactions

Herb	Interacting drug	Possible effects
Aloe	Cardiac glycosides, antiarrhythmics	May lead to hypokalemia, which may potentiate cardiac glycosides and antiarrhythmics
	Thiazide diuretics, licorice, and other potassium-wasting drugs	Increases the effects of potassium wasting
	Orally administered drugs	Causes potential for decreased absorption of drugs because of more rapid GI transit time
Bilberry	Antiplatelets, anticoagulants	Decreases platelet aggregation
	Insulin, hypoglycemics	May increase serum insulin levels, causing hypoglycemia; increases effect with diabetes drugs
Capsicum	Antiplatelets, anticoagulants	Decreases platelet aggregation and increases fibrinolytic activity, prolonging bleeding time
	Nonsteroidal anti-inflammatory drugs (NSAIDs)	Stimulates GI secretions to help protect against NSAID-induced GI irritation
	Angiotensin-converting enzyme inhibitors	May cause cough
	Theophylline	Increases absorption of theophylline, possibly leading to higher serum levels or toxicity
	Monoamine oxidase (MAO) inhibitors	Decreases the effects resulting from the increased catecholamine secretion

(continued)

Herb-drug interactions *(continued)*

Herb	Interacting drug	Possible effects
Capsicum *(continued)*	Central nervous system (CNS) depressants, such as opioids, benzodiazepines, barbiturates	Increases sedative effect
	Histamine-2 (H_2) receptor antagonists, proton pump inhibitors	Causes potential for decreased effectiveness because of increased acid secretion
Chamomile	Drugs requiring GI absorption	May delay drug absorption
	Anticoagulants	May enhance anticoagulant therapy and prolong bleeding time (if warfarin constituents)
	Iron	May reduce iron absorption because of tannic acid content
Echinacea	Immunosuppressants	May counteract immunosuppressant drugs
	Hepatotoxics	May increase hepatotoxicity with drugs known to elevate liver enzyme levels
	Warfarin	Increases bleeding time without an increased International Normalized Ratio (INR)
Evening primrose	Anticonvulsants	Lowers seizure threshold
Feverfew	Antiplatelets, anticoagulants	May decrease platelet aggregation and increase fibrinolytic activity

Herb-drug interactions *(continued)*

Herb	Interacting drug	Possible effects
Garlic	Antiplatelets, anticoagulants	Enhances platelet inhibition, leading to increased anticoagulation
	Insulin, other drugs causing hypoglycemia	May increase serum insulin levels, causing hypoglycemia, an additive effect with antidiabetics
	Antihypertensives	Causes potential for additive hypotension
	Antihyperlipidemics	May have additive lipid-lowering properties
Ginger	Chemotherapy	May reduce nausea associated with chemotherapy
	H_2-receptor antagonists, proton pump inhibitors	Causes potential for decreased effectiveness because of increased acid secretion by ginger
	Antiplatelets, anticoagulants	Inhibits platelet aggregation by antagonizing thromboxane synthase and enhancing prostacyclin, leading to prolonged bleeding time
	Calcium channel blockers	May increase calcium uptake by myocardium, leading to altered drug effects
	Antihypertensives	May antagonize antihypertensive effect
Ginkgo	Antiplatelets, anticoagulants	May enhance platelet inhibition, leading to increased anticoagulation
	Anticonvulsants	May decrease effectiveness of anticonvulsants
	Drugs known to lower seizure threshold	May further reduce seizure threshold

(continued)

Herb-drug interactions *(continued)*

Herb	Interacting drug	Possible effects
Ginseng	Stimulants	May potentiate stimulant effects
	Warfarin	May antagonize warfarin, resulting in a decreased INR
	Antibiotics	May enhance the effects of some antibiotics (Siberian ginseng)
	Anticoagulants, antiplatelets	Decreases platelet adhesiveness
	Digoxin	May falsely elevate digoxin levels
	MAO inhibitors	Potentiates action of MAO inhibitors
	Hormones, anabolic steroids	May potentiate effects of hormone and anabolic steroid therapies (estrogenic effects of ginseng may cause vaginal bleeding and breast nodules)
	Alcohol	Increases alcohol clearance, possibly by increasing activity of alcohol dehydrogenase
	Furosemide	May decrease diuretic effect of furosemide
	Antipsychotics	May stimulate CNS activity
Goldenseal	Heparin	May counteract anticoagulant effect of heparin
	Diuretics	Increases diuretic effect
	H_2-receptor antagonists, proton pump inhibitors	Causes potential for decreased effectiveness because of increased acid secretion by goldenseal

Herb-drug interactions *(continued)*

Herb	Interacting drug	Possible effects
Goldenseal *(continued)*	General anesthetics	May potentiate hypotensive action of general anesthetics
	CNS depressants, such as opioids, barbiturates, benzodiazepines	Increases sedative effect
Grapeseed	Warfarin	Increases the effects and INR caused by tocopherol content of grapeseed
Green tea	Warfarin	Decreases effectiveness resulting from vitamin content of green tea
Hawthorn berry	Digoxin	Causes additive positive inotropic effect, with potential for digoxin toxicity
Kava	CNS stimulants or depressants	May hinder therapy with CNS stimulants
	Benzodiazepines	May result in comalike states
	Alcohol	Potentiates the depressant effect of alcohol and other CNS depressants
	Levodopa	Decreases the effectiveness of levodopa
Licorice	Digoxin	Causes hypokalemia, which predisposes to digoxin toxicity
	Hormonal contraceptives	Increases fluid retention and potential for increased blood pressure resulting from fluid overload
	Corticosteroids	Causes additive and enhanced effects of the corticosteroids
	Spironolactone	Decreases the effects of spironolactone

(continued)

Herb-drug interactions *(continued)*

Herb	Interacting drug	Possible effects
Ma huang	MAO inhibitors	Potentiates MAO inhibitors
	CNS stimulants, caffeine, theophylline	Causes CNS stimulation
	Digoxin	Increases the risk of arrhythmias
	Hypoglycemics	Decreases hypoglycemic effect because of hyperglycemia caused by ma huang
Melatonin	CNS depressants (such as opioids, barbiturates, benzodiazepines)	Increases sedative effects
Milk thistle	Drugs causing diarrhea	Increases bile secretion and typically causes loose stools; may increase effect of other drugs commonly causing diarrhea; also causes liver membrane-stabilization and antioxidant effects leading to protection from liver damage from various hepatotoxic drugs, such as acetaminophen, phenytoin, ethanol, phenothiazines, butyrophenones
Nettle	Anticonvulsants	May increase sedative adverse effects and risk of seizure
	Opioids, anxiolytics, hypnotics	May increase sedative adverse effects
	Warfarin	Decreases effectiveness resulting from vitamin K content of aerial parts of nettle
	Iron	May reduce iron absorption because of tannic acid content

Herb-drug interactions *(continued)*

Herb	Interacting drug	Possible effects
Passion flower	CNS depressants (such as opioids, barbiturates, benzodiazepines)	Increases sedative effect
St. John's wort	Selective serotonin reuptake inhibitors (SSRIs), MAO inhibitors, nefazodone, trazodone	Causes additive effects with SSRIs, MAO inhibitors, and other antidepressants, potentially leading to serotonin syndrome, especially when combined with SSRIs
	Indinavir; human immunodeficiency virus protease inhibitors (PIs); nonnucleoside reverse transcriptase inhibitors (NNRTIs)	Induces cytochrome P450 metabolic pathway, which may decrease therapeutic effects of drugs using this pathway for metabolism (use of St. John's wort and PIs or NNRTIs should be avoided because of the potential for subtherapeutic antiretroviral levels and insufficient virologic response that could lead to resistance or class cross-resistance)
	Opioids, alcohol	Enhances the sedative effect of opioids and alcohol
	Photosensitizing drugs	Increases photosensitivity
	Sympathomimetic amines (such as pseudoephedrine)	Causes additive effects
	Digoxin	May reduce serum digoxin concentrations, decreasing therapeutic effects
	Reserpine	Antagonizes the effects of reserpine

(continued)

Herb-drug interactions *(continued)*

Herb	Interacting drug	Possible effects
St. John's wort *(continued)*	Hormonal contraceptives	Increases breakthrough bleeding when taken with hormonal contraceptives; also decreases the contraceptive's effectiveness
	Theophylline	May decrease serum theophylline levels, making the drug less effective
	Anesthetics	May prolong the effect of anesthesia drugs
	Cyclosporine	Decreases cyclosporine levels below therapeutic levels, threatening transplanted organ rejection
	Iron	May reduce iron absorption because of tannic acid content
	Warfarin	Has the potential to alter INR; reduces the effectiveness of anticoagulant, requiring increased dosage of drug
Valerian	Sedative hypnotics, CNS depressants	Enhances the effects of sedative hypnotic drugs
	Alcohol	Increases sedation with alcohol (although debated)
	Iron	May reduce iron absorption because of tannic acid content

Drugs that shouldn't be crushed

Many drug forms, such as slow-release, enteric-coated, encapsulated beads, wax-matrix, sublingual, and buccal forms, are designed to release their active ingredients over a certain period or at preset intervals after administration. The disruptions caused by crushing these drug forms can dramatically affect the absorption rate and increase the risk of adverse reactions.

Other reasons not to crush these drug forms include such considerations as taste, tissue irritation, and unusual formulation—for example, a capsule within a capsule, a liquid within a capsule, or a multiple-compressed tablet. Avoid crushing the following drugs, listed by brand name, for the reasons noted beside them.

Accutane (irritant)
Aciphex (delayed release)
Adalat CC (sustained release)
Advicor (extended release)
Aggrenox (extended release)
Allegra D (extended release)
Amnesteem (irritant)
Arthrotec (delayed release)
Asacol (delayed release)
Augmentin XR (extended release)
Avinza (extended release)
Azulfidine EN-tabs (enteric coated)
Biaxin XL (extended release)
Bisacodyl (enteric coated)
Bontril Slow-Release (slow release)
Breonesin (liquid filled)
Brexin LA (slow release)
Bromfed (slow release)
Bromfed PD (slow release)
Calan SR (sustained release)
Carbatrol (extended release)
Cardizem CD, LA, SR (slow release)
Cartia XT (extended release)
Ceclor CD (slow release)
Ceftin (strong, persistent taste)
Charcoal Plus DS (enteric coated)
Chloral Hydrate (liquid within a capsule, taste)
Chlor-Trimeton Allergy 8-hour and 12-hour (slow release)
Choledyl SA (slow release)
Cipro XR (extended release)
Claritin-D 12-hour (slow release)
Claritin-D 24-hour (slow release)
Colace (liquid within a capsule)
Colazal (granules within capsules must reach the colon intact)
Colestid (protective coating)
Compazine Spansules (slow release)
Concerta (extended release)
Congress SR (sustained release)
Contact 12-Hour Maximum-Strength (slow release)
Cotazym-S (enteric coated)
Covera-HS (extended release)
Creon (enteric coated)
Cytovene (irritant)
Dallergy, Dallergy-Jr (slow release)
Deconamine SR (slow release)
Depakene (slow release, mucous membrane irritant)
Depakote (enteric coated)
Depakote ER (extended release)
Desyrel (taste)
Dexedrine Spansule (slow release)
Diamox Sequels (slow release)
Dilacor XR (extended release)

(continued)

Drugs that shouldn't be crushed *(continued)*

Dilatrate-SR (slow release)
Diltia XT (extended release)
Dimetapp Extentabs (slow release)
Ditropan XL (slow release)
Dolobid (irritant)
Drisdol (liquid filled)
Dristan (protective coating)
Drixoral (slow release)
Dulcolax (enteric coated)
DynaCirc CR (slow release)
Easprin (enteric coated)
Ecotrin (enteric coated)
Ecotrin Maximum Strength (enteric coated)
E.E.S. 400 Filmtab (enteric coated)
Effexor XR (extended release)
Emend (hard gelatin capsule)
E-Mycin (enteric coated)
Entex LA (slow release)
Entex PSE (slow release)
Eryc (enteric coated)
Ery-Tab (enteric coated)
Erythrocin Stearate (enteric coated)
Erythromycin Base (enteric coated)
Eskalith CR (slow release)
Extendryl Jr., SR (slow release)
Feldene (mucous membrane irritant)
Feosol (enteric coated)
Feratab (enteric coated)
Fergon (slow release)
Fero-Folic 500 (slow release)
Fero-Grad-500 (slow release)
Ferro-Sequel (slow release)
Feverall Children's Capsules, Sprinkle (taste)
Flomax (slow release)
Fumatinic (slow release)
Geocillin (taste)
Glucophage XR (extended release)
Glucotrol XL (slow release)
Guaifed (slow release)
Guaifed-PD (slow release)
Guaifenex LA (slow release)
Guaifenex PSE (slow release)
Humibid DM, LA (slow release)
Hydergine LC (liquid within a capsule)
Hytakerol (liquid filled)
Iberet (slow release)
ICAPS Plus (slow release)
ICAPS Time Release (slow release)
Imdur (slow release)
Inderal LA (slow release)
Indocin SR (slow release)
InnoPran XL (extended release)
Ionamin (slow release)
Isoptin SR (sustained release)
Isosorbide Dinitrate Sublingual (sublingual)
Isordil Sublingual (sublingual)
Isordil Tembid (slow release)
Isosorbide Dinitrate Sublingual (sublingual)
Kaon-Cl (slow release)
K-Dur (slow release)
Klor-Con (slow release)
Klotrix (slow release)
K-Tab (slow release)
Levbid (slow release)
Levsinex Timecaps (slow release)
Lithobid (slow release)
Macrobid (slow release)
Mestinon Timespans (slow release)
Metadate CD, ER (extended release)
Methylin ER (extended release)
Micro-K Extencaps (slow release)
Motrin (taste)
MS Contin (slow release)
Mucinex (extended release)

Drugs that shouldn't be crushed *(continued)*

Naprelan (slow release)	Slow FE (slow release)
Nexium (sustained release)	Slow-K (slow release)
Niaspan (extended release)	Slow-Mag (slow release)
Nitroglyn (slow release)	Sorbitrate (sublingual)
Nitrong (slow release)	Sotret (irritant)
Nitrostat (sublingual)	Sudafed 12-Hour (slow release)
Norflex (slow release)	Sustaire (slow release)
Norpace CR (slow release)	Tegretol-XR (extended release)
Oramorph SR (slow release)	Ten-K (slow release)
OxyContin (slow release)	Tenuate Dospan (slow release)
Pancrease (enteric coated)	Tessalon Perles (slow release)
Pancrease MT (enteric coated)	Theobid Duracaps (slow release)
Paxil CR (controlled release)	Theochron (slow release)
PCE (slow release)	Theoclear LA (slow release)
Pentasa (controlled release)	Theolair-SR (slow release)
Phazyme (slow release)	Theo-Sav (slow release)
Phazyme 95 (slow release)	Theospan-SR (slow release)
Phenytex (extended release)	Theo-24 (slow release)
Plendil (slow release)	Theovent (slow release)
Prelu-2 (slow release)	Thorazine Spansules (slow release)
Prevacid, Prevacid SoluTab (delayed release)	Tiazac (sustained release)
Prilosec (slow release)	Topamax (taste)
Prilosec OTC (delayed release)	Toprol XL (extended release)
Pro-Banthine (taste)	T-Phyl (slow release)
Procanbid (slow release)	Trental (slow release)
Procardia (delayed absorption)	Trinalin Repetabs (slow release)
Procardia XL (slow release)	Tylenol Extended Relief (slow release)
Protonix (delayed release)	Uniphyl (slow release)
Proventil Repetabs (slow release)	Vantin (taste)
Prozac Weekly (slow release)	Verelan, Verelan PM (slow release)
Quibron T/SR (slow release)	Volmax (slow release)
Quinidex Extentabs (slow release)	Voltaren (enteric coated)
Respaire SR (slow release)	Voltaren-XR (extended release)
Respbid (slow release)	Wellbutrin SR (sustained release)
Risperdal M-Tab (delayed release)	Xanax XR (extended release)
Ritalin-LA, -SR (slow release)	Zerit XR (extended release)
Rondec-TR (slow release)	Zomig-ZMT (delayed release)
Sinemet CR (slow release)	ZORprin (slow release)
Slo-Bid Gyrocaps (slow release)	Zyban (slow release)
Slo-Niacin (slow release)	Zyrtec-D 12-hour (extended release)
Slo-Phyllin GG, Gyrocaps (slow release)	

Dialyzable drugs

The amount of a drug removed by dialysis differs among patients and depends on several factors, including the patient's condition, the drug's properties, length of dialysis and dialysate used, rate of blood flow or dwell time, and purpose of dialysis. This table shows the effect of hemodialysis on selected drugs.

Drug	Level reduced by hemodialysis
acetaminophen	Yes (may not affect toxicity)
acetazolamide	No
acyclovir	Yes
allopurinol	Yes
alprazolam	No
amikacin	Yes
amiodarone	No
amitriptyline	No
amlodipine	No
amoxicillin	Yes
amoxicillin and clavulanate potassium	Yes
amphotericin B	No
ampicillin	Yes
ampicillin and sulbactam sodium	Yes
aspirin	Yes
atenolol	Yes
azathioprine	Yes
aztreonam	Yes
captopril	Yes
carbamazepine	Yes
carbenicillin	Yes
carmustine	No
cefaclor	Yes
cefadroxil	Yes
cefamandole	Yes
cefazolin	Yes
cefepime	Yes
cefonicid	Yes (only by 20%)
cefoperazone	Yes
cefotaxime	Yes
cefotetan	Yes (only by 20%)
cefoxitin	Yes
cefpodoxime	Yes
ceftazidime	Yes
ceftibuten	Yes
ceftizoxime	Yes
ceftriaxone	No
cefuroxime	Yes
cephalexin	Yes
cephalothin	Yes
cephradine	Yes
chloral hydrate	Yes
chlorambucil	No
chloramphenicol	Yes (very small amount)
chlordiazepoxide	No
chloroquine	No
chlorpheniramine	No No
chlorpromazine	No
chlorthalidone	Yes
cimetidine	Yes
ciprofloxacin	Yes (only by 20%)
cisplatin	No
clindamycin	No
clofibrate	No
clonazepam	No
clonidine	No
clorazepate	No
cloxacillin	No
codeine	No
colchicine	No
cortisone	No

Dialyzable drugs *(continued)*

Drug	Level reduced by hemodialysis	Drug	Level reduced by hemodialysis
co-trimoxazole	Yes	glipizide	No
cyclophosphamide	Yes	glyburide	No
		guanfacine	No
diazepam	No	haloperidol	No
diazoxide	Yes	heparin	No
diclofenac	No	hydralazine	No
dicloxacillin	No	hydrochlorothiazide	No
didanosine	Yes		
digoxin	No	hydroxyzine	No
diltiazem	No	ibuprofen	No
diphenhydramine	No	imipenem and cilastatin	Yes
dipyridamole	No	imipramine	No
disopyramide	Yes	indapamide	No
doxazosin	No	indomethacin	No
doxepin	No	insulin	No
doxorubicin	No	irbesartan	No
doxycycline	No	iron dextran	No
enalapril	Yes	isoniazid	Yes
erythromycin	Yes (only by 20%)	isosorbide	Yes
ethacrynic acid	No	isradipine	No
ethambutol	Yes (only by 20%)	kanamycin	Yes
ethchlorvynol	Yes	ketoconazole	No
ethosuximide	Yes	ketoprofen	Yes
famciclovir	Yes	labetalol	No
famotidine	No	levofloxacin	No
fenoprofen	No	lidocaine	No
flecainide	No	lisinopril	Yes
fluconazole	Yes	lithium	Yes
flucytosine	Yes	lomefloxacin	No
fluorouracil	Yes	lomustine	No
fluoxetine	No	loracarbef	Yes
flurazepam	No	loratadine	No
foscarnet	Yes	lorazepam	No
fosinopril	No	mechlorethamine	No
furosemide	No		
gabapentin	Yes	mefenamic acid	No
ganciclovir	Yes	meperidine	No
gemfibrozil	No	mercaptopurine	Yes
gemifloxacin	Yes	meropenem	Yes
gentamicin	Yes	methadone	No

(continued)

Dialyzable drugs *(continued)*

Drug	Level reduced by hemodialysis	Drug	Level reduced by hemodialysis
methicillin	No	perindopril	Yes
methotrexate	Yes	phenobarbital	Yes
methyldopa	Yes	phenylbutazone	No
methylprednisolone	No	phenytoin	No
metoclopramide	No	piperacillin	Yes
metolazone	No	piperacillin and tazobactam	Yes
metoprolol	No	piroxicam	No
metronidazole	Yes	prazosin	No
mexiletine	Yes	prednisone	No
mezlocillin	Yes	primidone	Yes
miconazole	No	procainamide	Yes
midazolam	No	promethazine	No
minocycline	No	propoxyphene	No
minoxidil	Yes	propranolol	No
misoprostol	No	protriptyline	No
morphine	No	pyridoxine	Yes
nabumetone	No	quinapril	No
nadolol	Yes	quinidine	Yes
nafcillin	No	quinine	Yes
naproxen	No	ranitidine	Yes
nelfinavir	Yes	rifampin	No
netilmicin	Yes	rofecoxib	No
nifedipine	No	salsalate	Yes
nimodipine	No	sertraline	No
nitrofurantoin	Yes	sotalol	Yes
nitroglycerin	No	stavudine	Yes
nitroprusside	Yes	streptomycin	Yes
nizatidine	No	sucralfate	No
norfloxacin	No	sulbactam	Yes
nortriptyline	No	sulfamethoxazole	Yes
ofloxacin	Yes	sulindac	No
olanzapine	No	temazepam	No
omeprazole	No	theophylline	Yes
oxacillin	No	ticarcillin	Yes
oxazepam	No	ticarcillin and clavulanate	Yes
paroxetine	No	timolol	No
penicillin G	Yes		
pentamidine	No		
pentazocine	Yes		

Medications & I.V.s

Dialyzable drugs *(continued)*

Drug	Level reduced by hemodialysis	Drug	Level reduced by hemodialysis
tobramycin	Yes	valacyclovir	Yes
tocainide	Yes	valproic acid	No
tolbutamide	No	valsartan	No
topiramate	Yes	vancomycin	Yes
trazodone	No	verapamil	No
triazolam	No	warfarin	No
trimethoprim	Yes	zolpidem	No

Pharmacokinetics in older adults

Differences in the way older people absorb, distribute, metabolize, and eliminate drugs can alter the effects of medications. The age-related differences are listed below.

Absorption

- Change in quality and quantity of digestive enzymes
- Increased gastric pH
- Decreased number of absorbing cells
- Decreased GI motility
- Decreased intestinal blood flow
- Decreased GI emptying time

Distribution

- Decreased cardiac output and reserve
- Decreased blood flow to target tissues, liver, and kidneys
- Decreased distribution space and area
- Decreased lean body mass
- Increased adipose stores
- Decreased plasma protein (decreases protein-binding drugs)
- Decreased total body water

Metabolism

- Decreased microsomal metabolism of drug
- Decreased hepatic biotransformation

Elimination

- Decreased renal excretion of drug
- Decreased glomerular filtration
- Decreased renal tubular secretion

Drugs causing confusion in older adults

These drug classes can cause confusion in older adults:

- antiarrhythmics
- anticholinergics
- antiemetics
- antihistamines
- antihypertensives
- antiparkinsonian agents
- antipsychotics
- diuretics
- histamine blockers
- opioid analgesics
- sedative-hypnotics
- tranquilizers.

Medications associated with falls

This table highlights some classes of drugs that are commonly prescribed for older patients and the possible adverse effects of each that may increase a patient's risk of falling.

Drug class	Adverse effects
Alcohol	• Intoxication • Motor incoordination • Agitation • Sedation • Confusion
Antidiabetic drugs	• Acute hypoglycemia
Antihypertensives	• Hypotension
Antipsychotics	• Orthostatic hypotension • Muscle rigidity • Sedation
Benzodiazepines and antihistamines	• Excessive sedation • Confusion • Paradoxical agitation • Loss of balance
Diuretics	• Hypovolemia • Orthostatic hypotension • Electrolyte imbalance
Hypnotics	• Excessive sedation • Ataxia • Poor balance • Confusion • Paradoxical agitation
Opioids	• Hypotension • Sedation • Motor incoordination • Agitation
Tricyclic antidepressants	• Orthostatic hypotension

Adverse reactions misinterpreted as age-related changes

Some conditions result from aging, others from drug therapy; however, some can result from aging and drug therapy. This chart indicates drug classes and their associated adverse reactions.

	Adverse reactions					
Drug classifications	Agitation	Anxiety	Arrhythmias	Ataxia	Changes in appetite	Confusion
Alpha$_1$-adrenergic blockers		●				
Angiotensin-converting enzyme inhibitors						●
Antianginals	●	●	●			●
Antiarrhythmics			●			
Anticholinergics	●	●	●			●
Anticonvulsants	●		●	●	●	●
Antidepressants, tricyclic	●	●	●	●	●	●
Antidiabetics, oral						
Antihistamines					●	●
Antilipemics						
Antiparkinsonians	●	●		●	●	●
Antipsychotics	●	●	●	●	●	●
Barbiturates	●	●	●			●
Benzodiazepines	●			●		●
Beta-adrenergic blockers		●	●			
Calcium channel blockers		●	●			
Corticosteroids		●				●
Diuretics						●
Nonsteroidal anti-inflammatory drugs		●				●
Opioids	●	●				●
Skeletal muscle relaxants	●	●		●		●
Thyroid hormones			●		●	

Adverse reactions

	Constipation	Depression	Difficulty breathing	Disorientation	Dizziness	Drowsiness	Edema	Fatigue	Hypotension	Insomnia	Memory loss	Muscle weakness	Restlessness	Sexual dysfunction	Tremors	Urinary dysfunction	Vision changes
	●	●			●	●	●	●	●	●				●		●	●
	●	●			●			●	●	●				●			●
					●		●	●	●	●			●	●		●	●
	●		●		●		●	●	●								
	●	●		●	●	●		●	●		●	●	●			●	●
	●	●	●		●	●	●	●	●	●					●	●	●
	●		●	●	●	●		●	●	●			●	●	●	●	●
					●			●									
	●			●	●	●		●							●	●	●
	●				●			●		●		●		●		●	●
	●	●		●	●	●		●	●	●		●			●	●	●
	●	●			●	●		●	●	●			●	●	●	●	●
			●	●			●		●	●			●				
	●	●	●	●	●	●		●		●	●	●			●	●	●
		●	●		●			●	●		●			●	●	●	●
	●		●		●		●	●	●	●				●		●	●
		●					●	●		●		●					●
					●			●	●			●				●	
	●	●			●	●	●	●		●		●					●
	●	●	●	●	●	●		●	●	●	●		●	●		●	●
		●			●	●		●	●	●					●		
										●					●		

Preventing adverse drug reactions in older patients

A drug's action in the body and its interaction with body tissues (pharmacodynamics) change significantly in older people. In this chart, you'll find the information you need to help prevent adverse drug reactions in your older patients.

Pharmacology	Indications
Adrenergics, direct- and indirect-acting • Exert excitatory actions on the heart, glands, and vascular smooth muscle and peripheral inhibitory actions on smooth muscles of the bronchial tree	• Hypotension • Cardiac stimulation • Bronchodilation • Shock
Adrenocorticoids, systemic • Stimulate enzyme synthesis needed to decrease the inflammatory response	• Inflammation • Immunosuppression • Adrenal insufficiency • Rheumatic and collagen diseases • Acute spinal cord injury
Alpha-adrenergic blockers • Block the effects of peripheral neurohormonal transmitters (norepinephrine, epinephrine) on adrenergic receptors in various effector systems	• Peripheral vascular disorders • Hypertension • Benign prostatic hyperplasia
Aminoglycosides • Inhibit bacterial protein synthesis	• Infection caused by susceptible organisms
Angiotensin-converting enzyme (ACE) inhibitors • Prevent the conversion of angiotensin I to angiotensin II • Decrease vasoconstriction and adrenocortical secretion of aldosterone	• Hypertension • Heart failure

Special considerations

• An older patient may be more sensitive to therapeutic and adverse effects of some adrenergics and may require lower doses.

• These drugs may aggravate hyperglycemia, delay wound healing, or contribute to edema, insomnia, or osteoporosis in an older patient.
• Decreased metabolic rate and elimination may cause increased plasma levels and increase the risk of adverse effects. Monitor the older patient carefully.

• Hypotensive effects may be more pronounced in an older patient.
• These drugs should be administered at bedtime to reduce potential for dizziness or light-headedness.

• The older patient may have decreased renal function and thus be at greater risk for nephrotoxicity, ototoxicity, and superinfection (common).

• Diuretic therapy should be discontinued before ACE inhibitors are started to reduce the risk of hypotension.
• An older patient may need lower doses because of impaired drug clearance.

(continued)

Preventing adverse drug reactions in older patients *(continued)*

Pharmacology	Indications
Anticholinergics	
• Exert antagonistic action on acetylcholine and other cholinergic agonists within the parasympathetic nervous system	• Hypersecretory conditions • GI tract disorders • Sinus bradycardia • Dystonia and parkinsonism • Perioperative use • Motion sickness
Antihistamines	
• Prevent access and subsequent activity of histamine	• Allergy • Pruritus • Vertigo • Nausea and vomiting • Sedation • Cough suppression • Dyskinesia
Barbiturates	
• Decrease presynaptic and postsynaptic excitability, producing central nervous system (CNS) depression	• Seizure disorders • Sedation (including preanesthesia) • Hypnosis
Benzodiazepines	
• Act selectively on polysynaptic neuronal pathways throughout the CNS; synthetically produced sedative-hypnotic	• Seizure disorders • Anxiety, tension, insomnia • Surgical adjuncts for conscious sedation or amnesia • Skeletal muscle spasm, tremor
Beta-adrenergic blockers	
• Compete with beta agonists for available beta-receptor sites; individual agents differ in their ability to affect beta receptors	• Hypertension • Angina • Arrhythmias • Glaucoma • Myocardial infarction (MI) • Migraine prophylaxis

Special considerations

- These drugs should be used cautiously in an older adult, who may be more sensitive to the effects of these drugs; a lower dosage may be indicated.

- An older patient is usually more sensitive to the adverse effects of antihistamines; he's especially likely to experience a greater degree of dizziness, sedation, hypotension, and urine retention.

- An older patient and a patient receiving subhypnotic doses may experience hyperactivity, excitement, or hyperanalgesia. Use with caution.

- These drugs should be used cautiously in an older patient, who's sensitive to the drugs' CNS effects; parenteral administration is more likely to cause apnea, hypotension, bradycardia, and cardiac arrest.

- Increased bioavailability or delayed metabolism in the older patient may require a lower dosage; an older patient may also experience enhanced adverse effects.

(continued)

Preventing adverse drug reactions in older patients *(continued)*

Pharmacology	Indications
Calcium channel blockers	
• Inhibit calcium influx across the slow channels of myocardial and vascular smooth muscle cells, causing dilation of coronary arteries, peripheral arteries, and arterioles and slowing cardiac conduction	• Angina • Arrhythmias • Hypertension
Cardiac glycosides	
• Directly increase myocardial contractile force and velocity, atrioventricular node refractory period, and total peripheral resistance • Indirectly depress sinoatrial node and prolong conduction to the atrioventricular node	• Heart failure • Arrhythmias • Paroxysmal atrial tachycardia or atrioventricular junctional rhythm • MI • Cardiogenic shock • Angina
Cephalosporins	
• Inhibit bacterial cell wall synthesis, causing rapid cell lysis	• Infection caused by susceptible organisms
Coumadin derivatives	
• Interfere with the hepatic synthesis of vitamin K–dependent clotting factors II, VII, IX, and X, decreasing the blood's coagulation potential	• Treatment for or prevention of thrombosis or embolism
Diuretics, loop	
• Inhibit sodium and chloride reabsorption in the ascending loop of Henle and increase excretion of potassium, sodium, chloride, and water	• Edema • Hypertension
Diuretics, potassium-sparing	
• Act directly on the distal renal tubules, inhibiting sodium reabsorption and potassium excretion	• Edema • Hypertension • Diagnosis of primary hyperaldosteronism

Special considerations

• These drugs should be used cautiously in an older patient because the half-life of calcium channel blockers may be increased as a result of decreased clearance.

• These drugs should be used cautiously in an older patient with renal or hepatic dysfunction or with electrolyte imbalance that may predispose him to toxicity.

• Because the older patient commonly has impaired renal function, he may require a lower dosage.
• An older patient is more susceptible to superinfection and coagulopathies.

• An older patient has an increased risk of hemorrhage because of altered hemostatic mechanisms or age-related hepatic and renal deterioration.

• An older or debilitated patient is more susceptible to drug-induced diuresis and can quickly develop dehydration, hypovolemia, hypokalemia, and hyponatremia, which may cause circulatory collapse.

• An older patient may need a smaller dosage because of his susceptibility to drug-induced diuresis and hyperkalemia.

(continued)

Preventing adverse drug reactions in older patients *(continued)*

Pharmacology	Indications
Diuretics, thiazide and thiazide-like	
• Interfere with sodium transport, thereby increasing renal excretion of sodium, chloride, water, potassium, and calcium	• Edema • Hypertension • Diabetes insipidus
Estrogens	
• Promote development and maintenance of the female reproductive system and secondary sexual characteristics; inhibition of the release of pituitary gonadotropins	• Moderate to severe vasomotor symptoms of menopause • Atrophic vaginitis • Carcinoma of the breast and prostate • Prophylaxis of postmenopausal osteoporosis
Histamine-2 (H_2) receptor antagonists	
• Inhibit histamine's action at H_2 receptors in gastric parietal cells, reducing gastric acid output and concentration, regardless of the stimulatory agent or basal conditions	• Duodenal ulcer • Gastric ulcer • Hypersecretory states • Reflux esophagitis • Stress ulcer prophylaxis
Insulin	
• Increases glucose transport across muscle and fat-cell membranes to reduce blood glucose levels • Promotes conversion of glucose to glycogen • Stimulates amino acid uptake and conversion to protein in muscle cells • Inhibits protein degradation • Stimulates triglyceride formation and lipoprotein lipase activity; inhibits free fatty acid release from adipose tissue	• Diabetic ketoacidosis • Diabetes mellitus • Diabetes mellitus inadequately controlled by diet and oral antidiabetic agents • Hyperkalemia
Iron supplements, oral	
• Are needed in adequate amounts for erythropoiesis and efficient oxygen transport; essential component of hemoglobin	• Iron deficiency anemia

Special considerations

- Age-related changes in cardiovascular and renal function make the older patient more susceptible to excessive diuresis, which may lead to dehydration, hypovolemia, hyponatremia, hypomagnesemia, and hypokalemia.

- A postmenopausal woman on long-term estrogen therapy has an increased risk of developing endometrial cancer.

- These drugs should be used cautiously in an older patient because of his increased risk of developing adverse reactions, particularly those affecting the CNS.

- Insulin is available in many forms that differ in onset, peak, and duration of action; the physician will specify the individual dosage and form.
- Blood glucose measurement is an important guide to dosage and management.
- The older patient's diet and his ability to recognize hypoglycemia are important.
- A source of diabetic teaching should be provided, especially for the older patient, who may need follow-up home care.

- Iron-induced constipation is common among older patients; stress proper diet to minimize constipation.
- An older patient may also need higher doses due to reduced gastric secretions and because achlorhydria may lower his capacity for iron absorption.

(continued)

Medications & I.V.s

Preventing adverse drug reactions in older patients *(continued)*

Pharmacology	Indications
Nitrates • Relax smooth muscle; generally used for vascular effects (vasodilation)	• Angina pectoris • Acute MI
Nonsteriodal anti-inflammatory drugs (NSAIDs) • Interfere with prostaglandins involved with pain; anti-inflammatory action that contributes to analgesic effect	• Pain • Inflammation • Fever
Opioid agonists • Act at specific opiate receptor–binding sites in the CNS and other tissues; alteration of pain perception without affecting other sensory functions	• Analgesia • Pulmonary edema • Preoperative sedation • Anesthesia • Cough suppression • Diarrhea
Opioid agonists-antagonists • Act, in theory, on different opiate receptors in the CNS to a greater or lesser degree, thus yielding slightly different effects	• Pain
Opioid antagonists • Act differently, depending on whether an opioid agonist has been administered previously, the actions of that opioid, and the extent of physical dependence on it	• Opioid-induced respiratory depression • Adjunct in treating opiate addiction
Penicillins • Inhibit bacterial cell-wall synthesis, causing rapid cell lysis; most effective against fast-growing susceptible organisms	• Infection caused by susceptible organisms

Special considerations

- Severe hypotension and cardiovascular collapse may occur if nitrates are combined with alcohol.
- Transient dizziness, syncope, or other signs of cerebral ischemia may occur; instruct the older patient to take nitrates while sitting.

- A patient older than age 60 may be more susceptible to the toxic effects of NSAIDs because of decreased renal function; these drugs' effects on renal prostaglandins may cause fluid retention and edema, a drawback for a patient with heart failure.

- Lower doses are usually indicated for older patients, who tend to be more sensitive to the therapeutic and adverse effects of these drugs.

- Lower doses may be indicated in patients with renal or hepatic dysfunction to prevent drug accumulation.

- These drugs are contraindicated for opioid addicts, in whom they may produce an acute abstinence syndrome.

- An older patient (and others with low resistance from immunosuppressants or radiation therapy) should be taught the signs and symptoms of bacterial and fungal superinfection.

(continued)

Preventing adverse drug reactions in older patients *(continued)*

Pharmacology	Indications
Phenothiazines • Believed to function as dopamine antagonists, blocking postsynaptic dopamine receptors in various parts of the CNS; antiemetic effects resulting from blockage of the chemoreceptor trigger zones	• Psychosis • Nausea and vomiting • Anxiety • Severe behavior problems • Tetanus • Porphyria • Intractable hiccups • Neurogenic pain • Allergies and pruritus
Salicylates • Decrease formation of prostaglandins involved in pain and inflammation	• Pain • Inflammation • Fever
Serotonin-reuptake inhibitors • Inhibit reuptake of serotonin; have little or no effect on other neurotransmitters	• Major depression • Obsessive-compulsive disorder • Bulimia nervosa
Sulfonamides • Inhibit folic acid biosynthesis needed for cell growth	• Bacterial and parasitic infections • Inflammation
Tetracyclines • Inhibit bacterial protein synthesis	• Bacterial, protozoal, rickettsial, and fungal infections • Sclerosing agent
Thrombolytic enzymes • Convert plasminogen to plasmin for promotion of clot lysis	• Thrombosis, thromboembolism

Special considerations

- An older patient needs a lower dosage because he's more sensitive to these drugs' therapeutic and adverse effects, especially cardiac toxicity, tardive dyskinesia, and other extrapyramidal effects.
- Dosage should be titrated to patient response.

- A patient older than age 60 with impaired renal function may be more susceptible to these drugs' toxic effects.
- The effect of salicylates on renal prostaglandins may cause fluid retention and edema, a significant disadvantage for a patient with heart failure.

- These drugs should be used cautiously in a patient with hepatic impairment.

- These drugs should be used cautiously in an older patient, who's more susceptible to bacterial and fungal superinfection, folate deficiency anemia, and renal and hematologic effects because of diminished renal function.

- Some older patients have decreased esophageal motility; administer tetracyclines with caution and monitor for local irritation from slowly passing oral forms.

- Patients age 75 and older are at greater risk for cerebral hemorrhage because they're more apt to have preexisting cerebrovascular disease.

(continued)

Preventing adverse drug reactions in older patients *(continued)*

Pharmacology	Indications
Thyroid hormones	
• Have catabolic and anabolic effects • Influence normal metabolism, growth and development, and every organ system; vital to normal CNS function	• Hypothyroidism • Nontoxic goiter • Thyrotoxicosis • Diagnostic use
Thyroid hormones antagonists	
• Inhibit iodine oxidation in the thyroid gland through a block of iodine's ability to combine with tyrosine to form thyroxine	• Hyperthyroidism • Preparation for thyroidectomy • Thyrotoxic crisis • Thyroid carcinoma
Tricyclic antidepressants	
• Inhibit neurotransmitter reuptake, resulting in increased concentration and enhanced activity of neurotransmitters in the synaptic cleft	• Depression • Obsessive-compulsive disorder • Enuresis • Severe, chronic pain

Special considerations

- In a patient older than age 60, the initial hormone replacement dose should be 25% less than the recommended dose.

- Serum thyroid stimulating hormone should be monitored as a sensitive indicator of thyroid hormone levels. Dosage adjustment may be required.

- Lower doses are indicated in an older patient because he's more sensitive to both the therapeutic and adverse effects of tricyclic antidepressants.

Therapeutic drug monitoring guidelines

Drug	Laboratory test monitored	Therapeutic ranges of test
Aminoglycoside antibiotics (amikacin, gentamicin, tobramycin)	Amikacin peak Amikacin trough Gentamicin/ tobramycin peak Gentamicin/ tobramycin trough Creatinine	20 to 30 mcg/ml 1 to 8 mcg/ml 4 to 12 mcg/ml < 2 mcg/ml 0.6 to 1.3 mg/dl
Angiotensin-converting enzyme inhibitors (benazepril, captopril, enalapril, enalaprilat, fosinopril, lisinopril, moexipril, quinapril, ramipril, trandolapril)	White blood cell (WBC) count with differential Creatinine Blood urea nitrogen (BUN) Potassium	***** 0.6 to 1.3 mg/dl 5 to 20 mg/dl 3.5 to 5 mEq/L
Amphotericin B	Creatinine BUN Electrolytes (especially potassium and magnesium) Liver function Complete blood count (CBC) with differential and platelets	0.6 to 1.3 mg/dl 5 to 20 mg/dl Potassium: 3.5 to 5 mEq/L Magnesium: 1.5 to 2.5 mEq/L Sodium: 135 to 145 mEq/L Chloride: 98 to 106 mEq/L * *****

Note: ***** For those areas marked with asterisks, the following values can be used:

Hemoglobin: Women: 12 to 16 g/dl; Men: 13 to 18 g/dl
Hematocrit: Women 37% to 48%; Men: 42% to 52%
Red blood cell count (RBC): 4 to 5.5 × 10^6/mm^3
WBC count: 5 to 10 × 10^3/mm^3
Differential: Neutrophils: 45% to 74%
Bands: 0% to 8%
Lymphocytes: 16% to 45%
Monocytes: 4% to 10%
Eosinophils: 0% to 7%
Basophils: 0% to 2%

Medications & I.V.s

Monitoring guidelines

Wait until administering third dose to check drug levels. Obtain blood for peak level 30 minutes after I.V. infusion ends or 60 minutes after I.M. administration. For trough levels, draw blood just before next dose. Dosage may need to be adjusted accordingly. Recheck after three doses. Monitor creatinine and BUN levels and urine output for signs of decreasing renal function. Monitor urine for increased proteins, cells, and casts.

Monitor WBC count with differential before therapy, monthly during first 3 to 6 months, and then periodically for first year. Monitor renal function and potassium level periodically.

Monitor creatinine, BUN, and electrolyte levels at least weekly during therapy. Monitor blood counts and liver function test results regularly during therapy.

(continued)

* For those areas marked with an asterisk, the following values can be used:
Alanine aminotransferase: 7 to 56 units/L
Aspartate aminotransferase: 5 to 40 units/L
Alkaline phosphatase: 17 to 142 units/L
Lactate dehydrogenase: 60 to 220 units/L
Gamma glutamyl transferase (GGT): < 40 units/L
Total bilirubin: 0.2 to 1 mg/dl

Therapeutic drug monitoring guidelines *(continued)*

Drug	Laboratory test monitored	Therapeutic ranges of test
Antibiotics	WBC with differential Cultures and sensitivities	*****
Biguanides (metformin)	Creatinine Fasting glucose Glycosylated hemoglobin CBC	0.6 to 1.3 mg/dl 70 to 110 mg/dl 5.5% to 8.5% of total hemoglobin *****
Carbamazepine	Carbamazepine CBC with differential Liver function BUN Platelet count	4 to 12 mcg/ml ***** * 5 to 20 mg/dl 150 to 450 × $10^3/mm^3$
Clozapine	WBC with differential	*****
Corticosteroids (cortisone, hydrocortisone, prednisone, prednisolone, triamcinolone, methylprednisolone, dexamethasone, betamethasone)	Electrolytes (especially potassium) Fasting glucose	Potassium: 3.5 to 5 mEq/L Magnesium: 1.7 to 2.1 mEq/L Sodium: 135 to 145 mEq/L Chloride: 98 to 106 mEq/L Calcium: 8.6 to 10 mg/dl 70 to 110 mg/dl

Note: ***** For those areas marked with asterisks, the following values can be used:

Hemoglobin: Women: 12 to 16 g/dl; Men: 13 to 18 g/dl
Hematocrit: Women 37% to 48%; Men: 42% to 52%
Red blood cell count (RBC): 4 to 5.5 × $10^6/mm^3$
WBC count: 5 to 10 × $10^3/mm^3$
Differential: Neutrophils: 45% to 74%
Bands: 0% to 8%
Lymphocytes: 16% to 45%
Monocytes: 4% to 10%
Eosinophils: 0% to 7%
Basophils: 0% to 2%

Monitoring guidelines

Results of specimen cultures and sensitivities will determine cause of infection and best treatment. Monitor WBC count with differential weekly during therapy.

Check renal function and hematologic values before starting therapy and at least annually thereafter. If patient has impaired renal function, don't use metformin because it may cause lactic acidosis. Monitor response to therapy by evaluating fasting glucose and glycosylated hemoglobin levels periodically. A patient's home monitoring of glucose levels helps monitor compliance and response.

Monitor blood counts and platelet count before therapy, monthly during first 2 months, and then yearly. Liver function, BUN, and urinalysis results should be checked before and periodically during therapy.

Obtain WBC count with differential before starting therapy, weekly during therapy, and 4 weeks after discontinuing drug.

Monitor electrolyte and glucose levels regularly during long-term therapy.

(continued)

* For those areas marked with an asterisk, the following values can be used:
Alanine aminotransferase: 7 to 56 units/L
Aspartate aminotransferase: 5 to 40 units/L
Alkaline phosphatase: 17 to 142 units/L
Lactate dehydrogenase: 60 to 220 units/L
Gamma glutamyl transferase (GGT): < 40 units/L
Total bilirubin: 0.2 to 1 mg/dl

Therapeutic drug monitoring guidelines *(continued)*

Drug	Laboratory test monitored	Therapeutic ranges of test
Digoxin	Digoxin	0.8 to 2 ng/ml
	Electrolytes (especially potassium, magnesium, and calcium)	Potassium: 3.5 to 5 mEq/L Magnesium: 1.7 to 2.1 mEq/L Sodium: 135 to 145 mEq/L Chloride: 98 to 106 mEq/L Calcium: 8.6 to 10 mg/dl
	Creatinine	0.6 to 1.3 mg/dl
Diuretics	Electrolytes	Potassium: 3.5 to 5 mEq/L Magnesium: 1.7 to 2.1 mEq/L Sodium: 135 to 145 mEq/L Chloride: 98 to 106 mEq/L Calcium: 8.6 to 10 mg/dl
	Creatinine	0.6 to 1.3 mg/dl
	BUN	5 to 20 mg/dl
	Uric acid	2 to 7 mg/dl
	Fasting glucose	70 to 110 mg/dl
Erythropoietin	Hematocrit	Women: 36% to 48% Men: 42% to 52%
	Serum ferritin	10 to 383 mg/ml
	Transferrin saturation	220 to 400 mg/dl
	CBC with differential	*****
	Platelet count	150 to 450 $\times$ 10^3/mm^3
Ethosuximide	Ethosuximide	40 to 100 mcg/ml
	Liver function	*
	CBC with differential	*****
Gemfibrozil	Lipids	Total cholesterol: < 200 mg/dl Low-density lipoprotein (LDL): < 130 mg/dl

Note: ***** For those areas marked with asterisks, the following values can be used:

Hemoglobin: Women: 12 to 16 g/dl; Men: 13 to 18 g/dl
Hematocrit: Women 37% to 48%; Men: 42% to 52%
Red blood cell count (RBC): 4 to 5.5 $\times$ 10^6/mm^3
WBC count: 5 to 10 $\times$ 10^3/mm^3
Differential: Neutrophils: 45% to 74%
Bands: 0% to 8%
Lymphocytes: 16% to 45%
Monocytes: 4% to 10%
Eosinophils: 0% to 7%
Basophils: 0% to 2%

Medications & I.V.s

Monitoring guidelines
Check digoxin levels just before next dose or minimum of 6 to 8 hours after last dose. To monitor maintenance therapy, check drug levels at least 1 to 2 weeks after therapy is initiated or changed. Adjust therapy based on entire clinical picture, not solely based on drug levels. Also, check electrolyte levels and renal function periodically during therapy.
To monitor fluid and electrolyte balance, perform baseline and periodic determinations of electrolyte, calcium, BUN, uric acid, and glucose levels.
After therapy is initiated or changed, monitor hematocrit twice weekly for 2 to 6 weeks until it's stabilized in target range and maintenance dose is determined. Monitor hematocrit regularly thereafter.
Check drug level 8 to 10 days after therapy is initiated or changed. Periodically monitor CBC with differential and results of liver function tests and urinalysis.
Therapy is usually withdrawn after 3 months if response is inadequate.

(continued)

* For those areas marked with an asterisk, the following values can be used:
Alanine aminotransferase: 7 to 56 units/L
Aspartate aminotransferase: 5 to 40 units/L
Alkaline phosphatase: 17 to 142 units/L
Lactate dehydrogenase: 60 to 220 units/L
Gamma glutamyl transferase (GGT): < 40 units/L
Total bilirubin: 0.2 to 1 mg/dl

Therapeutic drug monitoring guidelines *(continued)*

Drug	Laboratory test monitored	Therapeutic ranges of test
Gemfibrozil *(continued)*		High-density lipoprotein (HDL): Women: 40 to 75 mg/dl Men: 37 to 70 mg/dl Triglycerides: 10 to 160 mg/dl
	Liver function	*
	Serum glucose	70 to 100 mg/dl
	CBC	*****
Heparin	Partial thromboplastin time (PTT)	1.5 to 2.5 times control
	Hematocrit	*****
	Platelet count	150 to 450 × 10^3/mm^3
3-hydroxy-3-methylglutaryl coenzyme A reductase inhibitors (fluvastatin, lovastatin, pravastatin, simvastatin)	Lipids	Total cholesterol: < 200 mg/dl LDL: < 130 mg/dl HDL: Women: 40 to 75 mg/dl Men: 37 to 70 mg/dl Triglycerides: 10 to 160 mg/dl
	Liver function	*
Insulin	Fasting glucose	70 to 110 mg/dl
	Glycosylated hemoglobin	5.5% to 8.5% of total hemoglobin
Isotretinoin	Pregnancy test	Negative
	Liver function	*

Note: ***** For those areas marked with asterisks, the following values can be used:

Hemoglobin: Women: 12 to 16 g/dl; Men: 13 to 18 g/dl
Hematocrit: Women 37% to 48%; Men: 42% to 52%
Red blood cell count (RBC): 4 to 5.5 × 10^6/mm^3
WBC count: 5 to 10 × 10^3/mm^3
Differential: Neutrophils: 45% to 74%
Bands: 0% to 8%
Lymphocytes: 16% to 45%
Monocytes: 4% to 10%
Eosinophils: 0% to 7%
Basophils: 0% to 2%

Monitoring guidelines

The patient must be fasting to measure triglyceride levels. Obtain blood counts periodically during first 12 months.

When drug is given by continuous I.V. infusion, check PTT every 4 hours in early stages of therapy and daily thereafter. When drug is given by deep subcutaneous injection, check PTT 4 to 6 hours after injection and daily thereafter.

Perform liver function tests at baseline, 6 to 12 weeks after therapy is initiated or changed, and approximately every 6 months thereafter. If adequate response isn't achieved within 6 weeks, consider changing therapy.

Monitor response to therapy by evaluating glucose and glycosylated hemoglobin levels. Glycosylated hemoglobin level is a good measure of long-term control. A patient's home monitoring of glucose levels helps measure compliance and response.

Use serum or urine pregnancy test with sensitivity of at least 25 international units/ml. Perform one test before therapy and a second test during second day of menstrual cycle before therapy begins or at least

(continued)

* For those areas marked with an asterisk, the following values can be used:
Alanine aminotransferase: 7 to 56 units/L
Aspartate aminotransferase: 5 to 40 units/L
Alkaline phosphatase: 17 to 142 units/L
Lactate dehydrogenase: 60 to 220 units/L
Gamma glutamyl transferase (GGT): < 40 units/L
Total bilirubin: 0.2 to 1 mg/dl

Therapeutic drug monitoring guidelines *(continued)*

Drug	Laboratory test monitored	Therapeutic ranges of test
Isotretinoin *(continued)*	Lipids	Total cholesterol: < 200 mg/dl LDL: < 130 mg/dl HDL: Women: 40 to 75 mg/dl Men: 37 to 70 mg/dl Triglycerides: 10 to 160 mg/dl
	CBC with differential	*****
	Platelet count	150 to 450 × $10^3/mm^3$
Linezolid	CBC with differential and platelets	*****
	Cultures and sensitivities	
	Platelet count	150 to 450 × $10^3/mm^3$
	Liver function	*
	Amylase	35 to 118 international units/L
	Lipase	10 to 150 units/L
Lithium	Lithium	0.6 to 1.2 mEq/L
	Creatinine	0.6 to 1.3 mg/dl
	CBC	*****
	Electrolytes (especially potassium and sodium)	Potassium: 3.5 to 5 mEq/L Magnesium: 1.7 to 2.1 mEq/L Sodium: 135 to 145 mEq/L Chloride: 98 to 106 mEq/L
	Fasting glucose	70 to 110 mg/dl
	Thyroid function tests	Thyroid-stimulating hormone (TSH): 0.2 to 5.4 microunits/ml Triiodothyronine (T_3): 80 to 200 ng/dl Thyroxine(T_4): 5.4 to 11.5 mcg/dl

Note: ***** For those areas marked with asterisks, the following values can be used:

Hemoglobin: Women: 12 to 16 g/dl; Men: 13 to 18 g/dl
Hematocrit: Women 37% to 48%; Men: 42% to 52%
Red blood cell count (RBC): 4 to 5.5 × $10^6/mm^3$
WBC count: 5 to 10 × $10^3/mm^3$
Differential: Neutrophils: 45% to 74%
Bands: 0% to 8%
Lymphocytes: 16% to 45%
Monocytes: 4% to 10%
Eosinophils: 0% to 7%
Basophils: 0% to 2%

Monitoring guidelines

11 days after the last unprotected act of sexual intercourse, whichever is later. Repeat pregnancy tests monthly. Obtain baseline liver function tests and lipid levels; repeat every 1 to 2 weeks until a response is established (usually 4 weeks).

Obtain baseline CBC with differential and platelet count. Repeat weekly, especially if patient receives more than 2 weeks of therapy. Monitor liver function test results and amylase and lipase levels during therapy.

Checking lithium levels is crucial to safe use of the drug. Obtain lithium levels immediately before next dose. Monitor levels twice weekly until they are stable. When at a steady state, levels should be checked weekly; when the patient is receiving the appropriate maintenance dose, levels should be checked every 2 to 3 months. Monitor creatinine, electrolyte, and fasting glucose levels; CBC; and thyroid function test results before therapy is initiated and periodically during therapy.

(continued)

* For those areas marked with an asterisk, the following values can be used:
Alanine aminotransferase: 7 to 56 units/L
Aspartate aminotransferase: 5 to 40 units/L
Alkaline phosphatase: 17 to 142 units/L
Lactate dehydrogenase: 60 to 220 units/L
Gamma glutamyl transferase (GGT): < 40 units/L
Total bilirubin: 0.2 to 1 mg/dl

Therapeutic drug monitoring guidelines *(continued)*

Drug	Laboratory test monitored	Therapeutic ranges of test
Methotrexate	Methotrexate	Normal elimination: ~ 10 micromol 24 hours postdose ~ 1 micromol 48 hours postdose < 0.2 micromol 72 hours postdose
	CBC with differential	*****
	Platelet count	150 to 450 × $10^3/mm^3$
	Liver function	*
	Creatinine	0.6 to 1.3 mg/dl
Nonnucleoside reverse transcriptase inhibitors (nevirapine, delavirdine, efavirenz)	Liver function	*
	CBC with differential and platelets	*****
	Lipids (efavirenz)	Total cholesterol: < 200 mg/dl LDL: < 130 mg/dl HDL: Women: 40 to 75 mg/dl Men: 37 to 70 mg/dl Triglycerides: 10 to 160 mg/dl
	Amylase	35 to 118 international units/L
Phenytoin	Phenytoin	10 to 20 mcg/ml
	CBC	*****

Note: ***** For those areas marked with asterisks, the following values can be used:

Hemoglobin: Women: 12 to 16 g/dl; Men: 13 to 18 g/dl
Hematocrit: Women 37% to 48%; Men: 42% to 52%
Red blood cell count (RBC): 4 to 5.5 × $10^6/mm^3$
WBC count: 5 to 10 × $10^3/mm^3$
Differential: Neutrophils: 45% to 74%
Bands: 0% to 8%
Lymphocytes: 16% to 45%
Monocytes: 4% to 10%
Eosinophils: 0% to 7%
Basophils: 0% to 2%

Monitoring guidelines

Monitor methotrexate levels according to dosing protocol. Monitor CBC with differential, platelet count, and liver and renal function test results more frequently when therapy is initiated or changed and when methotrexate levels may be elevated, such as when the patient is dehydrated.

Obtain baseline liver function tests and monitor results closely during first 12 weeks of therapy. Continue to monitor them regularly during therapy. Check CBC with differential and platelet count before therapy and periodically during therapy. Monitor lipid levels during efavirenz therapy. Monitor amylase level during efavirenz and delavirdine therapy.

Monitor phenytoin levels immediately before next dose and 7 to 10 days after therapy is initiated or changed. Obtain CBC at baseline and monthly early in therapy. Watch for toxic effects at therapeutic levels. Adjust measured level for hypoalbuminemia or renal impairment, which can increase free drug levels.

(continued)

* For those areas marked with an asterisk, the following values can be used:
Alanine aminotransferase: 7 to 56 units/L
Aspartate aminotransferase: 5 to 40 units/L
Alkaline phosphatase: 17 to 142 units/L
Lactate dehydrogenase: 60 to 220 units/L
Gamma glutamyl transferase (GGT): < 40 units/L
Total bilirubin: 0.2 to 1 mg/dl

Therapeutic drug monitoring guidelines *(continued)*

Drug	Laboratory test monitored	Therapeutic ranges of test
Potassium chloride	Potassium	3.5 to 5 mEq/L
Procainamide	Procainamide	3 to 10 mcg/ml (procainamide)
	N-acetylprocainamide (NAPA)	10 to 30 mcg/ml (combined procainamide and NAPA)
	CBC	*****
	Liver function	*
	Antinuclear antibody titer	Negative
Protease inhibitors (amprenavir, indinavir, lopinavir, nelfinavir, ritonavir, saquinavir)	Fasting glucose	70 to 110 mg/dl
	Liver function	*
	CBC with differential	*****
	Lipids	Total cholesterol: < 200 mg/dl LDL: < 130 mg/dl HDL: Women: 40 to 75 mg/dl Men: 37 to 70 mg/dl Triglycerides: 10 to 160 mg/dl
	Amylase	35 to 118 international units/L
	Creatine kinase (CK)	Women: 20 to 170 international units/L Men: 30 to 220 international units/L

Note: ***** For those areas marked with asterisks, the following values can be used:

Hemoglobin: Women: 12 to 16 g/dl; Men: 13 to 18 g/dl
Hematocrit: Women 37% to 48%; Men: 42% to 52%
Red blood cell count (RBC): 4 to 5.5 × 10^6/mm^3
WBC count: 5 to 10 × 10^3/mm^3
Differential: Neutrophils: 45% to 74%
Bands: 0% to 8%
Lymphocytes: 16% to 45%
Monocytes: 4% to 10%
Eosinophils: 0% to 7%
Basophils: 0% to 2%

Medications & I.V.s

Monitoring guidelines

After oral replacement therapy is initiated, check level weekly until it's stable and every 3 to 6 months thereafter.

Measure procainamide levels 6 to 12 hours after continuous infusion is started or immediately before next oral dose. Combined (procainamide and NAPA) levels can be used as an index of toxicity in patients with renal impairment. Obtain a CBC periodically during longer-term therapy.

Obtain baseline glucose level, liver function test results, CBC with differential, and lipid, CK, and amylase levels. Monitor during therapy.

(continued)

* For those areas marked with an asterisk, the following values can be used:
Alanine aminotransferase: 7 to 56 units/L
Aspartate aminotransferase: 5 to 40 units/L
Alkaline phosphatase: 17 to 142 units/L
Lactate dehydrogenase: 60 to 220 units/L
Gamma glutamyl transferase (GGT): < 40 units/L
Total bilirubin: 0.2 to 1 mg/dl

Therapeutic drug monitoring guidelines *(continued)*

Drug	Laboratory test monitored	Therapeutic ranges of test
Quinidine	Quinidine CBC Liver function Creatinine Electrolytes (especially potassium)	2 to 6 mcg/ml ***** * 0.6 to 1.3 mg/dl Potassium: 3.5 to 5 mEq/L Magnesium: 1.7 to 2.1 mEq/L Sodium: 135 to 145 mEq/L Chloride: 98 to 106 mEq/L
Sulfonylureas	Fasting glucose Glycosylated hemoglobin	70 to 110 mg/dl 4% to 7% of total hemoglobin
Theophylline	Theophylline	10 to 20 mcg/ml
Thiazolidinediones (rosiglitazone, pioglitazone)	Fasting glucose Glycosylated hemoglobin Liver function	70 to 110 mg/dl 4% to 7% of total hemoglobin *
Thyroid hormone	Thyroid function tests	TSH: 0.2 to 5.4 microunits/ml T_3: 80 to 200 ng/dl T_4: 5.4 to 11.5 mcg/dl
Valproate sodium, valproic acid, divalproex sodium	Valproic acid Liver function Ammonia PTT BUN Creatinine CBC with differential Platelet count	50 to 100 mcg/ml * 15 to 45 mcg/dl 10 to 14 seconds 5 to 20 mg/dl 0.6 to 1.3 mg/dl ***** 150 to 450 × 10^3/mm^3

Note: ***** For those areas marked with asterisks, the following values can be used:

Hemoglobin: Women: 12 to 16 g/dl; Men: 13 to 18 g/dl
Hematocrit: Women 37% to 48%; Men: 42% to 52%
Red blood cell count (RBC): 4 to 5.5 × 10^6/mm^3
WBC count: 5 to 10 × 10^3/mm^3
Differential: Neutrophils: 45% to 74%
Bands: 0% to 8%
Lymphocytes: 16% to 45%
Monocytes: 4% to 10%
Eosinophils: 0% to 7%
Basophils: 0% to 2%

Monitoring guidelines

Obtain levels immediately before next oral dose and 30 to 35 hours after therapy is initiated or changed. Obtain blood counts, liver and kidney function test results, and electrolyte levels periodically. With more specific assays, therapeutic levels are < 1 mcg/1 ml.

Monitor response to therapy by evaluating fasting glucose and glycosylated hemoglobin levels periodically. The patient should monitor glucose levels at home to help measure compliance and response.

Obtain theophylline levels immediately before next dose of sustained-release oral drug and at least 2 days after therapy is initiated or changed.

Monitor response by evaluating fasting glucose and glycosylated hemoglobin levels. Obtain baseline liver function test results, and repeat tests periodically during therapy.

Monitor thyroid function test results every 2 to 3 weeks until the appropriate maintenance dose is determined, and annually thereafter.

Monitor liver function test results, ammonia level, coagulation test results, renal function test results, CBC, and platelet count at baseline and periodically during therapy. Monitor liver function test results closely during first 6 months of therapy.

(continued)

* For those areas marked with an asterisk, the following values can be used:
Alanine aminotransferase: 7 to 56 units/L
Aspartate aminotransferase: 5 to 40 units/L
Alkaline phosphatase: 17 to 142 units/L
Lactate dehydrogenase: 60 to 220 units/L
Gamma glutamyl transferase (GGT): < 40 units/L
Total bilirubin: 0.2 to 1 mg/dl

Therapeutic drug monitoring guidelines *(continued)*

Drug	Laboratory test monitored	Therapeutic ranges of test
Vancomycin	Vancomycin Creatinine	20 to 40 mcg/ml (peak) 5 to 15 mcg/ml (trough) 0.6 to 1.3 mg/dl
Warfarin	International Normalized Ratio (INR)	For acute myocardial infarction, atrial fibrillation, treatment of pulmonary embolism, prevention of systemic embolism, tissue heart valves, valvular heart disease, or prophylaxis or treatment of venous thrombosis: 2 to 3 For mechanical prosthetic valves or recurrent systemic embolism: 3 to 4.5

Note: ***** For those areas marked with asterisks, the following values can be used:

Hemoglobin: Women: 12 to 16 g/dl; Men: 13 to 18 g/dl
Hematocrit: Women 37% to 48%; Men: 42% to 52%
Red blood cell count (RBC): 4 to 5.5 × 10^6/mm^3
WBC count: 5 to 10 × 10^3/mm^3
Differential: Neutrophils: 45% to 74%
Bands: 0% to 8%
Lymphocytes: 16% to 45%
Monocytes: 4% to 10%
Eosinophils: 0% to 7%
Basophils: 0% to 2%

Monitoring guidelines

Check vancomycin levels with third dose administered, at the earliest. Obtain peak levels 1½ to 2½ hours after a 1-hour infusion or when I.V. infusion is complete. Obtain trough levels within 1 hour of next dose administered. Renal function can be used to adjust dosing and intervals

Check INR daily, beginning 3 days after therapy is initiated. Continue checking it until therapeutic goal is achieved, and monitor it periodically thereafter. Also check levels 7 days after a change in warfarin dose or concomitant, potentially interacting therapy.Total bilirubin: 0.2 to 1 mg/dl.

* For those areas marked with an asterisk, the following values can be used:
Alanine aminotransferase: 7 to 56 units/L
Aspartate aminotransferase: 5 to 40 units/L
Alkaline phosphatase: 17 to 142 units/L
Lactate dehydrogenase: 60 to 220 units/L
Gamma glutamyl transferase (GGT): < 40 units/L
Total bilirubin: 0.2 to 1 mg/dl

Mixing insulins

When mixing insulin, always draw up clear insulin first, then cloudy. To mix insulins, follow these steps:

- Wipe the rubber top of the insulin vials with alcohol.
- Gently roll the cloudy insulin between your palms.
- Remove the needle cap.
- Pull out the plunger until the end of the plunger in the barrel aligns with the number of units of cloudy insulin that you need.
- Push the needle through the rubber top of the cloudy insulin bottle.
- Inject air into the bottle.
- Remove the needle.
- Pull out the plunger until the end of the plunger in the barrel aligns with the units of clear insulin that you need.
- Push the needle through the rubber top of the clear insulin bottle.
- Inject the air into the bottle.
- Without removing the needle, turn the bottle upside down.
- Withdraw the plunger until it aligns with the number of units of clear regular insulin that you need.
- Gently pull the needle out of the bottle.
- Push the needle into the cloudy insulin bottle without injecting the clear insulin into the bottle.
- Withdraw the plunger until you reach your total dosage of insulin in units (clear combined with cloudy).

Patient teaching

Applying learning domains to patient teaching

Understanding learning domains—cognitive, psychomotor, and affective—can make your teaching more precise and effective. By giving consideration to each domain as you prepare to teach, you'll be better able to identify what the patient needs and is ready to learn. This will help you develop effective teaching strategies and determine appropriate expected outcomes, which allow you to evaluate what the patient has actually learned.

Within each domain, learning can take place on several progressively complex levels. You'll want to assess what your patient is capable of understanding and what his functional ability is before targeting a specific level within a domain. The information below will help you identify the specific learning levels within each domain. (An example of a patient outcome is given for each level.)

Cognitive domain

Knowledge: Recalling information. *(The patient can identify signs and symptoms of hypoglycemia.)*
Comprehension: Understanding information and being able to draw conclusions. *(The patient can state the relationship between ostomy care and skin integrity.)*
Application: Adapting rules to specific problems. *(The patient uses sterile technique when giving himself a subcutaneous injection.)*
Analysis: Breaking down concepts into separate elements and identifying the relationships among them. *(The patient can distinguish cancer facts from myths.)*
Synthesis: Reassembling elements to create new concepts. *(The patient can use food exchange lists to develop weekly meal plans.)*
Evaluation: Appraising the value of material for a given purpose. *(The patient can judge the effectiveness of muscle relaxation to relieve stress.)*

Psychomotor domain

Perception: Becoming aware of stimuli through the senses. *(The patient can recognize the difference between a fast and slow pulse.)*
Set: Readiness for a specific action or experience. *(The patient correctly places his fingers over his wrist before taking his pulse.)*
Guided response: Performing a procedure. *(The patient changes his dressing correctly.)*
Mechanism: Learning a behavior to the point of habit. *(The patient can calibrate temperature with an oral glass thermometer without instruction.)*
Complex overt response: Performing a complex motor pattern. *(The patient can measure blood pressure accurately within 4 mm Hg of the expert's finding.)*

Applying learning domains to patient teaching
(continued)

Adaptation: Altering a motor response to solve new problems. *(The patient can adapt principles of applying a disposable colostomy pouch to applying a reusable pouch.)*

Affective domain

Receiving: Attending to and allowing continuation of a stimulus. *(The patient allows nongastric tube placement.)*

Responding: Reacting voluntarily to a stimulus. *(The patient cooperates with urinary catheter insertion.)*

Valuing: Accepting the preferred value of behavior to the point of acting it out. *(The patient accepts activity limitations that surgery has imposed.)*

Organization: Systematizing a behavior framework based on values. *(The patient organizes a schedule that includes relaxation time.)*

Value characterization: Expressing feelings that portray philosophy of life. *(The patient participates in a support group for cancer survivors.)*

Saving time for teaching

Teaching patients what they need to know is time-consuming—there's too much to cover and seldom enough time. This is especially true with critically ill patients; teaching is commonly delayed until they're more medically stable. Try the method below to make teaching effective, even when time is tight:

- List the patient's learning needs.
- Rank them: most important first, next most important second, and so on.
- Write your teaching to-do list based on this ranking.

This method helps you distinguish the patient's learning needs from his nursing care needs. It also helps you organize your time or quickly redirect your actions after an interruption.

To simplify ranking the patient's learning needs, classify each learning need as:

- *Immediate* (one that must be met promptly such as teaching the patient who's being discharged in 2 hours) or *long range*
- *Survival* (life-dependent such as teaching the warning signs of adrenal crisis) or *related to well-being* (good to know but not essential such as describing the effects of stress in cardiovascular disease)
- *Specific* (related to the patient's disorder, medication, or treatment such as preparing him for upcoming coronary artery bypass) or *general* (teaching that's done for every patient such as explaining hospital visiting hours).

After you have classified the patient's learning needs, establish priorities and gather available teaching materials.

Four steps to take before teaching

Follow these four steps to prepare for effective teaching. First, set teaching outcomes for your patient. Last, form a statement of his readiness, willingness, and ability to achieve those outcomes—your "teaching diagnosis." In between, collect and evaluate data. You may discover more areas for teaching based on what your patient and his family want to learn. If so, reassess, and modify your outcomes accordingly to create a workable teaching plan.

1. Set teaching outcomes.

- What must the patient learn?
- What does the health care team want him to learn?
- When should teaching occur?

2. Collect data.

- What do patient and family interviews tell you about learning needs, outcomes, and response?
- What does the patient's chart reveal?
- What information can the health care team give?
- How does the patient learn best?

3. Evaluate data.

- What does the patient want to learn?
- Do his goals conflict with his family's or the health care team's goals?
- Determine learning barriers, such as language or literacy level.
- What factors can promote learning?
- Does the patient use the Internet to access information?

4. Establish a teaching diagnosis.

- What is the patient ready, willing, and able to learn?
- Do the patient, his family, and health care team confirm your findings?
- Do you need to set new teaching outcomes?

Teaching tips

You can make your teaching more effective if you give careful thought to the words you choose and the way you organize your teaching points. These tips can help:

Word choice

- Use language appropriate to your patient's age, educational level, cultural background, and language ability. Select simple words with few syllables, make your sentences short, and use action verbs.
- Express complex medical and scientific concepts in layman's terms. Use analogies to make your meaning clear. Whenever possible, avoid complex clinical terms and abbreviations.
- Choose specific rather than general words when giving instructions. This applies particularly to directions for the patient's medications and self-care.

Organization

- To enhance clarity, break your information into large, distinct categories. You might say to the patient, "I have three important things to tell you. Number one is…" This is a good teaching technique whether you're in the patient's room or in a lecture room.
- Use examples and hypothetical cases to humanize your teaching.
- State your most important points first and last. Commonly, the first and last points are remembered best.
- Repeat important points, and don't be afraid to repeat them again if you suspect that the patient hasn't grasped them.
- Ask for feedback to clarify understanding. Be aware of nonverbal cues from your patient that may indicate his degree of learning and comprehension.

Documenting teaching: A legal safeguard

Protecting yourself from litigation is one of the most compelling reasons for you to create clear, complete documentation of all of your patient teaching efforts. The courts recognize the patient's right to informed consent—that is, to have appropriate information when making decisions about his health care. This puts the burden of decision on the patient, but it also makes you responsible for helping him make an intelligent choice.

Nurse practice acts in many states hold nurses responsible for patient teaching. The Joint Commission has set national standards for documentation that the courts use as guidelines. So, if a patient claims he was harmed by inadequate teaching and your documentation falls short of these standards, the courts may decide that you provided substandard nursing care—even if you taught the patient thoroughly.

Delegate wisely

Of course, dietitians, physical therapists, and others also do patient teaching. However, nurses commonly do the referring to ancillary staff members, making nurses ultimately responsible for the teaching outcomes. So document each referral and what you expect that person to teach, and delegate only to those qualified to teach. Remember: Licensed practical nurses aren't taught the fundamentals of patient teaching—it's beyond the scope of their practice. However, they can reinforce what you have already taught the patient, as long as you follow up, evaluate, and document what the patient understands.

Document what you don't teach

Keep in mind that documenting what you didn't teach is just as important as documenting what you did teach. For example, you'll have to postpone or redirect your teaching if it causes the patient too much stress or if he decides that he would rather have you teach a family member instead. Just make sure you record your teaching attempts and the cause for delay.

A last caution

As health care agencies and consumer groups become more educated about patients' rights to information, careless patient teaching may become a common ground for lawsuits against nurses. To avoid litigation, document what is taught, the patient's response to teaching, and the patient's understanding of what was taught.

Tips for improving drug compliance

Some older adults habitually forget to take their prescribed medication or take it incorrectly. They may even fail to have their prescriptions filled. If you know your patient hasn't been following his medication regimen as ordered, ask him why he's been unable to comply with it. Then, try these tips to help improve compliance.

Coping with costs

An older adult may not be able to afford his medications. Refer the patient to a social worker who can explore payment options and assistance programs.

Maintaining a schedule

Some older adults may take many medications, each with a different dosage schedule. Whenever possible, ask the health care provider to substitute formulations that can be taken less often.

If possible, suggest that the patient choose a regular time for taking his medication, such as just after a meal or at bedtime, so that it's part of his daily routine. Or suggest that he use a check-off system or a commercial device as a reminder.

Dealing with physical limitations

If the patient has difficulty reading labels, suggest that he use a magnifying glass. Tell him that many pharmacies provide large-print labels; he may want to ask about this when he fills his prescription.

If the patient has limited mobility or can no longer drive, he may have difficulty obtaining his medication. Review community resources that can help, such as delivery systems, transportation services, or home care agencies.

Preventing drug interactions

Adverse effects and noncompliance can stem from drug interactions. Review all the medications the patient is taking, and point out potential interactions. Advise the patient to review all medications with the pharmacist every time he has a new prescription filled.

Teaching topics: Acute coronary syndrome

- Definition of acute coronary syndrome (ACS) specific to how it affects the patient: unstable angina, non-ST-segment elevation myocardial infarction (MI), or ST-segment elevation MI
- Causes of ACS: atherosclerosis, thrombosis, or coronary artery spasm or stenosis
- Risk factor analysis (see *CAD risk factors,* pages 336 and 337)
- Signs and symptoms: chest pain, fatigue, anxiety, nausea, vomiting, diaphoresis, dyspnea
- Diagnostic tests, such as cardiac markers, electrocardiography, echocardiography, perfusion imaging, or cardiac catheterization
- Medication use and possible adverse effects
- Treatment options: percutaneous coronary intervention, intra-aortic balloon pump
- Surgical repair such as coronary artery bypass
- Preoperative and postoperative care: coughing and deep-breathing exercises, incentive spirometry, sequential compression stockings, mechanical ventilation, hemodynamic monitoring, pain management, wound care, activity recommendations
- Smoking cessation
- Activity recommendations: regular exercise schedule
- Dietary recommendations: low calorie (for weight reduction), low fat, low cholesterol
- Cardiac rehabilitation
- Potential complications: myocardial necrosis, cardiac arrhythmia, death
- Follow-up care

CAD risk factors

A risk factor is defined as any factor—whether arising from one's genes, environment, personal habits, or lifestyle choices—that can be used to predict a person's probability of developing a particular disease. Risk factors for coronary artery disease (CAD) have been studied and followed for more than 50 years through the Framingham Heart Study. In patients with CAD and angina, decreasing or eliminating specific risk factors is seen as a way to deter further disease progression. Intervention is possible after risk factors are identified. Some risk factors (such as age, sex, and family history) aren't modifiable; other risk factors (such as smoking and obesity) can be reduced or eliminated with treatments and lifestyle modifications.

Risk factors	Relationship to CAD
Major independent	
Cigarette or tobacco use	Smoking doubles the risk of cardiovascular disease and increases mortality by 50% in patients with a myocardial infarction.
High blood pressure	A strong relationship exists between hypertension and CAD. Hypertension is defined as an abnormally high blood pressure—that is, a systolic reading of 140 mm Hg or higher or a diastolic reading of 90 mm Hg or higher.
Elevated low-density lipoprotein (LDL) cholesterol levels	An elevated LDL cholesterol level is a well-established risk in CAD. Control of LDL cholesterol level is a cornerstone in the treatment of heart disease.
Advancing age	Men older than age 45 and women older than age 55 are at increased risk for heart disease.
Low high-density lipoprotein (HDL) cholesterol levels	A low level of HDL, or "good," cholesterol is an independent risk, regardless of the total cholesterol value. A level below 35 mg/dl is considered significant. An HDL level of greater than 60 mg/dl is considered protective and a "negative" risk factor.

CAD risk factors *(continued)*

Risk factors	Relationship to CAD
Diabetes mellitus	Type I and type II diabetes increase the risk of heart disease, so it's important to keep the diabetes under good control to decrease the risk of developing heart disease. Diabetes is characterized by a fasting glucose level of greater than 126 mg/dl.
Other	
Obesity	Obesity is a risk factor for heart disease. It's characterized by a body mass index of 30 or higher.
Abdominal obesity	Patients who have the apple shape, who carry weight in the trunk, are at higher risk than those who have the pear shape, who carry weight in the hips. The apple shape may be an indicator of insulin resistance.
Physical inactivity	Americans are becoming increasingly sedentary and aren't getting enough daily exercise to stay healthy, creating an increased risk of heart disease.

Teaching topics: Anaphylaxis

- Definition of anaphylaxis
- Cause of the anaphylactic reaction
- Signs and symptoms: swelling and difficulty breathing
- Potential complications: brain damage, death
- Identification of, and ways to avoid exposure to, the allergen
- Use of Epi-Pen
- Wearing medical identification jewelry to identify allergy

Teaching topics: Aneurysm

- Definition of aneurysm
- Information on specific type of aneurysm affecting the patient, such as cerebral or abdominal
- Causes of the aneurysm, such as congenital defect or hypertension
- Diagnostic tests: computed tomography scan, magnetic resonance imaging
- Signs and symptoms (based on type of aneurysm), such as headache or retroperitoneal pain
- Medication use and possible adverse effects
- Surgical repair, such as resection, clipping, or bypass
- Preoperative and postoperative care: coughing and deep-breathing exercises, incentive spirometry, sequential compression stockings, mechanical ventilation, hemodynamic monitoring, pain management, wound care, activity recommendations
- Potential complications: rupture, death
- Follow-up care

Teaching topics: Arrhythmia

- Explanation of normal cardiac conduction
- Information on the specific type of arrhythmia affecting the patient such as atrial fibrillation
- Diagnostic tests, such as electrocardiography or electrophysiologic studies
- Signs and symptoms (based on type of arrhythmia), such as palpitations or chest pain
- Smoking cessation
- Activity recommendations: regular exercise program
- Medication use and possible adverse effects
- Dietary recommendations: low-fat, low-cholesterol diet; potassium supplements; limited caffeine intake
- How to take a pulse
- Procedure options: cardioversion, radioablation
- Surgical options: pacemaker or implantable cardioverter-defibrillator (ICD), if indicated
- Preoperative and postoperative care: coughing and deep-breathing exercises, incentive spirometry, cardiac monitoring, wound care
- Potential complications: stroke, myocardial infarction, death
- Medical identification jewelry (for pacemaker or ICD)
- Follow-up care

Teaching about drugs for arrhythmias

Drug	Adverse reactions
Antiarrhythmics	
amiodarone (Cordarone)	• Watch for diaphoresis, dyspnea, lethargy, tingling in the extremities, weight loss or gain, and yellow eyes or fingernails. • Other reactions include corneal microdeposits, hyperthyroidism or hypothyroidism, photophobia, and bluish pigmentation.
disopyramide (Norpace)	• Watch for ankle edema, dizziness, drowsiness, excessive hunger, hypotension, impotence, irregular heart rate, rapid weight gain, shortness of breath, urine retention, and weakness. • Other reactions include anorexia, constipation, and mouth, nose, and eye dryness.
flecainide (Tambocor)	• Watch for ankle edema, chest pain, dizziness, irregular heart rate, shortness of breath, vision disturbances, and weight gain. • Other reactions include fatigue, headache, nausea, and palpitations.
mexiletine (Mexitil)	• Watch for ataxia, blurred vision, confusion, dizziness, headache, nystagmus, and tremors. • Other reactions include anorexia, constipation, and nausea.

Teaching points

• Tell the patient to take a missed dose any time in the same day or to skip it entirely. Warn him not to take a double dose.
• Advise him to have an eye examination if his vision changes.
• Tell him that limiting sun exposure will prevent sunburn and skin discoloration. Suggest using sunblock with a skin protection factor of at least 15 when outdoors.
• Stress the importance of keeping follow-up appointments to monitor thyroid, pulmonary, and liver function.

• Tell the patient who experiences excessive hunger, weakness, drowsiness, and shakiness to eat sweets or drink a sugar-containing beverage and then call his health care provider at once.
• Instruct him to rise slowly from a sitting or lying position to prevent dizziness or fainting from hypotension.
• Tell him to avoid operating machinery until he no longer experiences adverse reactions to the drug.
• Urge him to avoid alcohol, which can reduce blood pressure.
• Instruct him to take the drug on an empty stomach—1 hour before or 3 hours after a meal for faster absorption. Tell him to take the drug with meals if stomach upset occurs.
• Tell him to take a missed dose as soon as possible, but warn him not to take a double dose.

• Tell the patient to take a missed dose as soon as possible, but warn him not to take a double dose.
• Teach him how to take his pulse. Advise him to report an unusually high or low rate or a new irregularity.
• Warn against driving or using machinery if dizziness occurs.
• Instruct the patient to weigh himself at least every other day and to report sudden weight gain.
• If the patient has a permanent pacemaker, explain that the device may need modification after flecainide takes effect.

• Tell the patient that he can help relieve nausea by taking the medicine with food or antacids.
• Instruct the patient to take a missed dose as soon as possible, but warn him not to take a double dose.

(continued)

Teaching about drugs for arrhythmias *(continued)*

Drug	Adverse reactions
procainamide (Procan SR, Pronestyl)	• Watch for anorexia, nausea, and systemic lupus-like syndrome (chills and fever, joint pain, malaise, and rash). • Other reactions include bitter taste, diarrhea, and dizziness.
propafenone (Rhythmol)	• Watch for dizziness, nausea, vomiting, shortness of breath, edema, and signs of cardiac arrhythmias. • Other reactions include anxiety, fatigue, insomnia, blurred vision, abdominal pain or cramps, constipation or diarrhea, dyspepsia, arthralgia, or rash.
Anticoagulants	
heparin	• Watch for bleeding, increased bruising, and hypersensitivity reactions. • Other reactions include fever, chills, rhinitis, mild pain, and hematomas.
warfarin (Coumadin)	• Watch for signs of bleeding, fever, diarrhea, jaundice, or rash. • Other reactions include headache, nausea, vomiting, mouth ulcerations, melena, dermatitis, and alopecia.

Teaching points

- Advise him to reduce GI symptoms by taking procainamide with food.
- Inform him that although the tablet's shell may appear in the stool, the drug has been absorbed.
- Tell him to take a missed dose as soon as possible, but warn him not to take a double dose.

- Stress the importance of taking the drug exactly as prescribed.
- Tell the patient not to double the dose if he misses one, but to take the next dose at the usual time.
- Tell the patient not to crush, chew, or open the extended-release capsules.

- Instruct the patient and his family to watch for signs of bleeding or bruising and to notify the prescriber immediately if any occur.
- Tell the patient to avoid over-the-counter (OTC) drugs containing aspirin, other salicylates, or drugs that may interact with heparin unless ordered by the prescriber.

- Stress the importance of complying with the prescribed dosage and follow-up appointments. Tell the patient to carry a card that identifies his increased risk of bleeding.
- Tell the patient and his family to watch for signs of bleeding or abnormal bruising and to call the prescriber at once if they occur.
- Tell him to avoid OTC drugs containing aspirin, other salicylates, or drugs that may interact with warfarin unless ordered by the prescriber.
- Tell the patient to read food labels. Food, nutritional supplements, and multivitamins that contain vitamin K may impair anticoagulation.
- Tell him to use an electric razor when shaving and a soft toothbrush.

(continued)

Teaching about drugs for arrhythmias *(continued)*

Drug	Adverse reactions
Beta-adrenergic blockers	
acebutolol (Sectral) **atenolol** (Tenormin) **esmolol** (Brevibloc) **labetalol** (Trandate) **metoprolol** (Lopressor) **nadolol** (Corgard) **pindolol** (Visken) **propranolol** (Inderal) **timolol** (Blocadren)	• Watch for bradycardia, depression, dizziness, dyspnea, rash, and wheezing. • Other reactions include diarrhea, fatigue, headache, impotence, insomnia, nasal stuffiness, nausea, vivid dreams and nightmares, and vomiting.
Calcium channel blockers	
diltiazem (Cardizem) **verapamil** (Calan, Isoptin)	• Watch for ankle edema, bradycardia, chest pain, dyspnea, fainting, and tachycardia. • Other reactions include constipation, dizziness, flushing, headache, and nausea.

Patient teaching

Teaching points

- Teach the patient to take his pulse before taking the drug and to notify his health care provider if the rate falls below 50 beats/minute.
- If the patient complains of insomnia, suggest that he take the drug no later than 2 hours before bedtime.
- Instruct him to take labetalol, metoprolol, and propranolol with food to increase drug absorption.
- If the patient takes one dose daily, instruct him to take a missed dose within 8 hours. If he takes two or more doses each day, instruct him to take a missed dose as soon as possible, but warn him not to take a double dose.
- Warn against suddenly discontinuing the drug. He must taper the dosage, as directed, to avoid serious complications.

- Tell the patient to rise slowly from a sitting or lying position to minimize dizziness.
- Explain that the drug won't relieve acute chest pain. He must continue to use sublingual nitroglycerin, if prescribed.
- Reassure him that he can continue to eat and drink calcium-containing foods in reasonable amounts.
- Teach him to prevent constipation by increasing his fluid and fiber intake and by using a bulk laxative, as necessary.
- Advise him to limit alcohol intake to avoid dizziness.
- Tell him to take a missed dose within 4 hours, but warn him not to take a double dose.

(continued)

Teaching about drugs for arrhythmias *(continued)*

Drug	Adverse reactions
Cardiac glycosides	
digoxin (Lanoxicaps, Lanoxin)	• Watch for abdominal pain, anorexia, blurred vision, color vision changes, diplopia, dizziness, drowsiness, fatigue, headache, irregular heart rate, malaise, and nausea.

Teaching points

- Teach the patient to take his pulse before taking digoxin and to report an unusually low, high, or irregular pulse rate.
- Tell him to establish a daily routine for taking digoxin.
- Instruct him to take a missed dose within 12 hours, but warn him not to take a double dose.
- Warn him not to take another person's tablets; different generic digoxin tablets are absorbed at different rates.
- Tell the patient not to take this drug with liquid antacids, kaolin-pectin mixtures (Kaopectate), or cholestyramine (Questran) because doing so may decrease absorption. Separating the administration times by 2 hours will help avoid this interaction.

Teaching topics: Arterial occlusive disease

- Major causes of reduced arterial blood flow: atherosclerosis and arteriosclerosis
- Signs and symptoms of occlusion: intermittent claudication, pain, arterial ulcers
- Diagnostic tests: arteriography, ultrasonography
- Smoking cessation
- Weight reduction
- Activity recommendations: regular exercise program, especially walking
- Medication use and possible adverse effects
- Dietary recommendations: low fat orientation
- Skin assessment for arterial ulcers: wound care if present
- Surgical options: atherectomy, embolectomy, stent placement, bypass surgery, amputation
- Preoperative and postoperative care: coughing and deep-breathing exercises, incentive spirometry, pain management, cardiac monitoring, wound care
- Potential complications: arterial ulcer, infection, embolism
- Support group and community resource information with amputation
- Follow-up care

Teaching topics: Brain cancer

- Explanation of the specific type of malignant brain tumor affecting the patient
- Diagnostic tests: computed tomography scan, magnetic resonance imaging, angiography
- Signs and symptoms of increased intracranial pressure (ICP): headache, vision changes, confusion, respiratory depression
- Smoking cessation
- Safety measures
- Medication use and possible adverse effects
- Treatment options: chemotherapy, radiation therapy; Ommaya reservoir, brachytherapy
- Surgical options: craniotomy, craniectomy
- Preoperative and postoperative care: pain management, hemodynamic monitoring, ICP monitoring, wound care, potential mechanical ventilation
- Potential complications: tumor recurrence, metastasis, coma
- Support group and community resource information; hospice information if appropriate
- Follow-up care

Teaching about brain surgery

The prospect of brain surgery can make your patient anxious and frightened. Offer support and clarify the surgeon's explanation of the surgery. As appropriate, discuss a craniotomy or craniectomy.

Craniotomy

For a craniotomy, a large incision is made in the skull, exposing the cranial (skull) cavity. Then a bone flap is formed that may be completely removed or remain attached to muscle during surgery. Next, an incision is made into the dura to open it in the opposite direction. Then the tumor is removed, and the dura, skull, and skin flap are sutured back into place.

Be sure to review safety measures if the bone flap is completely removed.

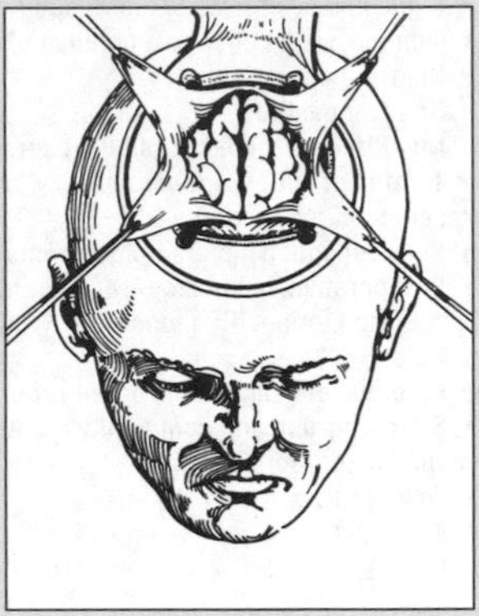

Craniectomy

For a craniectomy, a tiny skull portion—the size of a burr hole (smaller than a dime or about the size of the little fingertip) is made. If necessary, the opening is enlarged with a bone forceps. Then the tumor is removed. The detached bone plug may be frozen for later replacement.

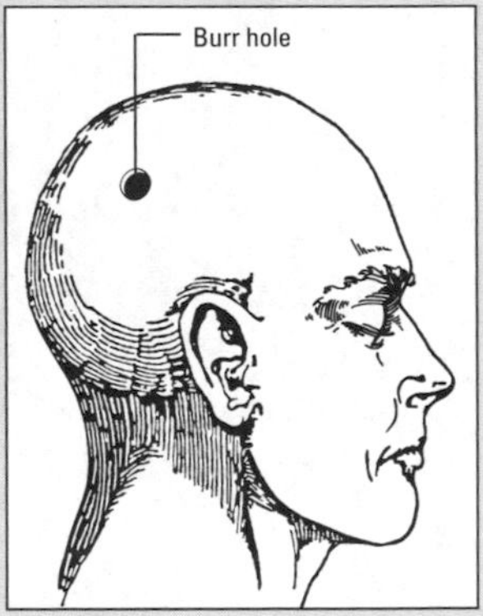

Patient teaching

Teaching topics: Laryngeal cancer

- Explanation of the specific type of laryngeal cancer affecting the patient
- Diagnostic tests: endoscopy, computed tomography scan, magnetic resonance imaging, biopsy
- Signs and symptoms of tumor pressure on larynx: hoarseness, difficulty swallowing or breathing
- Smoking cessation
- Medication use and possible adverse effects
- Treatment options: chemotherapy, radiation therapy
- Surgical options (see *Teaching about laryngeal cancer surgery*, pages 352 and 353)
- Preoperative and postoperative care: coughing and deep-breathing exercises, incentive spirometry, sequential compression stockings, pain management, hemodynamic monitoring, wound care, potential mechanical ventilation, tracheostomy care
- Dietary changes: tube feedings progressing to thickened foods and soft foods
- Aspiration precautions
- Alternate methods of communication (See *Teaching about alternative speech methods*, pages 354 and 355)
- Potential complications: metastasis, aspiration pneumonia, airway occlusion
- Support group and community resource information; hospice information if appropriate
- Follow-up care

Teaching about laryngeal cancer surgery

For most laryngeal cancer patients, treatment includes surgery. Use the information that follows to help the patient and his family understand the purpose, extent, and effects of the planned surgery.

Endoscopy with laser surgery

Explain that endoscopy with laser surgery, performed during laryngoscopy, uses a laser beam to remove a glottic tumor that's confined to a small area—usually a single true vocal cord. Tell the patient that the laser beam will effectively eliminate the cancerous growth, that he'll retain his voice, and that he can resume his usual activities shortly after the procedure.

Laryngofissure

Inform the patient that a laryngofissure removes larger glottic tumors confined to a single vocal cord. The surgeon makes an incision in the thyroid cartilage and removes the diseased vocal cord.

Tell the patient that after surgery, he'll have a temporary tracheostomy and his voice may be hoarse but that hoarseness will abate as scar tissue replaces the vocal cord.

Vertical hemilaryngectomy

Explain that a vertical hemilaryngectomy removes a widespread tumor. This procedure involves excision of about one-half of the thyroid cartilage and the subglottic cartilage, one false cord, and one true cord. Then the surgeon rebuilds the area with strap muscles.

Tell the patient that he'll have a temporary tracheostomy. Reassure him that postoperative hoarseness will subside as scar tissue replaces the vocal cord.

Horizontal supraglottic laryngectomy

Explain that a horizontal supraglottic laryngectomy removes a large supraglottic tumor. The top of the larynx (the epiglottis, hyoid bone, and false vocal cords) is removed, leaving the true vocal cords intact.

Tell the patient that he'll have a temporary tracheostomy to ensure a patent airway until swelling subsides. Also explain that he won't lose his voice, but that he may have swallowing difficulties without the epiglottis.

Total laryngectomy

Inform the patient that a total laryngectomy removes the vocal cords, epiglottis, hyoid bone, cricoid cartilage, and two or three tracheal rings. Neighboring areas may also be removed, depending on the tumor's extent.

Explain that the surgeon must remove the vocal cords and create a permanent tracheostomy and a laryngeal stoma. Reassure the patient that although he will lose his voice, speech therapy will be provided to explore appropriate alternatives that will allow him to communicate.

Radical neck dissection

Explain that when cancer spreads to surrounding tissues and glands, the cervical chain of lymph nodes, sternomastoid muscle, fascia, and internal jugular vein are also removed.

Because this operation leaves the patient with little muscle control and support for the head and neck, teach him exercises to strengthen accessory support muscles.

Because radical neck dissection disfigures the face and neck, you'll need to provide strong emotional support along with your teaching before surgery and throughout the recovery period.

Teaching about alternative speech methods

Let your patient know that the speech pathologist can teach him new ways to speak. Then review the possibilities discussed here.

Esophageal speech

The patient talks by drawing air in through his mouth, trapping it in the upper esophagus, and releasing it slowly while forming words with his mouth. With training and practice, a highly motivated patient can master esophageal speech in about 1 month. Inform the patient that his speech will be choppy at first but will become smoother and more easily understood as he gains skill.

Because esophageal speech requires strength, an elderly patient or a patient with asthma or emphysema may find it too physically demanding to learn. Because it also requires frequent sessions with a speech pathologist, a chronically ill patient may find esophageal speech overwhelming.

Artificial larynges

The throat vibrator and the Cooper-Rand device are the two basic artificial larynges. Both types vibrate to produce speech that's easy to understand, despite sounding monotonous and mechanical.

Tell the patient he can operate a throat vibrator by holding it in place against his neck. A pulsating disc in the device vibrates the throat tissue as the patient forms words with his mouth. The throat vibrator device may be difficult to use immediately after surgery, when the patient's neck wounds still feel sore.

The Cooper-Rand device vibrates sounds piped into the patient's mouth through a thin tube, which the patient positions in the corner of his mouth. Easy to use, this device may be preferred immediately after surgery.

Surgically implanted prostheses

Most surgical implants generate speech by vibrating when the patient manually closes the tracheostomy, forcing air upward. One such device is the Blom-Singer indwelling low-pressure voice prosthesis. This prosthesis enables the patient to speak in a normal voice within just a few hours after it's inserted through an incision in the stoma. The surgeon may implant the device when radiation therapy ends or within a few days (or even years) after laryngectomy.

To speak, the patient covers his stoma while exhaling. Exhaled air travels through the trachea, then passes through an airflow port on the bottom of the prosthesis, and exits through a slit at the esophageal end of the prosthesis, creating the vibrations needed to produce sound.

Not all patients are eligible for tracheoesophageal puncture, the procedure needed to insert the prosthesis. Considerations include the extent of the laryngectomy; pharyngoesophageal muscle status; stomal size and location; and the patient's mental and emotional status, visual and auditory acuity, hand-eye coordination, bimanual dexterity, and self-care skills.

Teaching topics: Lung cancer

- Explanation of the specific type of lung cancer the patient has
- Diagnostic tests: bronchoscopy, computed tomography scan, magnetic resonance imaging, biopsy
- Signs and symptoms of tumor pressure in lungs: shortness of breath, hemoptysis, fatigue
- Smoking cessation
- Medication use and possible adverse effects
- Treatment options: chemotherapy, radiation therapy
- Surgical options (see *Teaching about lung cancer surgery*)
- Preoperative and postoperative care: coughing and deep-breathing exercises, incentive spirometry, sequential compression stockings, pain management, hemodynamic monitoring, chest tube, wound care, oxygen therapy with potential mechanical ventilation, frequent repositioning
- Potential complications: metastasis, respiratory failure
- Support group and community resource information; hospice information if appropriate
- Follow-up care

Teaching about lung cancer surgery

If your patient has operable lung cancer and is scheduled for surgery, discuss the type of operation he'll have. Explain how his particular procedure will be performed.

Lobectomy

A lobectomy removes a cancerous lobe from the lung.

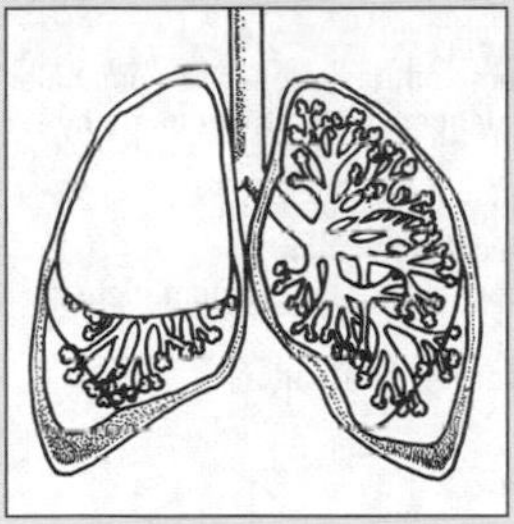

Segmentectomy

A segmentectomy removes one or more lung segments, preserving functional, healthy tissue.

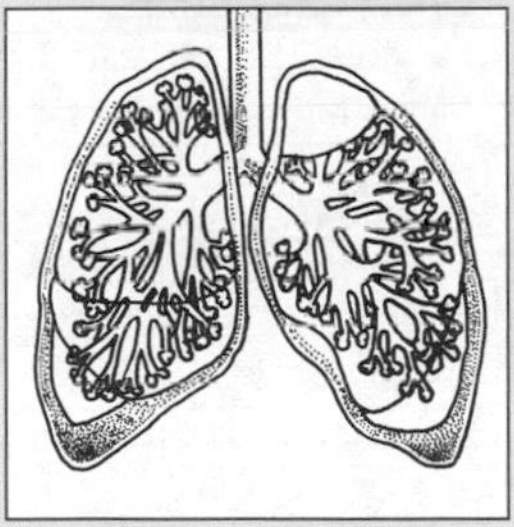

Wedge resection

A wedge resection removes lung tissue without regard to segmental planes. This operation is reserved for small cancers in patients with poor pulmonary reserve.

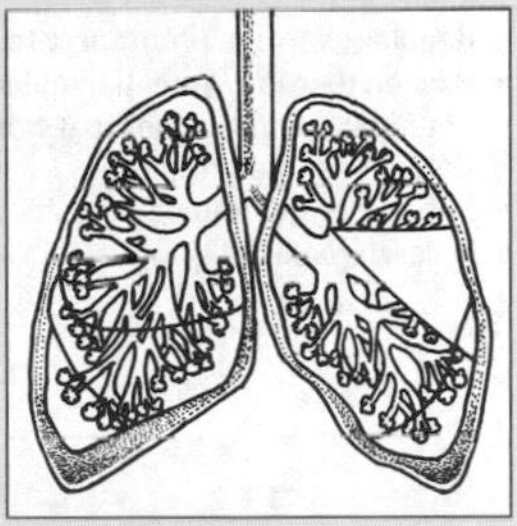

Pneumonectomy

A pneumonectomy removes the entire cancerous lung.

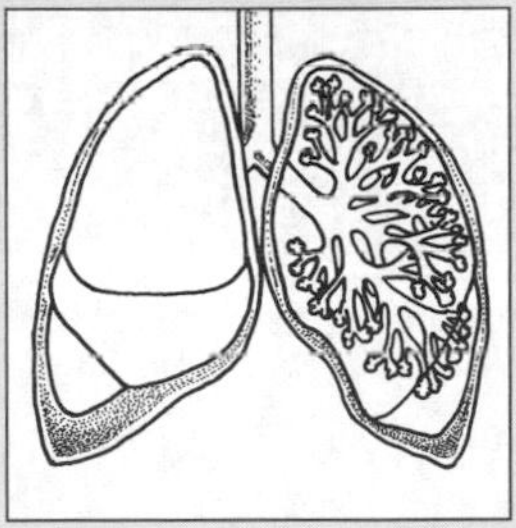

Teaching topics: Chronic obstructive lung disease

- Explanation of the specific type of lung disease affecting the patient
- Diagnostic tests: chest X-ray, computed tomography scan, arterial blood gas analysis, pulmonary function tests
- Signs and symptoms of exacerbation: shortness of breath, anxiety, cough, mucus production
- Identification of triggers for asthma
- Smoking cessation
- Medication use and possible adverse effects; proper use of inhaler
- Dietary recommendations: well-balanced diet with adequate hydration
- Regular exercise program with frequent rest periods
- Oxygen therapy; potential mechanical ventilation
- Potential complications: respiratory failure, status asthmaticus, spontaneous pneumothorax
- Support group and community resource information
- Follow-up care

Teaching topics: Deep vein thrombosis

- Explanation of deep vein thrombosis (DVT)
- Major causes and risk factors for DVT (see *DVT risk factors*)
- Signs and symptoms of occlusion: pain, swelling, redness
- Diagnostic tests: Doppler ultrasonography, venography
- Medication use and possible adverse effects
- Prophylaxis: leg movement, with ambulation, if possible; sequential compression stockings and antiembolism stockings while in bed; avoidance of tight clothing, crossing legs, remaining immobile for long periods of time, such as when traveling
- Adequate hydration with avoidance of alcohol
- Smoking cessation
- Treatment option: vena cava filter (to prevent pulmonary embolus)
- Potential complications: prolonged bleeding (due to medication), pulmonary emboli, stroke
- Follow-up care

DVT risk factors

Certain conditions increase the risk of deep vein thrombosis (DVT) formation. These risk factors include:

- immobility
- trauma
- surgery, especially knee or hip replacement
- radiation therapy
- personal or family history of blood clots or a coagulation disorder
- history of an inflammatory disorder
- infection
- pregnancy
- hormonal contraceptive use (especially coupled with smoking)
- obesity
- history of hypertension
- history of cancer
- smoking
- travel with prolonged sitting
- having a central venous catheter in place.

Teaching topics: Diabetes mellitus

- Explanation of the specific type of diabetes affecting the patient
- Diagnostic tests: capillary glucose testing, serum blood glucose levels, glycosylated hemoglobin test, ophthalmic examination, urinalysis
- Signs and symptoms of hypoglycemia and hyperglycemia: weakness, cool, clammy skin, confusion, decreased level of consciousness, seizures
- Smoking cessation
- Medication use and possible adverse effects; proper injection technique, if appropriate
- Dietary recommendations: prescribed calorie and carbohydrate intake
- Regular exercise program
- Self-testing for capillary glucose level
- Skin care and assessment for poor wound healing
- Potential complications: neuropathies, sexual dysfunction, retinopathy, infection, hypoglycemia, diabetic ketoacidosis
- Support group and community resource information
- Follow-up care

Teaching topics: GI bleeding

- Explain the source of the GI bleeding affecting the patient
- Causes of GI bleeding
- Diagnostic tests: hemoglobin level, hematocrit, endoscopy, stools for occult blood
- Signs and symptoms of GI bleeding: bright red blood in vomitus or stools, melena, coffee ground emesis or nasogastric (NG) drainage, pallor, weakness
- Need for fluid resuscitation: I.V. fluids and blood products
- Medication use and possible adverse effects
- Dietary recommendations: non-spicy, nonirritating foods
- Treatment options: NG decompression, endoscopic therapy, selective arterial embolization, transjugular intrahepatic portosystemic shunt (with variceal bleeding)
- Surgical options: gastrectomy, vagotomy
- Preoperative and postoperative care: coughing and deep-breathing exercises, incentive spirometry, sequential compression stockings, NG tube drainage monitoring, hemodynamic monitoring
- Lifestyle modifications: stress reduction, smoking cessation, alcohol cessation; acquaint patient with relevant support cessation programs and support groups
- Potential complications: hemorrhage, aspiration, hypovolemic shock
- Follow-up care

Teaching topics: Head injury

- Explain the type of head injury affecting the patient (see *Classifying head injuries*)
- Diagnostic tests: skull X-ray, computed tomography scan, magnetic resonance imaging
- Signs and symptoms of increased intracranial pressure (ICP): headache, vision changes, confusion, respiratory depression
- Medication use and possible adverse effects
- Treatment options: burr holes, intraventricular drain
- Surgical options: hematoma removal
- Preoperative and postoperative care: sequential compression stockings, ICP monitoring, hemodynamic monitoring, pain management, possible mechanical ventilation
- Safety measures (for confused patient)
- Activity restrictions (based on type of head injury)
- Wound care, if appropriate
- Physical and occupational therapy based on type of head injury
- Potential complications: hemorrhage, brain injury, neurologic deficits
- Rehabilitation based on neurologic deficits
- Follow-up care

Classifying head injuries

Tell the patient and his family that health care providers use varying classification systems for head injuries.

Explain that classification may be based on the severity of the injury (mild, moderate, severe); the type of injury (concussion, contusion, laceration); the mechanism of injury (direct impact, acceleration, deceleration); or skull integrity (open or closed). As shown in the illustrations below, head injuries may also be classified by cerebral involvement—focal or diffuse.

Focal head injury

If the patient has a focal head injury, inform him that cerebral damage, which usually results from direct impact, is well delineated. Examples include hematomas, concussions, contusions, and skull fractures. Focal injuries can cause permanent deficits. However, complications may be moderated if the patient's injury (for example, from a skull fracture) also falls in the open head trauma class because the open skull accommodates cerebral swelling.

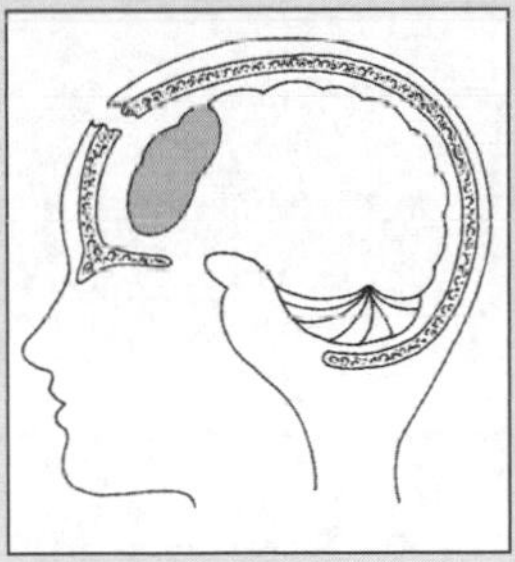

Diffuse head injury

Many brain areas are damaged in a diffuse injury. Typical causes include an indirect blow to the head or a combination of direct and indirect impacts. Examples are concussions and diffuse axonal injuries in which axons tear as the brain jostles against the skull. These injuries are associated with closed head injury and rarely cause outward signs of trauma. However, generalized swelling and increased intracranial pressure may occur inside the skull.

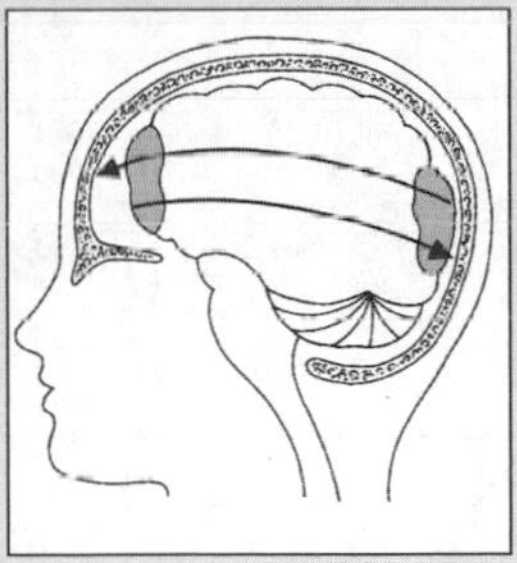

Teaching topics: Heart failure

- Explanation of heart failure and how it affects cardiac function
- Causes of heart failure: coronary artery disease, myocardial infarction, hypertension, valvular disease
- Signs and symptoms: dyspnea, orthopnea, wheezing, cough with pink sputum, weight gain, edema, palpitations
- Diagnostic tests: chest X-ray, blood test (B-type natriuretic peptide), echocardiography
- Medication use and possible adverse effects
- Oxygen therapy
- Smoking cessation
- Activity recommendations: adequate rest with avoidance of overexertion
- Dietary recommendations: low sodium, fluid restricted
- Daily weight record
- Potential complications: pulmonary edema, pneumonia
- Follow-up care

Teaching topics: Hypertension

- Explanation of hypertension, with a review of normal and high blood pressure and the factors that affect blood pressure
- Signs and symptoms (see *Hypertension signs and symptoms*)
- Medication use and possible adverse effects
- Activity recommendations: regular exercise program
- Dietary recommendations: low calorie, low carbohydrate (if weight loss needed), low sodium
- Home blood pressure monitoring
- Lifestyle modifications: stress reduction, smoking
sation
- Surgical options (based on cause of hypertension)
excision of pheochromocytoma
- Preoperative and postoperative care: coughing ar
breathing exercises, incentive spirometry, sequentia
stockings, frequent blood pressure monitoring
- Potential complications: myocardial infarction, str
age
- Follow-up care

Hypertension signs and symptoms

Tell the patient and his family that hypertension is called "the silent killer" because most people have no signs or symptoms. Explain, however, that some patients do experience signs and symptoms, including:

- headache, especially in the morning
- dizziness, faintness, numbness, weakness
- vision changes, nosebleeds
- chest pain, palpitations, shortness of breath
- leg pain, leg edema
- muscle cramps
- increased urination, bloody urine.

CHF Teachings

Teaching about antihypertensives

Drug	Adverse reactions
Angiotensin-converting enzyme inhibitors	
captopril (Capoten) **enalapril** (Vasotec) **lisinopril** (Prinivil, Zestril) **quinapril** (Accupril) **ramipril** (Altace)	• Watch for chest pain, diaphoresis, dyspnea, fever, mouth sores, orthostatic hypotension, persistent cough, rapid heart rate, rash, severe diarrhea and vomiting, and sore throat. • Other reactions include altered taste, dizziness, fatigue, headache, and palpitations.
Beta-adrenergic blockers	
acebutolol (Sectral) **atenolol** (Tenormin) **carvedilol** (Coreg) **esmolol** (Brevibloc) **labetalol** (Trandate) **metoprolol** (Lopressor) **nadolol** (Corgard) **propranolol** (Inderal) **sotalol** (Betapace)	• Watch for depression, dizziness, dyspnea, rash, very slow heart rate, and wheezing. • Other reactions include decreased libido, diarrhea, fatigue, headache, insomnia, nasal stuffiness, nausea, nightmares, vivid dreams, and vomiting.
Calcium channel blockers	
diltiazem (Cardizem) **nicardipine** (Cardene) **nifedipine** (Procardia) **nimodipine** (Nimotop) **verapamil** (Calan, Isoptin)	• Watch for ankle edema, chest pain, dyspnea, fainting, and very slow or fast heart rate. • Other reactions include constipation, dizziness, flushing, headache, and nausea.

Teaching points

• Instruct the patient to take a missed dose as soon as he remembers, but not to take a double dose.
• Advise him to rise slowly from a sitting or lying position to minimize hypotension.
• Instruct him to limit his intake of high-potassium foods.
• Tell him to report fever, sore throat, or other signs and symptoms of infection.

• If the patient takes one dose daily, instruct him to take a missed dose within 8 hours. If he takes two or more doses daily, tell him to take a missed dose as soon as possible. He should never take a double dose.
• Warn him against suddenly discontinuing the drug. To avoid serious complications, the dosage must be tapered.
• Teach him to check his pulse before taking the drug and to report if his pulse rate falls below 60 beats/minute.
• Advise him to take the drug no later than 2 hours before bedtime to avoid insomnia.
• Suggest that he take the drug with food to increase its absorption.

• Instruct the patient to take a missed dose as soon as he remembers, but not to take a double dose.
• Tell him to rise slowly from a sitting or lying position to minimize dizziness.
• Reassure him that he can continue to eat and drink reasonable amounts of calcium-containing foods.
• Suggest that he increase his fluid and fiber intake and use a bulk laxative to prevent constipation.
• Advise him to limit alcohol intake.

(continued)

Teaching about antihypertensives *(continued)*

Drug	Adverse reactions
Thiazide and thiazide-like diuretics *(continued)*	
polythiazide (Renese) **quinethazone** (Hydromox) **trichlormethiazide** (Diurese)	
Vasodilators	
hydralazine (Apresoline)	• Watch for chest pain, numbness, palpitations, rapid heart rate, systemic lupus erythematosus–like syndrome (fever, joint pain, malaise, skin rash), and tingling. • Other reactions include anorexia, diarrhea, headache, nasal stuffiness, and nausea.
minoxidil (Loniten)	• Watch for distended neck veins, dyspnea, edema, rapid heart rate, and weight gain. • Other reactions include lengthening and darkening of fine body hair.

Patient teaching

Teaching points

- Instruct the patient to record his weight daily to monitor fluid loss.
- Tell him to avoid large doses of calcium supplements.

- If the patient is taking four doses per day and he misses a dose, tell him to take the missed dose no later than 2 hours before his next scheduled dose. Warn him not to take a double dose.
- Advise him to take the drug on an empty stomach—either 1 hour before or 3 hours after a meal.

- Tell the patient to take a missed dose within 8 hours of the scheduled time. Warn him not to take a double dose.
- Suggest that he remove unwanted hair by shaving or using a depilatory.
- If a beta-adrenergic blocker has been ordered to control reflex tachycardia or a diuretic to control sodium and water retention, remind the patient to take all drugs on schedule to ensure their safety and effectiveness.
- Instruct him to weigh himself at least every other day and to report sudden weight gain.

Teaching topics: Hypothermia

- Explanation of hypothermia
- Causes of hypothermia
- Signs and symptoms of hypothermia, based on degree of hypothermia (see *Hypothermia signs and symptoms*)
- Medication use and possible adverse effects
- Warmed fluid resuscitation
- Oxygen therapy; potential mechanical ventilation
- Treatment options: warming techniques (hyperthermia blanket, warm baths); hemodialysis; peritoneal, gastric, and mediastinal lavage
- Lifestyle modifications: environmental adjustment for temperature, appropriate outer wear, alcohol cessation
- Potential complications: cardiac arrhythmia, frostbite, death
- Community support information
- Follow-up care

Hypothermia signs and symptoms

Hypothermia is defined as a core body temperature below 95° F (35° C). It may be classified as mild (89.6° to 95° F [32° to 35° C]), moderate (86° to 89.6° F [30° to 32° C]), or severe (77° to 86° F [25° to 30° C]). This chart highlights the major signs and symptoms associated with each classification.

Classification	Signs and symptoms
Mild hypothermia (89.6° to 95° F)	• Severe shivering • Slurred speech • Amnesia
Moderate hypothermia (86° to 89.6° F)	• Unresponsiveness • Peripheral cyanosis • Muscle rigidity
Severe hypothermia (77° to 86° F)	• Unresponsiveness • Absence of palpable pulses • No audible heart sounds • Dilated pupils • Rigor-mortis-like state • Loss of deep tendon reflexes

Teaching topics: Pneumonia

- Explanation of the specific type of pneumonia affecting the patient
- Causes and risk factors for pneumonia: aspiration, bacterial, viral, community acquired, hospital acquired
- Diagnostic tests: chest X-ray, sputum culture, arterial blood gas analysis, white blood cell count, bronchoscopy
- Signs and symptoms (see *Pneumonia signs and symptoms*, pages 378 to 380)
- Oxygen therapy; potential mechanical ventilation
- Medication use and possible adverse effects
- Treatment options: coughing and deep-breathing exercises, incentive spirometry, chest physiotherapy
- Dietary recommendations: high-calorie diet with adequate hydration
- Activity recommendations: minor activity with frequent rest periods
- Smoking cessation
- Prevention measures: pneumococcal and influenzae vaccinations, proper hand washing and tissue disposal
- Potential complications: respiratory failure, bacteremia, septic shock
- Community resource information
- Follow-up care

Pneumonia signs and symptoms

Here's an overview of the various types of pneumonia, including their causative agents and common assessment findings.

Type	Assessment findings
Aspiration pneumonia	• Fever • Crackles • Dyspnea • Hypotension • Tachycardia • Cyanosis • Chest X-ray with infiltrates
Community-acquired pneumonia	
Streptococcal pneumonia (pneumococcal pneumonia)	• Sudden onset of single shaking chill • Fever of 102° to 104° F (38.9° to 40° C) • History of previous upper respiratory infection • Pleuritic chest pain • Severe cough • Rust-colored sputum • Areas of consolidation on chest X-ray (usually lobar) • Elevated white blood cell (WBC) count • Sputum culture possibly positive for gram-positive *S. pneumoniae*
Haemophilus influenzae	• Insidious onset • History of upper respiratory tract infection 2 to 6 weeks earlier • Fever • Chills • Dyspnea • Productive cough • Nausea and vomiting • Chest X-ray with infiltrates in one or more lobes
Mycoplasma pneumonia	• Insidious onset • Sore throat • Nasal congestion • Ear pain • Headache • Low-grade fever • Pleuritic pain • Erythema rash • Pharyngitis

Pneumonia signs and symptoms *(continued)*

Type	Assessment findings
Viral pneumonia	• Initially beginning as upper respiratory infection • Cough (initially nonproductive; later, purulent sputum) • High fever • Chills • Malaise • Dyspnea • Substernal pain • Moist crackles • Cyanosis • Frontal headache • Chest X-ray with diffuse bilateral bronchopneumonia radiating from hilus • Normal to slightly elevated WBC count
Legionnaires' disease	• Flulike symptoms • Malaise • Headache within 24 hours • Fever • Shaking chills • Progressive dyspnea • Mental confusion • Anorexia • Nausea, vomiting • Myalgia • Chest X-ray with patchy infiltrates, consolidation, and possible effusion
Hospital-acquired pneumonia	
Klebsiella pneumonia	• Fever • Recurrent chills • Rusty, bloody viscous sputum • Cyanosis of lips and nail beds • Shallow grunting respirations • Severe pleuritic chest pain • Chest X-ray typically with consolidation in upper lobe • Elevated WBC count • Sputum culture and Gram stain possibly positive for gram-negative cocci, Klebsiella

(continued)

Pneumonia signs and symptoms *(continued)*

Type	Assessment findings
Pseudomonas pneumonia	• Fever • Chills • Confusion • Delirium • Green, foul-smelling sputum • Chest X-ray with diffuse consolidation
Staphylococcal pneumonia (may also be community acquired)	• Cough • Chills • High fever of 102° to 104° F • Pleuritic pain • Progressive dyspnea • Bloody sputum • Tachypnea • Hypoxemia • Chest X-ray with multiple abscesses and infiltrate; empyema • Elevated WBC count • Sputum culture and Gram stain possibly positive for gram-positive staphylococci

Teaching topics: Pulmonary embolism

- Explanation of pulmonary embolus (PE)
- Major causes and risk factors for PE (see *DVT risk factors*, page 359)
- Signs and symptoms: shortness of breath, chest pain, anxiety, cough with blood-tinged sputum
- Diagnostic tests: spiral computed tomography scan, ventilation-perfusion scan, arterial blood gas analysis, pulmonary angiogram
- Oxygen therapy: potential mechanical ventilation
- Medication use and possible adverse effects
- Treatment option: vena cava filter (if unable to have anticoagulants)
- Prophylaxis: leg movement, with ambulation, if possible; sequential compression stockings and antiembolism stockings while in bed; avoidance of tight clothing, crossing legs, remaining immobile for long periods such as when traveling
- Adequate hydration
- Smoking cessation
- Potential complications: prolonged bleeding, hemorrhage, respiratory failure, stroke
- Follow-up care

Teaching topics: Seizures

- Explanation of the specific type of seizure affecting the patient
- Diagnostic tests: computed tomography scan, positron emission tomography scan, magnetic resonance imaging, EEG
- Identification of triggers and preventive measures (see *Preventing seizures*)
- Safety measures
- Medication use and possible adverse effects
- Treatment options: vagus nerve stimulation
- Surgical options: lesion removal
- Dietary recommendations: well-balanced with adequate hydration but no alcohol
- Potential complications: injury, status epilepticus
- Support group and community resource information
- Follow-up care

Preventing seizures

Teach the patient to control factors that can precipitate a seizure.

- Instruct him to take his exact dose of medication at the times prescribed. Missing doses, doubling doses, or taking extra doses can cause a seizure.
- Advise him to eat balanced, regular meals. Explain that low blood glucose levels (hypoglycemia) and inadequate vitamin intake can lead to seizures.
- Teach him to be alert for odors that may trigger an attack. Advise him and his family to note any strong odors they notice at the time of a seizure.
- Caution him to limit his alcohol intake. He should check with the health care provider to find out whether he may drink any alcoholic beverages.
- Urge him to get enough sleep. Excessive fatigue can precipitate a seizure.
- Tell him to treat a fever early during an illness. If he can't reduce a fever, he should notify the health care provider.
- Help him learn to control stress. Suggest learning relaxation techniques such as deepbreathing exercises.
- Tell him to avoid his trigger factors; for example, flashing lights, hyperventilation, loud noises, heavy musical beats, video games, and television.

Teaching topics: Stroke

- Explanation of the specific type of stroke affecting the patient
- Diagnostic tests: computed tomography scan, positron emission tomography scan, magnetic resonance imaging, EEG
- Causes and risk factors of stroke (see *Stroke risk factors,* page 384)
- Signs and symptoms (see *Stroke signs and symptoms,* page 385)
- Safety measures
- Oxygen therapy
- Medication use and possible adverse effects
- Treatment options: physical therapy, occupational therapy, speech therapy
- Dietary recommendations: well-balanced diet with adequate hydration; aspiration precautions if appropriate
- Surgical options: embolectomy, carotid endarterectomy
- Preoperative and postoperative care: pain management, hemodynamic monitoring, intracranial pressure monitoring, wound care, potential mechanical ventilation
- Potential complications: aspiration pneumonia, injury, recurrent stroke, neurologic deficits
- Support group and community resource information
- Follow-up care

Stroke risk factors

Certain risk factors for stroke are controllable, and others are not. Teach the patient and his family about risk factors that increase the event of stroke. Changing one risk factor can reduce the chance of stroke.

Uncontrollable risk factors

- Age. Older than 55, the risk for stroke doubles with each decade.
- History of stroke. Family and personal history of stroke increases the risk of stroke.
- Race. African Americans have an increased risk of stroke.
- Gender. Although more men suffer from stroke, more women die from stroke.
- History of transient ischemic attack (TIA). One or more TIA increases the risk of stroke by 10 times.
- History of myocardial infarction.

Controllable risk factors

- High blood pressure
- Smoking
- Diabetes mellitus
- Carotid or other arterial disease
- Atrial fibrillation
- Heart disease
- Sickle cell disease
- High blood cholesterol level
- Poor diet
- Physical inactivity
- Obesity

Other risk factors

- Geographical location. More strokes occur in the southeastern United States.
- Socioeconomic status. Some evidence shows that strokes occur more among low-income people.
- Alcohol and drug abuse
- Clotting disorder or history of blood clots
- Migraines. Women with migraines with an aura have a 10 times greater risk of stroke.
- Birth control pills. Use of hormonal contraceptives doubles the risk of stroke.

Stroke signs and symptoms

Certain signs and symptoms are significant indicators of stroke. Teach the patient and his family to immediately report any of these signs or symptoms:

- Sudden numbness or weakness of the face, arm or leg, especially on one side of the body
- Sudden confusion, trouble speaking or understanding
- Sudden trouble seeing in one or both eyes
- Sudden trouble walking, dizziness, loss of balance or coordination
- Sudden, severe headache with no known cause

Appendices

Selected references

Index

Cardiac nursing

Cardiac nurses help patients with cardiovascular disease achieve and maintain optimal cardiac health. They work in such settings as cardiac intensive care units or critical care units, interventional cardiology units, cardiac catheterization and electrophysiology labs, cardiothoracic intensive care units, telemetry units, heart failure clinics, and cardiac rehabilitation units. Education requirements for all of these certifications are a current registered nurse (RN) license or on-the-job training or orientation. A critical care course may be required in some facilities.

Certification

Cardiac/vascular nurse certification (Registered Nurse, Board-Certified [RN, BC]) recognizes nurses who care for patients diagnosed with, or at risk for, cardiovascular disease.

Certifying body

American Nurses Credentialing Center

Examination

This is a 3½-hour examination consisting of 175 multiple-choice questions focusing on the care of the cardiac or vascular patient in acute and ambulatory care settings. Computer-based testing is offered year-round at more than 300 testing centers throughout the United States. Paper and pencil examinations are available in May and October.

Eligibility

Candidates must have:

- a diploma, associate, baccalaureate or higher nursing degree
- unrestricted RN or advanced practice registered nurse (APRN) licensure in the United States or its territories
- 2 years full-time practice
- 2,000 clinical hours caring for cardiac patients in the past 3 years
- 30 contact hours completed within the past 3 years.

Renewal

- Every 5 years
- Professional development requirements: complete minimum of two of five categories or double any single category
  - continuing education requirements: 75 contact hours (with 51% of education hours in your specialty)

– academic courses: 5 semester hour credits (course content applicable to your area of certification)
– presentations and lectures: 5 different presentations on your specialty
– publications and research: one published book article or chapter, one research project, development of one educational topic in media form (such as a CD, or completion of a master's thesis or doctoral dissertation)
– preceptorships: 120 hours

- 1,000 practice hours or option to retest

Web site

www.nursecredentialing.org

Certification

Critical care registered nurse (CCRN) is a certification that recognizes nurses who provide care for critically ill patients.

Certifying body

American Association of Critical Care Nurses (AACN)

Examination

This is a 3-hour examination consisting of 150 multiple-choice questions focusing on clinical judgment related to patient problems and nursing interventions. Computer-based testing is offered year-round at more than 100 testing centers throughout the United States. Paper and pencil examinations are available at the National Testing Institute.

Eligibility

Candidates must have:

- an unrestricted RN or APRN license in the United States or its territories
- 1,750 hours in direct bedside care during the previous 2 years, with 875 of those hours accrued in the year preceding application caring for the acutely or critically ill patient.

Renewal

- Every 3 years
- 100 continuing education recognition points (CERPs) or re-examination
- 432 practice hours within the 3 years, with 144 of those hours in the year preceding renewal
- Education and patient care: must focus on the care or supervision of care of the acutely or critically ill patient.

Web site

www.certcorp.org

Certification

Cardiac medicine certification (CMC) is a subspecialty certification that recognizes nurses who provide care for acutely ill cardiac patients. *Cardiac surgery certification* (CSC) is a subspecialty certification that recognizes nurses who provide care for acutely ill cardiac patients during the first 48 hours after surgery.

Certifying body

AACN

Examination

This is a 2-hour examination consisting of 90 multiple-choice questions focusing on clinical judgment related to patient problems and nursing interventions. Computer-based testing is offered year-round at more than 100 testing centers throughout the United States. Paper and pencil examinations are available at the National Testing Institute.

Eligibility

Candidates must have:

- unrestricted RN or APRN licensure in the United States or its territories
- 1,750 hours in direct bedside care during the previous 2 years, with 875 of those hours accrued in the year preceding application caring for the acutely ill cardiac patient (CMC), or cardiac surgery patients during first 48 hours after surgery (CSC)
- current nationally accredited clinical nursing specialty certification.

Renewal

- Every 3 years
- 25 category "A" CERPs
- 432 practice hours within the 3 years, with 144 of those hours in the year preceding renewal
- education and patient care must focus on the care of critically ill cardiac patients (CMC) or cardiac surgery patients in the first 48 hours after surgery (CSC).

Web site

www.certcorp.org

Critical care nursing

Critical care nurses help critically ill patients achieve and maintain optimal health. They work in such settings as general intensive care units, specialty critical care units (burns, neurological, cardiac, cardiothoracic, medical, surgical, trauma, pulmonary), and neonatal or pediatric intensive care units.

Education requirements

A current registered nurse (RN) license, on-the-job training, or orientation; critical care course may be required in some facilities.

Certification

Critical care registered nurse certification (CCRN) recognizes nurses who provide care for the critically ill patient.

Certifying body

American Association of Critical Care Nurses

Examination

This is a 3-hour examination consisting of 150 multiple-choice questions focusing on clinical judgment related to patient problems and nursing interventions. Computer-based testing is offered year-round at more than 100 testing centers throughout the United States. Paper and pencil examinations are available at the National Testing Institute.

Eligibility

Candidates must have:
- unrestricted RN or advanced practice registered nurse licensure in the United States or its territories
- 1,750 hours in direct bedside care during the previous 2 years, with 875 of those hours accrued in the year preceding application caring for the acutely or critically ill patients.

Renewal

- Every 3 years
- 100 continuing education recognition points or reexamination
- 432 practice hours within the 3 years, with 144 of those hours in the year preceding renewal
- Education and patient care: must focus on the care or supervision of care of the acutely or critically ill patient

Web site

www.certcorp.org

Emergency care nursing

Emergency nurses provide emergency service for patients of all ages to help restore optimal health in acute situations. They work in acute care facilities, emergency medical services, ambulance transport services, flight rescue, or transport.

Education requirements

A current RN license, on-the-job training, or orientation; critical care course or trauma course may be required in some facilities.

Certifications

Certified emergency nurse (CEN) recognizes nurses who provide emergency care for acutely ill patients.

Certifying body

Board of Certification for Emergency Nursing (BCEN)

Examination

This is a 3-hour examination consisting of 175 multiple-choice questions (150 scored and 25 nonscored pretest questions) focusing on:

- cardiovascular emergencies
- gastrointestinal emergencies
- obstetrical, gynecological, and genitourological emergencies
- maxillofacial and ocular emergencies
- neurological emergencies
- orthopedic emergencies and wound management
- psychological and social issues
- toxicological and environmental emergencies
- shock
- multisystem trauma
- communicable diseases
- professional issues.

The test is offered year-round at specified sites via computer.

Eligibility

Candidates must have:

- unrestricted RN or advanced practice registered nurse (APRN) licensure in the United States or its territories
- 2 years of experience in emergency nursing practice (recommended; not required).

Renewal

- Every 4 years
- 100 education hours, reexamination, or Internet-based testing

Web site

www.ena.org

Certification

Certified flight registered nurse (CFRN) recognizes nurses who provide emergency care and air transport for the acutely ill patient.

Certifying body

BCEN

Examination

This is a 3-hour examination consisting of 175 multiple-choice questions (150 scored and 25 nonscored pretest questions) focusing on the same issues listed for the CEN examination as well as knowledge of advanced airway care, transport considerations, safety issues, disaster management, and survival. This computer based test is offered year-round at specified testing sites.

Eligibility

Candidates must have:

- unrestricted RN or APRN licensure in the United States or its territories
- 2 years experience in flight nursing practice (recommended; not required).

Renewal

- Every 4 years
- 100 education hours or reexamination

Web site

www.ena.org

Certification

Certified transport registered nurse (CTRN) recognizes nurses who provide emergency care and ground transport for acutely ill patients.

Certifying body

BCEN

Examination

This is a 3-hour examination consisting of 155 multiple-choice questions (130 scored and 25 nonscored pretest questions) focusing on the same issues listed for the CEN examination as well as knowledge of advanced airway care, transport considerations, safety issues, disaster management, and survival. This computer-based test is offered year-round at specified testing sites.

Eligibility

Candidates must have:

- unrestricted RN or APRN licensure in the United States or its territories
- 2 years of experience in flight nursing practice (recommended; not required).

Renewal

- Every 4 years
- 100 education hours or reexamination

Web site

www.ena.org

Choosing liability insurance

To find professional liability coverage that fits your needs, compare the coverage of a number of different policies. Make sure your policy provides coverage for in-court and out-of-court malpractice suits and expenses and for defense of a complaint or disciplinary action made to or by your board of nursing. Understanding insurance policy basics will enable you to shop more aggressively and intelligently for the coverage you need. You should work with an insurance agent who's experienced in this type of insurance. If you already have professional liability insurance, the information below may help you better evaluate your coverage.

Type of coverage

Ask your insurance agent whether the policy covers only claims made before the policy expires (claims-made coverage) or if it covers any negligent act committed during the policy period, regardless of when it's reported (occurrence coverage). Keep in mind that the latter type offers better coverage.

Coverage limits

All malpractice insurance policies cover professional liability. Some also cover representation before your board of nursing, general personal liability, medical payments, assault-related bodily injury, and property damage.

The amount of coverage varies, as does your premium. Remember that professional liability coverage is limited to acts and practice settings specified in the policy. Make sure your policy covers your nursing role, whether you're a student, a graduate nurse, or a working nurse with advanced education and specialized skills.

Options

Check whether the policy would provide coverage for these incidents:

- negligence on the part of nurses under your supervision
- misuse of equipment
- errors in reporting or recording care
- failure to provide patient education
- errors in administering medication
- mistakes made while providing care in an emergency, outside your employment setting.

Also ask whether the policy provides protection if your employer sues you.

Definition of terms

Definition of terms can vary from policy to policy. If your policy includes restrictive definitions, you won't be covered for actions outside those guidelines. Therefore, for the best protection, seek the broadest definitions possible and ask the insurance company for examples of actions the company hasn't covered.

Duration of coverage

Insurance is an annual contract that can be renewed or canceled each year. Most policies specify how they can be canceled—for example, in writing by either you or the insurance company. Some contracts require a 30-day notice for cancellation. If the company is canceling the policy, you'll probably be given at least 10 days' notice.

Exclusions

Ask the insurer about exclusions—areas not covered by the insurance policy. For example: "This policy doesn't apply to injury arising out of performance of the insured of a criminal act" or "This policy doesn't apply to nurse anesthetists."

Other insurance clauses

All professional liability insurance policies contain "other insurance" clauses that address payment obligations when a nurse is covered by more than one insurance policy, such as the employer's policy and the nurse's personal liability policy.

- The *pro rata* clause states that two or more policies in effect at the same time will pay any claims in accordance with a proportion established in the individual policies.
- The *in excess* clause states that the primary policy will pay all fees and damages up to its limits, at which point the second policy will pay any additional fees or damages up to its limits.
- The *escape* clause relieves an insurance company of all liability for fees or damages if another insurance policy is in effect at the same time; the clause essentially states that the other company is responsible for all liability.

If you're covered by more than one policy, be alert for "other insurance" clauses and avoid purchasing a policy with an escape clause for liability.

Additional tips

Here's some additional information that will guide you in the purchase of professional liability insurance.

- The insurance application is a legal document. If you provide false information, it may void the policy.

- If you're involved in nursing administration, education, research, or advanced or nontraditional nursing practice, be especially careful in selecting a policy because many policies don't cover these activities.
- After selecting a policy that ensures adequate coverage, stay with the same policy and insurer, if possible, to avoid potential lapses in coverage that could occur when changing insurers.
- No insurance policy will cover you for acts outside of your scope of practice or licensure; nor will insurance cover you for intentional acts that you know will cause harm.
- Be prepared to uphold all obligations specified in the policy; failure to do so may void the policy and cause personal liability for any damages. Remember that an act of willful wrongdoing on your part renders the policy null and void and may lead to a breach-of-contract lawsuit.
- Check out the insurance company by calling your state division of insurance to inquire about the company's financial stability.

The ethics committee

The ethics committee addresses ethical issues regarding the clinical aspects of patient care. It provides a forum for the patient, his family, and health care providers to resolve difficult conflicts.

The functions of an ethics committee include:

- policy development (such as developing policies to guide deliberations over individual cases)
- education (such as inviting guest speakers to visit your health care facility and discuss ethical concerns)
- case consultation (such as debating the prognosis of a patient who's in a persistent vegetative state)
- addressing a single issue (such as reviewing all cases that involve a no-code, or do-not-resuscitate [DNR] order)
- addressing problems of a specific population group (for example, the American Academy of Pediatrics recommending that hospitals have a standing committee called the "infant bioethical review committee")
- addressing issues of organization ethics (such as business practice, marketing, admission, and reimbursement).

Pros and cons

Properly run, an ethics committee provides a safe outlet for venting opposing views on emotionally charged ethical conflicts. The committee process can help to lessen the bias that interferes with rational decision making. It allows for members of disparate disciplines, including physicians, nurses, clergy, social workers, hospital administrators, and ethicists, to express their views on treatment decisions.

Critics of the ethics committee think that committee decision making is too bureaucratic and slow to be useful in clinical crises. They also point out that one dominating committee member may intimidate others with opposing views. Furthermore, they contend that physicians may view the committee as a threat to their autonomy in patient-care decisions. For these reasons, many ethics committees use a "rapid response team" of committee members who are on call to respond quickly in emergent ethical dilemmas. The rapid response team usually consists of three or four committee members, including a physician, who have had special training in negotiation and mediation. The entire committee will retrospectively review each case.

Selection of committee members

Committee members should be selected for their ability to work cooperatively in a group. The American Hospital Association recommends the following ratio of committee members: one-third physicians, one-third nurses, and one-third others, including laypersons, clergy, and other health professionals. Joint Commission regulations require that nursing staff members participate in the hospital ethics committee.

The nurse's role on a hospital ethics committee

Because of the nurse's close contact with the patient, his family, and other members of the health care team, she's frequently in a position to identify ethical dilemmas such as when a family is considering a DNR order for a relative. In many cases, the nurse is the first to recognize conflicts among family members or between the physician and the patient or his family.

Before ethics committees were widely used, nurses had no official outlet for voicing their opinions in ethical debates. In many situations, physicians made ethical decisions about patient care behind closed doors. Nursing supervisors would frequently call meetings to alert nursing staff on treatment decisions and to discourage protest. Now, ethics committees provide nurses with a means to express their views, hear the opinions of others, and better understand the rationales behind ethical decisions.

National Organ Transplant Act

In response to widespread public interest in organ transplantation, Congress enacted the National Organ Transplant Act of 1984 (PL 98-507). This act:

- prohibits the sale of organs
- provides funding for grants to organ procurement agencies
- establishes a national organ-sharing system.

Task Force on Organ Transplantation

This act also convened the 25-member Task Force on Organ Transplantation, with members representing medicine, law, theology, ethics, allied health, the health insurance industry, and the general public.

Representatives from the Office of the Surgeon General, the National Institutes of Health, the Food and Drug Administration, and the Centers for Medicare & Medicaid Services were also appointed to the task force. This task force examined the medical, legal, ethical, economic, and social issues created by organ transplantation.

In its final report, the task force concluded that the best way to close the gap between the small number of organ donors and the large number of potential transplant recipients was to actively solicit donations from bereaved families. As a result, the task force recommended that all state legislatures introduce and enact legislation requiring health care professionals to present organ donation as an option to families ("required request").

Assertive approach

Required request policies are legally mandated in many states. This assertive approach to organ procurement has proved highly successful; as many as 80% of families given the option to become donor families ultimately do so. Significantly, studies show that organ donation can facilitate the grieving process and speed recovery for the bereaved family.

Selected references

All Things Nursing. Philadelphia: Lippincott Williams & Wilkins, 2008.

American Association of Critical Care Nurses. *AACN's Quick Reference to Critical Care Nursing Procedures.* Philadelphia: W.B. Saunders Co., 2007.

Dirkes, S., and Hodge, K. "Continuous Renal Replacement Therapy in the Adult Intensive Care Unit: History and Current Trends," *Critical Care Nurse* 27(2):61-66, 68-72, 74-80, April 2007.

Elkin, M., et al. *Nursing Interventions & Clinical Skills.* St. Louis: Mosby–Year Book, Inc., 2008.

Frakes, M. "Emergency Department Management of Severe Sepsis," *Advanced Emergency Nursing Journal* 29(3): 228-38, July-September 2007.

Hinkle, J., and Guanci, M. "Acute Ischemic Stroke Review," *Journal of Neuroscience Nursing* 39(5):285-93, 310, October 2007.

Holcomb, S. "Stopping the Destruction of Acute Pancreatitis," *Critical Care Nursing Quarterly* 37(6):42-47, July-September 2007.

Lien, Y., and Shapiro, J. "Hyponatremia: Clinical Diagnosis and Management," *The American Journal of Medicine* 120(8):653-58, August 2007.

Neiderman, M., and Brito, V. "Pneumonia in the Older Patient," *Clinics in Chest Medicine* 28(4):751-71, December 2007.

Nursing 2008 Drug Handbook. Philadelphia: Lippincott Williams & Wilkins, 2008.

Nursing Journal Series: Deciphering Diagnostic Tests. Philadelphia: Lippincott Williams & Wilkins, 2007.

Pagana, K., and Pagana, T. *Mosby's Diagnostic and Laboratory Test Reference,* 8th ed. St. Louis: Mosby–Year Book, Inc., 2007.

Sieggreen, M. "Recognize Acute Arterial Occlusion," *Nursing Critical Care* 2(5):50-59, September 2007.

Sims, J. "An Overview of Pulmonary Embolism," *Dimensions of Critical Care Nursing* 26(5):182-86, September-October 2007.

Steele, A., et al. "Nausea and Vomiting: Applying Research to Bedside Nursing," *AACN Advanced Critical Care* 18(1): 61-73, January-March 2007.

Taylor, C., et al. *Fundamentals of Nursing: The Art and Science of Nursing.* Philadelphia: Lippincott Williams & Wilkins, 2007.

Weber, J. *Nurse's Handbook of Health Assessment,* 6th ed. Philadelphia: Lippincott Williams & Wilkins, 2007.

Index

i refers to an illustration; t refers to a table.

i refers to an illustration; t refers to a table.

i refers to an illustration; t refers to a table.

i refers to an illustration; t refers to a table.

i refers to an illustration; t refers to a table.

i refers to an illustration; t refers to a table.

i refers to an illustration; t refers to a table.

i refers to an illustration; t refers to a table.

i refers to an illustration; t refers to a table.

i refers to an illustration; t refers to a table.

i refers to an illustration; t refers to a table.